National-Louis University
UNIVERSITY LIBRARY

LISLE CAMPUS
850 Warrenville Road
Lisle, Illinois 60532-1356

DEMCO

METHODS FOR DISASTER
MENTAL HEALTH RESEARCH

Methods for Disaster Mental Health Research

Edited by

FRAN H. NORRIS
SANDRO GALEA
MATTHEW J. FRIEDMAN
PATRICIA J. WATSON

THE GUILFORD PRESS
New York   London

© 2006 The Guilford Press
A Division of Guilford Publications, Inc.
72 Spring Street, New York, NY 10012
www.guilford.com

Printed in the United States of America

This book is printed on acid-free paper.

Last digit is print number: 9 8 7 6 5 4 3 2 1

Library of Congress Cataloging-in-Publication Data

Methods for disaster mental health research / edited by Fran H. Norris . . . [et al.].
    p. ; cm.
  Includes bibliographical references and index.
  ISBN-10: 1-59385-310-6 ISBN-13: 978-1-59385-310-5 (cloth : alk. paper)
  1. Post-traumatic stress disorder. 2. Disasters—Psychological aspects. I. Norris, Fran H.
  [DNLM: 1. Disasters. 2. Stress Disorders, Post-Traumatic. 3. Research—methods.
WM 170 M592 2006]
  RC552.P67M48 2006
  616.85′21—dc22

About the Editors

Fran H. Norris, PhD, a community/social psychologist, is a Research Professor in the Department of Psychiatry at Dartmouth Medical School, where she is affiliated with the National Center for PTSD and the National Consortium for the Study of Terrorism and Responses to Terrorism (START) headed by the University of Maryland. Dr. Norris has received numerous grants for research, research education, and professional development and has published extensively on the psychosocial consequences of disasters. She is the Deputy/Statistical Editor for the *Journal of Traumatic Stress* and received the 2005 Robert S. Laufer Award for Outstanding Scientific Achievement from the International Society for Traumatic Stress Studies.

Sandro Galea, MD, DrPH, is an Associate Professor of Epidemiology at the University of Michigan School of Public Health and a Research Affiliate of the Population Studies Center at the Institute for Social Research. His research focuses on the social and economic production of health, particularly mental health and behavior in urban settings, and he has an abiding interest in the social and health consequences of collectively experienced traumatic events. Dr. Galea completed his graduate training at the University of Toronto Medical School, at the Harvard University School of Public Health, and at the Columbia University Mailman School of Public Health.

Matthew J. Friedman, MD, PhD, is Executive Director of the U.S. Department of Veterans Affairs National Center for PTSD and Professor of Psychiatry and Pharmacology at Dartmouth Medical School. He has worked with patients with PTSD for more than 30 years and has written or edited 180 books, monographs, chapters, and peer-reviewed journal articles. Dr. Friedman is listed in *The Best Doctors in America*, is Past President of the International Society for Traumatic Stress Studies (ISTSS) and Chair of the scientific advisory board of the Anxiety Disorders Association of America, and has received many honors, including the ISTSS Lifetime Achievement Award.

Patricia J. Watson, PhD, is an educational specialist for the National Center for PTSD and Assistant Professor at Dartmouth Medical School in the Department of Psychiatry. She collaborates with the Substance Abuse and Mental Health Services Administration, the Centers for Disease Control and Prevention, and subject-matter experts to create publications for public and mental health interventions following large-scale terrorism, disaster, and pandemic flu. Dr. Watson received her doctorate in clinical psychology from Catholic University and completed a postgraduate fellowship in pediatric psychology at Harvard Medical School. Her areas of professional interest include science-to-service interventions in disaster/terrorism events, early intervention treatments for trauma, trauma in children and adolescents, and growth aspects of trauma.

Contributors

Apryl Alexander, BS, Department of Psychology, Virginia Tech, Blacksburg, Virginia

Lawrence Amsel, PhD, Center for Bioethics, College of Physicians and Surgeons, Columbia University, New York, New York

Charles C. Benight, PhD, Department of Psychology, University of Colorado at Colorado Springs, Colorado Springs, Colorado

John Boyle, PhD, Schulman, Ronca & Bucuvalas Inc., New York, New York

Evelyn J. Bromet, PhD, Department of Psychiatry, State University of New York at Stony Brook, Stony Brook, New York

Melissa J. Brymer, PsyD, National Center for Child Traumatic Stress, Department of Psychiatry and Biobehavioral Sciences, University of California, Los Angeles, Los Angeles, California

Michael Bucuvalas, PhD, Schulman, Ronca & Bucuvalas Inc., New York, New York

Franklin Carvajal, PhD, Department of Psychology, Virginia Tech, Blacksburg, Virginia

Sara Chapman, BS, Department of Psychology, Virginia Tech, Blacksburg, Virginia

Lauren Collogan, BA, New York Academy of Medicine, New York, New York

Carrie L. Elrod, PhD, Elrod and Associates, Buckhead, Georgia

Alan R. Fleischman, MD, New York Academy of Medicine, New York, New York

Matthew J. Friedman, MD, PhD, National Center for PTSD, Veterans Affairs Medical Center, White River Junction, Vermont

Carol S. Fullerton, PhD, Department of Psychiatry, Uniformed Services University of the Health Sciences, Bethesda, Maryland

Sandro Galea, MD, DrPH, Department of Epidemiology, University of Michigan School of Public Health, Ann Arbor, Michigan

Laura E. Gibson, PhD, The Behavior Therapy and Psychotherapy Center, Department of Psychology, University of Vermont, Burlington, Vermont

James M. Hadder, BS, Department of Psychology, Virginia Tech, Blacksburg, Virginia

Jessica L. Hamblen, PhD, National Center for PTSD, Veterans Affairs Medical Center, White River Junction, Vermont; Department of Psychiatry, Dartmouth Medical School, Hanover, New Hampshire

Johan M. Havenaar, MD, PhD, Department of Psychiatry, Utrecht University Hospital, Utrecht, The Netherlands

Eric Jones, PhD, Department of Anthropology, University of North Carolina at Greensboro, Greensboro, North Carolina

Russell T. Jones, PhD, Department of Psychology, Virginia Tech, Blacksburg, Virginia

Dean Kilpatrick, PhD, National Crime Victims Research and Treatment Center, Medical University of South Carolina, Charleston, South Carolina

Annette M. La Greca, PhD, Department of Psychology, University of Miami, Coral Gables, Florida

Fred Lerner, DLS, Veterans Affairs Medical Center, White River Junction, Vermont

Randall D. Marshall, MD, New York State Psychiatric Institute, College of Physicians and Surgeons, Columbia University, New York, New York

James E. McCarroll, PhD, Department of Psychiatry, Uniformed Services University of the Health Sciences, Bethesda, Maryland

Alexander C. McFarlane, MD, Center for Military and Veterans Health, Department of Psychiatry, University of Adelaide, Adelaide, Australia

Arthur D. Murphy, PhD, Department of Anthropology, University of North Carolina at Greensboro, Greensboro, North Carolina

Yuval Neria, PhD, New York State Psychiatric Institute, College of Physicians and Surgeons, Columbia University, New York, New York

Carol S. North, MD, Department of Psychiatry, University of Texas Southwestern Medical Center, Dallas, Texas

Fran H. Norris, PhD, National Center for PTSD, Veterans Affairs Medical Center, White River Junction, Vermont; Department of Psychiatry, Dartmouth Medical School, Hanover, New Hampshire

Lawrence A. Palinkas, PhD, School of Social Work, University of Southern California, Los Angeles, California

Julia L. Perilla, PhD, Department of Psychology, Georgia State University, Atlanta, Georgia

Betty Pfefferbaum, MD, JD, Department of Psychiatry, University of Oklahoma Health Sciences Center, Oklahoma City, Oklahoma

Heidi Resnick, PhD, National Crime Victims Research and Treatment Center, Medical University of South Carolina, Charleston, South Carolina

Craig S. Rosen, PhD, National Center for PTSD, VA Palo Alto Health Care System, Menlo Park, California; Department of Psychiatry, Stanford University School of Medicine, Palo Alto, California

William E. Schlenger, PhD, Behavioral Health Research Practice, Abt Associates, Inc., Research Triangle Park, North Carolina

Roxane Cohen Silver, PhD, Department of Psychology and Social Behavior, University of California, Irvine, Irvine, California

Alan M. Steinberg, PhD, National Center for Child Traumatic Stress, Department of Psychiatry and Biobehavioral Sciences, University of California, Los Angeles, Los Angeles, California

Jesse R. Steinberg, MA, Department of Philosophy, University of California, Santa Barbara, Santa Barbara, California

Eun Jung Suh, PhD, New York State Psychiatric Institute, College of Physicians and Surgeons, Columbia University, New York, New York

Farris Tuma, PhD, Traumatic Stress Disorders Research Program, National Institute of Mental Health, Bethesda, Maryland

Robert J. Ursano, MD, Department of Psychiatry, Uniformed Services University of the Health Sciences, Bethesda, Maryland

David Vlahov, PhD, Center for Urban Epidemiologic Studies, New York Academy of Medicine, New York, New York

Anka A. Vujanovic, BA, Department of Psychology, University of Vermont, Burlington, Vermont

Helena E. Young, PhD, National Center for PTSD, VA Palo Alto Health Care System, Menlo Park, California

Michael J. Zvolensky, PhD, Department of Psychology, University of Vermont, Burlington, Vermont

Preface

On average, a disaster occurs somewhere in the world each day. These events are almost always of high local interest. Occasionally they are also of national interest, and every now and then they capture the attention of the entire world. In this new century, we already have witnessed disasters so great that they were virtually incomprehensible. Events like the terrorist attacks of September 11, 2001, the southeast Asian tsunami of December 26, 2004, and Hurricane Katrina of August 29, 2005, galvanize concern, leaving policy makers, service providers, journalists, scientists, and the general public clamoring for information that can shed light on the implications of such catastrophes for the survivors, first responders, children and other special populations, the community at large, and entire societies. Interest in findings from research on the psychological consequences of disasters has never been more pronounced than it has been in recent years.

Past disaster mental health research has much to offer these various constituencies, but these recent events have also highlighted the shortcomings of the research. Although our confidence is growing that the extant literature provides us with reliable estimates of the burden of psychopathology among different groups after disasters, large gaps in knowledge remain. For example, research on intervention and treatment has seldom been conducted in the context of a disaster. Few of the studies that document the effects of disasters provide clear answers that can guide the prevention of disaster-related mental health problems. Also, most studies conducted after disasters have been atheoretical, limiting our ability to understand why disasters have documented mental health consequences in populations and, by inference, limiting our understanding of how we can mitigate these consequences.

Disaster research is different from research done in most other fields in that much of the work is motivated by a sense of urgency. Most researchers enter the field of disaster mental health when a significant event occurs in their home community and frequently do not have time to build research questions on a measured critical appraisal of the body of literature that is scattered across a variety of journals. Concerns about experimental designs and scientific rigor often take a back seat to provider beliefs, consumer demands, and clinical necessities. In many cases, especially following large-scale natural disasters, damage to the community's infrastructure makes fieldwork challenging. Legitimate concerns about ethical issues surrounding research with trauma survivors lead to additional compromises. Researchers and local public health and mental health authorities do not always know how to collaborate with each other and may fear that they do not and cannot speak the same language.

Because of these various issues, the editors of this volume applied for and received grants from the National Institute of Mental Health to increase the quality and utility of disaster mental health research through research education. Through these projects, we have created websites for rapid dissemination of disaster research findings and methods (www.redmh.org and www.disasterresearch.org), mentoring programs for new investigators, and various educational materials and presentations. This book was a direct outgrowth of these activities.

PURPOSE AND CONTENTS OF THIS BOOK

The purpose of this book is to educate the reader about research methods and strategies that can be used to study (1) the effects of disasters on mental health and related constructs or (2) the effectiveness or dissemination of interventions undertaken to prevent or reduce disaster-related mental health problems. Increased understanding of methodological issues and strategies is crucial to developing evidence-based findings that can inform public policy. The book focuses on research that is conducted in community settings using a public health approach. The book is oriented to novice disaster researchers in the fields of psychology, public health, and related disciplines, but we believe it also has something to offer experienced researchers. The text emphasizes the practical and logistical challenges of conducting disaster research as well as methodological and scientific issues. The authors, who are all experienced disaster researchers, are candid about the shortcomings and pitfalls of the particular approach they are describing and make extensive use of examples that illustrate successful approaches.

The book is divided into five parts. Part I provides an introduction to the field. McFarlane and Norris tackle the not-so-simple job of defining the parameters of this field of study and delineate the various features on which disasters vary. Norris and Elrod then provide a review of the empirical research on the psychosocial consequences of disasters that has been conducted over the past 25 years. They describe the methods that have predominated in the field and summarize findings on the magnitude and duration of effects and the influence of various risk and protective factors.

Part II addresses research fundamentals. Using a framework of "why, who, what, when, and how," North and Norris set the stage for the rest of the book by outlining how study goals dictate methodological choices. Benight, McFarlane, and Norris highlight theories and models that may guide the formulation of useful and significant questions about the development and prevention of mental health problems in the aftermath of disaster. Concluding this section, Fleischman, Collogan, and Tuma aim to increase awareness and understanding of the ethical issues surrounding disaster research and discuss the potential risks and benefits to research participants. This knowledge is essential for any researcher working in this field.

Part III describes the specific methods for sampling and data collection used in the field. Bromet and Havenaar introduce the reader to epidemiological approaches and designs and discuss the advantages of face-to-face procedures in epidemiological research. Their use of examples from research on the 1986 Chornobyl nuclear accident enriches their presentation notably. Galea, Bucuvalas, Resnick, Boyle, Vlahov, and Kilpatrick then provide a practical introduction to the use of telephone-based methods in disaster research. Drawing upon their extraordinary combined experience, these authors describe how these methods allow for the rapid assessment of large populations and offer particular advantages for researchers interested in the consequences of disasters. Schlenger and Silver describe the methods they used to conduct web-based nationwide surveys in the immediate aftermath of the September 11, 2001, terrorist attacks and show how these emerging methods can enhance the field of disaster research. Next, La Greca writes of the considerations surrounding efforts to conduct research on the effects of disasters and terrorism within schools. Schools are a logical setting in which to evaluate children's reactions to disasters, but they pose many methodological and practical challenges. Palinkas concludes this section by reminding us that quantitative and qualitative research traditions complement one another. He examines the rationale for using qualitative methods and outlines the types of methods that have been or might be used in disaster research.

Part IV shifts our attention to research for planning, policy, and service delivery. Galea and Norris examine a topic of high relevance for disaster-stricken communities: public mental health surveillance and monitoring.

The authors summarize the history and key concepts underlying public health surveillance, discuss the collection and analysis of surveillance data, and argue that public mental health surveillance can play a central role in mitigating the mental health consequences of disasters. Often drawing upon their experience in evaluating postdisaster crisis counseling programs, Rosen and Young then discuss the "precepts, pragmatics, and politics" of conducting mental health services and evaluation research in the aftermath of disaster. Gibson, Hamblen, Zvolensky, and Vujanovic summarize past research on evidence-based treatments for traumatic stress, giving particular attention to "gold-standard" studies. They also discuss the challenges of conducting treatment research in disaster settings. Finally, Marshall, Amsel, Neria, and Suh draw upon their experience in training clinicians in New York after the terrorist attacks of September 11, 2001, to discuss the critical problem of dissemination of evidence-based treatments. Their chapter is organized around the five key questions that dissemination studies must answer.

Part V addresses special challenges in disaster research. These challenges apply across the designs and modalities discussed in Parts III and IV. Steinberg, Brymer, Steinberg, and Pfefferbaum draw upon their tremendous international experience to outline the key issues in conducting disaster research with children and adolescents. They touch upon methodological issues in research design and selection of instruments, coordination of research efforts among research groups, a variety of ethical issues, and special considerations in regard to intervention outcome studies. Likewise, Fullerton, McCarroll, and Ursano draw upon their many years of research and policy experience to advise the reader on how to study military and uniformed service workers effectively. These groups are often first on the scene in the aftermath of disasters, and they bring special characteristics, histories, disaster experiences, and occupational cultures to the research context. Jones, Hadder, Carvajal, Chapman, and Alexander discuss the challenges and opportunities of conducting research with minority and marginalized communities. After outlining the reasons why this work is important, they identify three key barriers to this research (mistrust, access, culture/linguistics) and propose solutions that will help researchers to overcome these barriers. Finally, Murphy, Perilla, and Jones educate the reader about the process of conducting research in foreign countries. Reminding us of the various concerns to keep in mind when undertaking a project across cultural and national boundaries, they describe issues regarding collaboration, finances, language, validity, protection for human participants, engaging the study community, and being a guest researcher.

Matthew Friedman brings the book to a close by reviewing key themes that emerged throughout the text and forging an agenda for the future. This last chapter is followed by two appendices. The first, prepared by

Sandro Galea, contains brief descriptions of the various disasters that are mentioned throughout the text. The second, prepared by Fred Lerner, provides instruction about how to search the literature on disasters and traumatic stress effectively.

A few words are in order about topics that we elected not to include in this book. We did not include a chapter on assessment because many other sources of information are available, including the second edition of *Assessing Psychological Trauma and PTSD* (Wilson & Keane, 2004). In greater detail than was possible here, contributors to that volume describe various approaches to assessment, including standardized self-report measures, structured clinical interviews, and psychophysiological measures, and they addressed special topics, such as traumatic bereavement, substance use, and gender and developmental influences on assessment.

It should also be recognized that disaster mental health is but one topical area in a much broader, multidisciplinary field of study. Readers who are interested in field methods and other social science approaches for studying organized and organizational behavior are referred to Stallings's (2002) edited volume, *Methods of Disaster Research: Unique or Not?*

Finally, we limit our focus to research methods and say little about the host of challenges involved in providing direct mental health care to disaster victims. Interested readers are referred to a number of recent works addressing this topic (Green et al., 2003; Myers & Wee, 2005; National Institute of Mental Health, 2002; Ritchie, Watson, & Friedman, 2006; Ursano & Norwood, 2003).

SUPPLEMENTARY RESOURCES

This volume should be useful not only to individuals who seek to expand their own research skills but also to instructors who might offer seminars to students seeking graduate or professional degrees. Interested instructors will find supplementary materials that can be downloaded at no cost from www.redmh.org. These materials include a draft course syllabus, lecture outlines, a list of topics and controversies for further discussion and exploration, updated bibliographies and recommended reading lists, and a DVD in which expert disaster researchers share their personal experiences and opinions about past and future research. Instructors and other readers may also consult www.disasterresearch.org for guidance on preparing disaster research proposals. Alternatively, readers may contact Fran Norris or Sandro Galea, the first and second editors of this volume, respectively, for these materials.

The editors welcome readers' comments and suggestions. We sincerely hope that this book is helpful, maybe even inspiring, to investigators in this challenging, intriguing, and significant field of research.

REFERENCES

Green, B., Friedman, M., de Jong, J., Solomon, S., Keane, T., Fairbank, J. et al. (Eds). (2003). *Trauma interventions in war and peace: Prevention, practice, and policy.* New York: Kluwer/Plenum.

Myers, D., & Wee, D. (2005). *Disaster mental health services: A primer for practitioners.* New York: Brunner-Routledge.

National Institute of Mental Health. (2002). *Mental health and mass violence: Evidence based early psychological intervention for victims/survivors of mass violence: A workshop to reach consensus on best practices* (NIH Publication No. 02-5138). Washington, DC: U.S. Government Printing Office. [Note: this report is also available online at www.nimh.nih.gov/research/massviolence.pdf.]

Norris, F., Friedman, M., & Watson, P. (2002). 60,000 disaster victims speak, Part II: Summary and implications of the disaster mental health research. *Psychiatry, 65,* 240–260.

Ritchie, E. C., Watson, P. J., & Friedman, M. J. (Eds.). (2006). *Mental health interventions following mass violence and disasters: Strategies for mental health practice.* New York: Guilford Press.

Stallings, R. (Ed.). (2002). *Methods of disaster research: Unique or not?* Philadelphia: Xlibris.

Ursano, R., & Norwood, A. (Eds.) (2003). *Annual review of psychiatry. Vol. 22: Trauma and disaster responses and management.* Washington DC: American Psychiatric Press.

Wilson, J., & Keane, T. (Eds.). (2004). *Assessing psychological trauma and PTSD* (2nd ed.). New York: Guilford Press.

Contents

PART I. Introduction to the Field

CHAPTER 1   Definitions and Concepts in Disaster Research   3
Alexander C. McFarlane and Fran H. Norris

CHAPTER 2   Psychosocial Consequences of Disaster: 20
A Review of Past Research
Fran H. Norris and Carrie L. Elrod

PART II. Research Fundamentals

CHAPTER 3   Choosing Research Methods to Match Research Goals   45
in Studies of Disaster or Terrorism
Carol S. North and Fran H. Norris

CHAPTER 4   Formulating Questions about Postdisaster Mental Health   62
*Charles C. Benight, Alexander C. McFarlane,
and Fran H. Norris*

CHAPTER 5   Ethical Issues in Disaster Research   78
Alan R. Fleischman, Lauren Collogan, and Farris Tuma

PART III. Methods for Sampling and Data Collection

CHAPTER 6   Basic Epidemiological Approaches to Disaster Research: 95
Value of Face-to-Face Procedures
Evelyn J. Bromet and Johan M. Havenaar

Contents

CHAPTER 7   Telephone-Based Research Methods   111
            in Disaster Research
            Sandro Galea, Michael Bucuvalas, Heidi Resnick,
            John Boyle, David Vlahov, and Dean Kilpatrick

CHAPTER 8   Web-Based Methods in Disaster Research   129
            William E. Schlenger and Roxane Cohen Silver

CHAPTER 9   School-Based Studies of Children Following Disasters   141
            Annette M. La Greca

CHAPTER 10 Qualitative Approaches to Studying the Effects   158
            of Disasters
            Lawrence A. Palinkas

PART IV. Research for Planning, Policy, and Service Delivery

CHAPTER 11 Public Mental Health Surveillance and Monitoring   177
            Sandro Galea and Fran H. Norris

CHAPTER 12 Mental Health Services and Evaluation Research: 194
            Precepts, Pragmatics, and Politics
            Craig S. Rosen and Helena E. Young

CHAPTER 13 Evidence-Based Treatments for Traumatic Stress: 208
            An Overview of the Research with an
            Emphasis on Disaster Settings
            Laura E. Gibson, Jessica L. Hamblen, Michael J. Zvolensky,
            and Anka A. Vujanovic

CHAPTER 14 Strategies for Dissemination of   226
            Evidence-Based Treatments: Training Clinicians
            after Large-Scale Disasters
            Randall D. Marshall, Lawrence Amsel, Yuval Neria,
            and Eun Jung Suh

PART V. Special Challenges in Disaster Research

CHAPTER 15 Conducting Research with Children   243
            and Adolescents after Disaster
            Alan M. Steinberg, Melissa J. Brymer,
            Jesse R. Steinberg, and Betty Pfefferbaum

CHAPTER 16 Conducting Research with Military and   254
            Uniformed Services Workers
            Carol S. Fullerton, James E. McCarroll,
            and Robert J. Ursano

CHAPTER 17 Conducting Research in Diverse, Minority, and 265
            Marginalized Communities
            Russell T. Jones, James M. Hadder, Franklin Carvajal,
            Sara Chapman, and Apryl Alexander

CHAPTER 18 Conducting Research in Other Countries   278
            Arthur D. Murphy, Julia L. Perilla, and Eric Jones

CHAPTER 19 Disaster Mental Health Research: 289
            Challenges for the Future
            Matthew J. Friedman

APPENDIX 1 Disasters Mentioned in the Text   303
            Sandro Galea

APPENDIX 2 Searching the Traumatic Stress Literature   309
            Fred Lerner

            Index   317

METHODS FOR DISASTER
MENTAL HEALTH RESEARCH

PART I

Introduction to the Field

CHAPTER 1

Definitions and Concepts in Disaster Research

ALEXANDER C. MCFARLANE
and FRAN H. NORRIS

This chapter outlines some of the definitions and concepts that lie behind understanding the impact of disasters on the health and welfare of the affected communities. We first define varied meanings of the term *disaster* and the (fuzzy) boundaries of research that aims to understand the mental health consequences of these events. We then describe the traditional typology that has guided this field of study, noting distinctions among natural disasters, technological accidents, and sudden episodes of mass violence. Next, we describe other important characteristics of disasters and disaster exposure and conclude by elaborating on the temporal dimension of disaster impact and recovery. Chapter 2 (Norris & Elrod) then delves into the effects of disasters drawn from the research to date.

DEFINITIONS OF DISASTER AND BOUNDARIES OF THE FIELD

Although the word *disaster* may suggest a readily apparent meaning, it is actually difficult to define the term precisely. The original derivation of the word came from the Latin *dis astro* or "bad star" and implied a calamity blamed on an unfavorable position of the planet. The *Oxford English Dictionary* (1987) defines disaster as a "sudden or great misfortune; calamity; complete failure." Although consistent with the day-to-day informal usage of the term, this definition is highly inadequate because it fails to distinguish disasters from other adversities (Green, 1996). For the purposes of this book, we define a disaster as *a potentially traumatic event that is collectively experienced, has an acute onset, and is time-delimited; disasters may be attributed to natural, technological, or human causes.* The rationale for this definition follows.

Disasters as Potentially Traumatic Events

Not surprisingly, mental health researchers usually think of disasters as a particular type of traumatic event (see Figure 1). It is important to note that *disaster* is not a synonym for *trauma*; rather it is a category, an exemplar, of trauma. By classifying disasters as traumatic events, we imbue certain meanings that should be made explicit. The fourth edition of the American Psychiatric Association's (1994) *Diagnostic and Statistical Manual of Mental Disorders* defines a traumatic event as one in which both of the following were present: "(1) the person experienced, witnessed, or was confronted with an event or events that involved actual or threatened death or serious injury, or a threat to the physical integrity of self or others," and (2) the person's response involved intense fear, helplessness, or horror (pp. 427–428). By qualifying the term *traumatic events* with the adjective *potentially*, we acknowledge that while not every disaster will cause death or injury to self or others, certainly all disasters have the potential to do so.

Because disasters belong to a larger set of potentially traumatic events, it is useful to consider their place in the overall epidemiology of trauma and posttraumatic stress disorder (PTSD). Most of what is known about the mental health consequences of disasters has been derived from studies of specific groups of victims or workers or the communities in which they live. This is the type of research that is the focus of this book. However, research on the epidemiology of trauma and PTSD in general populations gives us different information that has both advantages and disadvantages relative to the primary mode of this research. The National Comorbidity Survey, a nationally representative mental health survey, determined that 19% of men and 15% of women in the United States had been exposed to a disaster, with respective conditional probabilities of lifetime PTSD being 3.7% and 5.4% (Kessler, Sonnega, Bromet, Hughes, & Nelson, 1995). Similarly, in a nationally representative sample of Australians, 20% of men and 13% of women reported that they had experienced a disaster at some point in their lives, but only 4 of the 158 past-year cases of PTSD were specifically attributable to these events (Creamer, Burgess, & McFarlane, 2001).

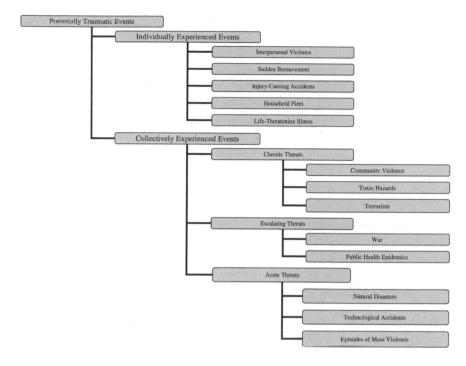

FIGURE 1.1. Classification of potentially traumatic events. Subordinate categories are illustrative, not exhaustive.

There are three important observations to make about such findings. First, the findings help to keep this area of research in perspective. Compared to the conditional probabilities of PTSD following interpersonal violence and some other forms of individually experienced trauma, the conditional probability of PTSD after disasters is relatively low. Accordingly, disasters account for only a small proportion of posttraumatic morbidity on a national level. Second, it is nonetheless important to keep in mind that percentages that seem quite small translate to large numbers when applied to a population. Third, national epidemiological studies are problematic in terms of the information they provide about disasters. Unlike most other types of trauma, major disasters are not evenly distributed. Minor flood and storm damage may be relatively common, but the major disasters that are of most concern occur less often. Typically, in broad surveys, a single question asks only whether the individual has experienced a disaster, with no definition or threshold given. It is likely that national epidemiologic findings under-estimate the lifetime prevalence of PTSD in specific disaster-affected communities.

Disasters as Collectively Experienced Events

The distinction between individually and collectively experienced events is important for our purposes (see Figure 1.1). Early disaster researchers Kinston and Rosser (1974) suggested that the term *disaster* be used to describe "massive collective stress." Disasters create stress for many people simultaneously. Almost all present-day definitions emphasize the collective nature of disaster exposure (Bolin, 1986; Quarantelli, 1986) but differ in the relative emphasis placed on the physical or social impacts of the agents (e.g., destruction, loss) or political phenomena (e.g., declarations).

Definitions Based on Collective Impacts

For many years, the International Federation of Red Cross and Red Crescent Societies has published the *World Disasters Report*, which provides an excellent example of a definition that emphasizes the physical or social impacts of collective crises. In this report, events are considered disasters if (1) 10 or more people are reported killed, (2) 100 or more people are reported affected, (3) an appeal for international assistance is issued, and/or (4) a state of emergency is declared (International Federation of Red Cross and Red Crescent Societies, 2000). The detailed reports allow statistics for subcategories of events to be compiled by country or global region, and have been instrumental in documenting that developing countries and Asia are at particular risk for disasters (DeGirolamo & McFarlane, 1996; Somasundarum, Norris, Asukai, & Murthy, 2003).

The Red Cross definition of *disaster*—based on severity of impact with little attention to the onset/duration of impact—includes public health epidemics, mass displacements, war, droughts, famine, natural disasters, and large accidents and fires. From a response perspective, this makes a good deal of sense. The same principles are often involved in planning and mounting relief efforts for disasters, war, and other collective traumas. Massive destruction and loss reliably follow in the wake of war, creating environments that share many qualities with those created by large-scale natural disasters. Overlap between political conflicts and mass displacement is quite salient, as modern warfare is increasingly driven by ethnic cleansing and religious bigotry. The active eviction of families from regions is used as a weapon of war. For example, in Kosovo, the refugee crisis meant that NATO troops were tied down because of the immediate needs to provide relief for the refugees and could not take a more active peacekeeping role until further logistical resources were mobilized. In addition, the communities into which refugees move are often destabilized.

Ongoing environmental hazards also have added to the global refugee crisis. As water and other natural resources become increasingly scarce, combined with climate change due to global warming, droughts, and other disasters, there will be increasing problems with refugee migration. The changing distribution of vector-borne disease will further complicate the boundaries between disaster, war, and epidemic. These modern humanitarian crises must be studied from multiple dimensions to characterize their full impact and ensure the development of optimal management strategies.

Political Definitions

As noted previously, some definitions of disaster focus on political declarations in addition to severity of impacts alone. Political definitions have much practical importance. Political definitions of disaster distinguish between large-scale accidents, emergencies, and disasters, a determination that is often made by the civil domain of government. Disaster declarations evoke certain instrumental powers that allow temporary suspension of normal civil administration and the rapid coordination of protective and relief efforts. A bus or plane crash will not be called a disaster unless it causes large numbers of dead and injured. Whether such an event is defined as a large-scale accident or disaster will also be determined by its impact on the surrounding community. The crash of an aircraft into a housing complex near an airport, killing passengers on the plane and residents on the ground, may well be deemed a disaster, whereas the crash of an aircraft in a remote region may not be considered a disaster by governmental entities. These differentiations are somewhat artificial, and many of the same principles apply in both settings. The mental health of survivors (or rescue workers) has often been studied after events that were not officially designated as major disasters; thus political considerations have not played a strong role in defining this field of research.

Proposing a definition that was related to but distinct from merely political ones, Quarantelli (1986) defined disaster as a consensus-type crisis occasion in which demands exceed capabilities. This definition is useful conceptually because it reminds us that the consequences of disasters follow not only from needs of the community but from the community's capacity to meet those needs. In smaller communities with fewer emergency relief resources, the threshold for an event to disrupt the capacity to manage and organize an effective response will be lower than in larger communities. However, the definition is broad and rather abstract for the purposes of defining the boundaries of a field of research.

Disasters as Acute-Onset, Time-Delimited Events

For building a knowledge base, it is important to define not only what is included in the phenomenon under study but also what is not. Because they are characterized by collective impacts and political considerations, disasters share much in common with stressors such as war, epidemics, and mass displacements, but they differ in temporal dimensions. Disregarding labels for a moment, we should consider the various ways in which collectively experienced traumas unfold. To do so, we rely largely on the notion of threat, which is the perceived possibility of future harm or loss. Actual harm/loss may or may not be preceded by a period of threat, and it may or may not be followed by a period of threat.

On this basis, we here differentiate between chronic, escalating, and acute threats as they describe collectively experienced events or mass trauma. The same typology could be used to distinguish among individually experienced events (e.g., ongoing domestic violence vs. a sudden single-episode assault), but that discussion is beyond the purposes of this chapter.

Sometimes, the course of the phenomenon is characterized by a prolonged, relatively constant period of threat. Actual harm/loss may or may not occur, and the threat subsides little or not at all. The event is not delimited, that is, neither the beginning nor the end of the event is easy to demark or define. Hypothetically, if one could chart the population's threat over time, it would be moderately high but relatively flat; kurtosis (peakedness) would be minimal. Such circumstances just barely adhere to the meaning of *event*, except that there is generally a point at which one first learns of or is confronted with the threat. We label these as *chronic* threats, with the connotation of a continuing, constant, unremitting threat of harm or loss. Many toxic hazards, ongoing community violence, and threat of terrorism (as opposed to a terrorist attack) might be examples of chronically threatening, collectively experienced, potentially traumatic events (see Figure 1.1).

Sometimes the course of the phenomenon begins with a period of escalating threat. There was a point at which the threat was absent, but it emerges and then grows over time. There will be a period in which harm or loss peaks, followed by a period of gradually declining threat. Hypothetically, if one could chart the threat over time, it might look like a classic normal, or bell-shaped, distribution. Of course, this description oversimplifies matters, as any or all of these periods may be prolonged, and the iterations may be cyclic rather than clearly phased. We label these as *escalating/peaking/diminishing* threats, or merely as escalating threats, for short. Many public health epidemics, political conflicts, and refugee crises adhere to a pattern like this.

Sometimes, the course of the phenomenon begins suddenly; the threat (or warning) period is short (no longer than a few days) or absent completely. As in the preceding case, there is also a period in which harm or loss peaks, but it is followed by a rapidly declining threat, a point when the worst is clearly over and the magnitude of the threat declines markedly.

Hypothetically, the course of threat over time is sharply peaked, radically changing from low to high and back to low, at least relative to the first two clusters. Many events, such as earthquakes, storms, accidents, and shooting sprees, follow a pattern like this. We label these as *acute onset, time-delimited* threats, or as acute threats for short. The descriptor *acute* carries the meaning of a short/sharp but severe course. In our use, the meaning is relative because, of course, the disruption following disasters may be long-lasting, but the period of peak danger is short-lived relative to chronic or escalating threats.

As might be evident, constructs like threat and duration are continuous rather than categorical, and words like *escalating* and *declining* and even *constant* cannot be easily or precisely defined. The scaling is undoubtedly multidimensional rather than unidimensional, as the preceding simplified grouping implies. Notwithstanding these difficulties, we believe the temporal dimension is the key to classification (at least for research purposes) and recommend reserving the term disaster for events of the third type: those with a relatively clear beginning and a relatively clear end. The exclusion of certain human experiences from the definition of disaster does not imply that the excluded events are less important. Certainly, worldwide, more people are affected by public health epidemics, such as the AIDS crisis, than are affected by natural or human-caused disasters (International Federation of Red Cross and Red Crescent Societies, 2000). Indeed, one could argue that the consequences of ongoing community violence, political violence, or environmental hazards are potentially more pathogenic than disasters. The point is simply that an area of study is defined in part by its boundaries, and the characteristic of sudden, forceful, but time-limited impact appears to define the boundaries of disasters reasonably well. We revisit some of the issues around the boundaries subsequently, after describing the primary types of disasters.

TRADITIONAL DISASTER
TYPOLOGY BY AGENT/CAUSE

Arising out of these definitions, various typologies of disaster have been proposed. Most commonly, distinctions are made according to the determinants or agents of the destruction, especially whether they were *natural* in origin, such as floods and earthquakes, or *human-caused*. Human-caused disasters can be further subdivided into *technological accidents* and *mass violence*. Technological accidents are disasters caused by neglect, carelessness, or failures of technology, such as mass transportation accidents or dam collapses, whereas mass violence refers to disasters caused by intent or malevolence, such as shooting sprees or peacetime terrorist attacks.

Technological disasters may be more difficult for individuals to tolerate than are natural disasters because of the meanings imparted to the events. Natural disasters possibly are able to be dismissed as acts of God. Technological accidents, on the other hand, represent callousness, carelessness, and insensitivity (Bolin, 1986). At times these failures involve frank negligence rather than simply failing to foresee a risk, the Bhopal (India) disaster being one such example. These technological disasters have the capacity to divide communities, particularly where one party is seen to represent a sector of privilege and wealth that is exercised with little concern for the welfare of the broader community. The historic 1889 disaster in Johnstown, Pennsylvania, was a dramatic example of this division. Technological disasters are frequently followed by lasting disputes and litigation concerning the allocation of blame that further fragment and politicize the community (Kroll-Smith & Couch, 1993).

However, the notion that, in general, technological accidents have greater mental health impact than do natural disasters has not withstood empirical test. A meta-analysis of the relationship between disasters and psychopathology in controlled studies (Rubonis & Bickman, 1991) came to the opposite conclusion—namely, that natural disasters resulted in greater rates of disorder. Norris et al. (2002) found no overall difference between the effects of the two types of disasters in their more recent and comprehensive review (see also Norris & Elrod, Chapter 2, this volume), although technological disasters had somewhat greater effects than did natural disasters when the analysis was limited to studies conducted in developed countries.

The differentiation between natural and technological forces might be somewhat illusory. For example, failure to comply with construction codes can lead to the collapse of buildings in earthquakes, with much greater resultant loss of life than would have been the case if the standards were adhered to. Without question, land-use policies in coastal regions, such as extensive development on barrier islands, contribute to the financial impact of "natural" disasters. The distinction between natural and technological disasters is especially blurred when disasters occur in developing countries. Overall, housing quality is poor relative to that found in the developed countries, so houses are less capable of withstanding the forces of water and wind. Lacking means for obtaining other property, families may "invade" flood plains, steep mountainsides, and other undesirable locations. Deadly mudslides are often the result of deforestation. Natural disasters, as well as technological accidents, are frequently politicized because of issues surrounding the availability and distribution of resources both within and between communities.

The evidence does suggest that disasters of mass violence are more likely to have serious mental health consequences than either natural disasters or technological accidents (see Norris & Elrod, Chapter 2, this vol-

ume). To perceive oneself as a victim of intentional harm is especially difficult and threatening. Several studies of peacetime (terrorist) bombings (e.g.,
North et al., 1999; Scott, Brooks, & McKinlay, 1995) and sniper attacks
(e.g., Creamer, Burgess, Buckingham, & McFarlane, 1993; Pynoos et al.,
1987) have documented quite severe effects on mental health. However, the
category of "mass violence" disasters is also difficult to define precisely.
Wildfires, for example, are typically classified as natural disasters, but they
may result from human intent (arson). Moreover, the boundaries between
acts of war and terrorism are not clear-cut. Terrorist attacks, such as occurred in Bali on October 12, 2002, and in New York City on September
11, 2001, target civilians, but in many regards terrorism is undeclared warfare fought by unconventional means. Generally, we classify terrorist events
as disasters when they meet the criteria of acute onset and time-limited
threat, that is, victims of these events had no anticipation of the events that
unfolded, in contrast to the combatants in a more typical armed conflict or
even civilians in a context of continued political conflict.

Bioterrorism is especially difficult to classify because the agents are
invisible and strange, the course of threat will vary depending upon the
extent of contagion or contamination, and the aftermath is potentially un-
bounded by time and space (Ursano, Norwood, Fullerton, Holloway, &
Hall, 2003). Depending upon the agent, bioterrorist incidents could begin
suddenly with a severe threat that lessens over time, but they could just as
easily behave like epidemics with an escalation of the threat once recognized. The nature of the impact of these events may be different as well,
with people being uncertain about their levels of exposure and fearful of infection or quarantine. Naturally occurring epidemics, like that associated
with severe acute respiratory syndrome (SARS), provide a glimpse into the
range of potential consequences, including stigma and isolation of direct
victims (extending even to medical professionals who have treated them)
and severe economic hardship for cities associated with the outbreak (e.g.,
Des Jarlais, Galea, Tracy, Tross, & Vlahov, 2006).

Considering the sum total of these issues, we may eventually find that
any agent-based nomenclature—differentiating natural disasters, technological accidents, and episodes of mass violence from one another as well as
from chronic hazards, epidemics, and war—has little descriptive or predictive
value. Describing specific incidents dimensionally according to time, space,
scope, magnitude, and mixture of causes will continue to be important.

OTHER CHARACTERISTICS OF DISASTERS
AND DISASTER EXPOSURE

Characteristics of disasters and disaster exposure are important determinants of the consequences of such events and may influence the nature of

the public sector's response. Here we will describe a few of the primary dimensions on which disasters (and other collective traumas) may be expected to vary.

Centripetal versus Centrifugal Disasters

Most disasters can be described as either centripetal or centrifugal (Lindy & Grace, 1986). This is an important way of typing disaster that is often overlooked. *Centripetal* refers to disasters that strike an extant community of people, and *centrifugal* to disasters that strike a group of people congregated temporarily. The former category might describe the prototypical disaster, where members of a geographically circumscribed community are struck by a disaster, such as a hurricane or earthquake. These disasters pose a risk to all those who live and work in these communities and may affect social and community functioning as well as psychological functioning. Moreover, the community that is harmed will also be called upon for rescue and recovery, creating a conflict between the role of victim and rescuer for many individuals. Centripetal disasters vary among themselves in the extent to which they are geographically circumscribed. For example, forest fires and tornadoes are events where there are typically clearly defined margins to the disaster. In contrast, events such as earthquakes and tropical storms have long gradients of exposure where the margins of the disaster are less precise.

Centrifugal disasters differ from centripetal disasters in two important ways: (1) they are highly concentrated and localized; and (2) they strike a group who happen to be congregated, often by chance. Mass transportation accidents, office tower explosions, and nightclub fires are good examples of centrifugal disasters. In these events, very few of the injured or dead may come from the locality of the disaster. The victims of mass transportation disasters are not always strangers (for example, there are examples of plane crashes where the plane was occupied by a group of travelers from the same community who were intentionally traveling together). Occasionally, these disasters have an international impact, with the survivors or the bereaved coming from many regions. One such example would be the 2002 Bali bombing, which killed more than 200 people. While a significant number of Balinese were killed, the bombing of a tourist venue meant that people from all around the world were killed or grievously injured. These distinctions have major implications for how rescues are mounted and the provision of services in the aftermath. Centrifugal disasters pose particular challenges for research with direct victims, so they have been studied less often than have centripetal disasters. The sinking of the Jupiter cruise ship and the Beverly Hills Supper Club fire are two examples of centrifugal disasters where survivors were studied (Green, Grace, & Gleser, 1985; Yule et al., 2000). Many studies of these events have focused on rescue/recovery workers (e.g., Dougall, Herberman, Delahanty, Inslicht, & Baum, 2000; Fullerton, Ursano, & Wang, 2004) or the broader community in which the disaster happened (e.g., Chung, Werrett, Farmer, Easthope, & Chung, 2000).

Onset and Duration Revisited

Although disasters by definition are acute stressors, they nonetheless vary in the *rapidity of onset*. The slower the onset, the longer is the warning period, which can save countless lives and reduce the prevalence of injuries. This characteristic is correlated with the centripetal–centrifugal distinction, as centrifugal disasters are almost always rapid in onset, whereas centripetal disasters sometimes are slower in onset, such as in the case of riverine floods. The impact of a disaster may be lessened by the anticipation and implementation of mitigation and protective strategies. As the threat emerges, there are also many actions by communities and individuals that can limit the destruction and protect life and property.

Similarly, although we have defined disasters as time-limited in character, they also vary in the relative *duration of the crisis*. Most disasters are characterized by an acute threat that is contained, and there is a relatively rapid restoration of order and safety. However, in some disasters, the postdisaster environment has many ongoing intrinsic threats to the individual and community, especially those where there is risk of epidemics or the income-earning infrastructure and housing have been destroyed. Further there are those where the nature of the danger is more insidious and difficult to identify and control. The implications of this prolonged threat are substantial because it may disrupt the development of a sense of safety. At the extreme end of this continuum, disasters become indistinguishable from chronic toxic hazards or ongoing political violence. Perhaps it might be said that an event can switch categories, beginning as a disaster and evolving into a chronic hazard.

The Times Beach contamination disaster (Robins et al., 1986) and the Chornobyl nuclear disaster, where a power reactor melted down and released toxic materials (Bromet et al., 2000), are illustrative of events that began as disasters but initiated a period of persisting threat. The invisible nature of chemical and radiation hazards has a number of implications. First, it is difficult to be immediately aware of exposure, as this occurs in an invisible manner. Second, when the hazard has been contained, it is hard to reassure the exposed community that the hazard is no longer a risk, especially if there is no visible evidence and there have been initial failures to warn of the risk, resulting in mistrust of the information given by the public authorities. Also, the harmful consequences of exposures are often slow to manifest, and there are long latency periods before diseases emerge, such as cancers and degenerative diseases. Genetic damage leading to congenital malformations remains an incipient fear for generations. Public distrust and fear of misinformation further erode the sense of safety in the community and maintain the sense of injustice, victimization, and loss. As is the case after all disasters, bringing an end to the sense of threat is critical to recovery.

Severity of Exposure at Population and Individual Levels

When studying the mental health impact of disasters, it is essential to characterize severity of exposure at both the population and individual levels. At the population level, an important characteristic is the *impact ratio*, the proportion of the population that is affected directly by the disaster. This characteristic emphasizes the proportion of persons directly affected rather than the absolute number of these persons, because the former may have more to do with the ability of the community to respond effectively. As the impact ratio increases, the mental health consequences of the disaster may likewise increase (Phifer & Norris, 1989). North and Norris (Chapter 3, this volume) discuss the implications of choosing research participants to represent severely exposed disaster victims or the general population of a disaster-stricken area.

Of course, from a psychological perspective, the extent of *terror and horror* associated with the disaster is especially important. Some disasters engender more fear, threat to life, and actual loss of life than do others. Although individual differences in severity of exposure typically are highly predictive of psychological outcomes (see Norris & Elrod, Chapter 2, this volume), there are important interactions between grief and traumatic psychopathology that are not yet thoroughly understood. In normal grief, the individual is able to revisit the memory of the person who died with a sense of longing and pain but also able to search positive memories. In disasters, the traumatic memories intrude and inhibit this normal process.

There are numerous challenges in conceptualizing the nature of individuals' disaster exposure. To begin with, losses can be in a series of domains, such as homes, the death and injury of friends and relatives, the destruction of community resources, and a loss of property that is involved in the generation of income and the provision of employment. Communities share losses in the natural, built, social, and economic environments. From an ecological perspective, an important question is this: When predicting individuals' psychological responses and recovery, do only their own losses matter, or are they influenced by the severity of losses and degree of recovery experienced by the community at large? If the exposure within a population is to be measured, these various dimensions must be scaled. Little work has been done examining the validity of such methods of scaling. Understanding of these matters is critical to the comparison of disaster studies. Equally, if information is to be used in making predictions about the likely effects of some recent event, estimates based on the degree of exposure are required.

Measurement of exposure is not a trivial issue, because researchers often underestimate the complexity of characterizing the experience of individuals. Van der Kolk et al. (1996) have argued that one of the primary characteristics of traumatic experiences is that they are events that challenge an individual's capacity to create a narrative of his or her experience and to integrate the traumatic experience with other events. As a consequence, traumatic memories are often not coherent stories and tend to consist of intense emotions or somatosensory impressions. Thus, these are events that test the capacity of language to capture and characterize experience. Hence, it is easy for researchers and clinicians alike to not fully embrace the horror and the helplessness that research data and patients' stories embody. This is a critical issue for the development of adequate methodologies and instruments to describe and characterize disaster experience.

Phases of Disaster

If the defining characteristics of disasters, relative to other collectively experienced potentially traumatic events, are their acute onset and time-limited threat, it follows that the temporal unfolding of a disaster is extremely important in planning services or research. In October 2001, an international panel of experts on trauma and mental health convened to determine best practices in disaster mental health (National Institute of Mental Health, 2002). As part of this effort, the group reached consensus on the differentiation of phases and identified the primary goals, behaviors, roles of helpers, and roles of mental health professionals that corresponded to each phase. Table 1.1 summarizes the main points of this guidance according to phases of *preincident, impact* (0–48 hours), *rescue* (0–1 week), *recovery* (1–4 weeks), and *return to life* (2 weeks–2 years). The table is relatively self-explanatory, and therefore we will not repeat the various points. We invite readers to reflect on this table, as thoughtful consideration of the identified roles and actions may help one to generate potential questions for research that are relevant to policymakers and practitioners. Myers and Wee (2005) also provide an excellent introduction to phased disaster mental health services that may be a good source of research ideas.

CONCLUSION

We have defined disasters as potentially traumatic events that are collectively experienced, have an acute onset, and are time-delimited. We have acknowledged that the boundaries of disaster research are not always clear and that there is considerable overlap between disasters and the larger set

TABLE 1.1. Guidance for Timing of Early Interventions

Phase	Preincident	Impact (0–48 hours)	Rescue (0–1 week)	Recovery (1–4 weeks)	Return to Life (2 weeks–2 years)
Goals	• Preparation • Improve coping	• Survival • Communication	• Adjustment	• Appraisal Planning	• Reintegration
Behavior	• Preparation versus denial	• Fight, flight, freeze, surrender, etc.	• Resilience versus exhaustion	• Grief, reappraisal, intrusive memories, narrative formation	• Adjustment versus phobias, PTSD, avoidance, depression, etc.
Role of helpers	• Prepare, train, gain knowledge.	• Rescue, protect	• Orient, provide for needs.	• Respond with sensitivity.	• Continue assistance.
Role of mental health professionals	*Prepare:* • Train, gain knowledge. • Collaborate. • Inform and influence policy. • Set structures for rapid assistance.	*Meet basic needs:* • Establish safety, security, survival. • Ensure food, shelter. • Provide orientation. • Facilitate communication with family, friends. • Assess environment for ongoing threat/toxins. *Provide psychological "first-aid":* • Provide support. • Keep families together. • Provide information. • Reduce arousal. *Monitor environment:* • Observe, listen. *Provide technical assistance/consultation:* • Improve capacity of organizations and caregivers.	*Needs assessment:* • Assess current status, how well needs are being addressed, and recovery environment. • Identify needs for interventions for individuals, groups, populations. *Triage:* • Clinical assessment. • Refer when indicated. • Identify vulnerable, high-risk individuals and groups. • Emergency hospitalization or outpatient treatment. *Outreach:* • Provide information about coping and recovery through established structures in community. *Foster resilience:* • Build natural supports. • Repair organizational fabric. • Educate.	*Monitor recovery environment:* • Observe, listen to those most affected. • Monitor environment for toxins. • Monitor past and ongoing threats. • Monitor services that are being provided. Continue relevant activities from earlier phases, by providing technical assistance, performing community outreach and fostering resilience.	*Treatment:* • Reduce or ameliorate symptoms or improve functioning via individual, family, or group psychotherapy, pharmacotherapy, or short-term or long-term hospitalization. Continue relevant activities from earlier phases, by providing technical assistance, performing community outreach, fostering resilience, and monitoring recovery environment.

Note. Summarized from National Institute of Mental Health (2002, Appendix B).

of collective crises, which includes war, public health epidemics, and mass displacements. Although this book primarily addresses methods that are useful for studying disasters, many of the fundamentals, methods, and challenges described in this volume have relevance for the study of escalating threats, such as political conflicts and epidemics, as well as for the study of chronic threats, such as toxic hazards and community violence.

We have also advised the reader to consider and describe the disaster under study in terms of several important attributes, including (1) whether it was centripetal or centrifugal and, if the former, the extent to which the impact was geographically circumscribed or diffuse; (2) the rapidity of the disaster's onset, extent of warning, and the duration of the period of threat; and (3) the severity of its impact, both in terms of the proportion of the population affected and the nature and magnitude of the stressors experienced by individuals and shared by the community. As these factors are considered and described in more standardized ways in future research, we may be able to determine whether these characteristics influence the mental health consequences of disasters more so than does their classification as natural disasters or technological accidents or episodes of mass violence.

We returned to temporal issues in concluding this chapter, this time through a practitioner's lens rather than through a researcher's lens. The two perspectives sometimes compete in the aftermath of disasters, but they do not have to, as each perspective has much to offer the other. Practitioners and researchers would undoubtedly agree that consequences and needs are changing rapidly and that data are perishable, meaning that disasters must be studied with minimal delay and with focused attention on the way that the event unfolds over time.

ACKNOWLEDGMENTS

Preparation of this chapter was supported by NH&MRC Program Grant No. 300403 to Alexander C. McFarlane and Grant No. R25 MH 068298 from the National Institute of Mental Health to Fran H. Norris.

REFERENCES

American Psychiatric Association. (1994). *Diagnostic and statistical manual of mental disorders* (4th ed.). Washington DC: Author.

Bolin, R. (1986). Disaster characteristics and psychosocial impacts. In B. Sowder & M. Lystad (Ed.), *Disasters and mental health: Selected contemporary perspectives* (pp. 3–28). Rockville, MD: National Institute of Mental Health.

Bromet, E., Goldgaber, D., Carlson, G., Panina, N., Golovakha, E., Gluzman, S., et al.

(2000). Children's well-being 11 years after the Chornobyl catastrophe. *Archives of General Psychiatry, 57,* 563–571.

Chung, M., Werrett, J., Farmer, S., Easthope, Y., & Chung, C. (2000). Responses to traumatic stress among community residents exposed to a train collision. *Stress Medicine, 16,* 17–25.

Creamer, M., Burgess, P., Buckingham, W., & Pattison, P. (1993). Posttrauma reactions following a multiple shooting: A retrospective study and methodological inquiry. In J. Wilson & B. Raphael (Eds.), *International handbook of traumatic stress syndromes* (pp. 201–212). New York: Plenum Press.

Creamer, M., Burgess, P. M., & McFarlane, A. C. (2001). Post-traumatic stress disorder: Findings from the Australian National Survey of Mental Health and Well-Being. *Psychological Medicine, 31*(7), 1237–1247.

De Girolamo, G., & McFarlane, A. (1996). The epidemiology of PTSD: A comprehensive review of the international literature. In A. Marsella, M. Friedman, E. Gerrity, & R. Surfield (Eds.), *Ethnocultural aspects of posttraumatic stress disorder: Issues, research, and clinical applications* (pp. 33–85). Washington, DC: American Psychological Association.

Des Jarlais, D., Galea, S., Tracy, M., Tross, S., & Vlahov, D. (2006). Stigmatization of newly emerging infectious diseases: AIDS and SARS. *American Journal of Public Health, 96*(3), 561–567.

Dougall, A., Herberman, H., Delahanty, D., Inslicht, S., & Baum, A. (2000). Similarity of prior trauma exposure as a determinant of chronic stress responding to an airline disaster. *Journal of Consulting and Clinical Psychology, 68,* 290–295.

Fullerton, C. S., Ursano, R. J., & Wang, L. (2004). Acute stress disorder, posttraumatic stress disorder, and depression in disaster or rescue workers. *American Journal of Psychiatry, 161,* 1370–1376.

Green, B. (1996). Cross-national and ethnocultural issues in disaster research. In A. Marsella, M. Friedman, E. Gerrity, & R. Surfield (Eds.), *Ethnocultural aspects of posttraumatic stress disorder: Issues, research, and clinical applications* (pp. 341–361). Washington, DC: American Psychological Association.

Green, B., Grace, M., & Gleser, G. (1985). Identifying survivors at risk: Long-term impairment following the Beverly Hills Supper Club fire. *Journal of Consulting and Clinical Psychology, 53,* 672–678.

International Federation of Red Cross and Red Crescent Societies (2000). *World disasters report: A focus on public health.* Dordrecht, The Netherlands: Martinus Nijhoff.

Kessler, R. C., Sonnega, A., Bromet, E., Hughes, M., & Nelson, C. B. (1995). Posttraumatic stress disorder in the National Comorbidity Survey. *Archives of General Psychiatry, 52*(12), 1048–1060.

Kinston, W., & Rosser, R. (1974). Disaster: Effects on mental and physical state. *Journal of Psychosomatic Research, 18,* 437–456.

Kroll-Smith, J., & Couch, S. (1993). Technological hazards: Social responses as traumatic stressors. In J. Wilson & B. Raphael (Eds.), *International handbook of traumatic stress syndromes* (pp. 79–91). New York: Plenum Press.

Lindy, J., & Grace, M. (1986). The recovery environment: Continuing stressor versus a healing psychosocial space. In B. Sowder & M. Lystad (Ed.), *Disasters and mental health: Selected contemporary perspectives* (pp.147–160). Rockville, MD: National Institute of Mental Health.

Myers, D., & Wee, D. (2005). *Disaster mental health services: A primer for practitioners.* New York: Brunner-Routledge.

National Institute of Mental Health. (2002). *Mental health and mass violence: Evidence-based early psychological intervention for victims/survivors of mass violence: A workshop to reach consensus on best practices* (NIH Pub. No. 02–5138). Washington, DC: U.S. Government Printing Office. Available online at www.nimh.nih.gov/publicat/massviolence.pdf

Norris, F., Friedman, M., Watson, P., Byrne, C., Diaz, E., & Kaniasty, K. (2002). 60,000 disaster victims speak: Part I. An empirical review of the empirical literature, 1981–2001. *Psychiatry, 65,* 207–239.

North, C., Nixon, S., Shariat, S., Mallonee, S., McMillen, J., Spitznagel, E., et al. (1999). Psychiatric disorders among survivors of the Oklahoma City bombing. *Journal of the American Medical Association, 282,* 755–762.

Oxford English Dictionary (1987). Oxford, UK: Oxford University Press.

Phifer, J., & Norris, F. (1989). Psychological symptoms in older adults following disaster: Nature, timing, duration, and course. *Journal of Gerontology, 44,* 207–217.

Pynoos, R., Frederick, C., Nader, K., Arroyo, W., Steinber, A., Eth, S., et al. (1987). Life threat and posttraumatic stress in school-age children. *Archives of General Psychiatry, 44,* 1057–1063.

Quarantelli, E. (1986). What is disaster? The need for clarification in definition and conceptualization in research. In B. Sowder & M. Lystad (Eds.) *Disasters and mental health: Selected contemporary perspectives* (pp. 49–81). Rockville, MD: National Institute of Mental Health.

Robins, L., Fischbach, R., Smith, E., Cottler, L., Solomon, S., & Goldring, E. (1986). Impact of disaster on previously assessed mental health. In J. Shore (Ed.), *Disaster stress studies: New methods and findings* (pp. 22–48). Washington, DC: American Psychiatric Press.

Rubonis, A., & Bickman, L. (1991). Psychological impairment in the wake of disaster: The disaster–psychopathology relationship. *Psychological Bulletin, 109,* 384–399.

Scott, R., Brooks, N., & McKinlay, W. (1995). Post-traumatic morbidity in a civilian community of litigants: A follow-up at 3 years. *Journal of Traumatic Stress, 8,* 403–418.

Somasundaram, D., Norris, F., Asukai, N, & Murthy, R. (2003). Natural and technological disasters. In B. Green, M. Friedman, J. de Jong, S. Solomon, T. Keane, J. Fairbank et al. (Eds.), *Trauma interventions in war and peace: Prevention, practice, and policy* (pp. 291–318). New York: Kluwer/Plenum.

Ursano, R., Norwood, A., Fullerton, C., Holloway, H., & Hall, M. (2003). Terrorism with weapons of mass destruction: Chemical, biological, nuclear, radiological, and explosive agents. In R. Ursano and A. Norwood (Eds.), *Annual review of psychiatry: Vol. 22. Trauma and disaster responses and management* (pp. 125–154). Washington, DC: American Psychiatric Press.

Van der Kolk, B., Pelcovitz, D., Roth, S., Mandel, F., McFarlane, A., & Herman, J. L. (1996). Dissociation, somatization, and affect dysregulation: The complexity of adaption of trauma. *American Journal of Psychiatry, 153,* 83–93.

Yule, W., Bolton, D., Udwin, O., Boyle, S., O'Ryan, D., & Nurrish, J. (2000). The long-term psychological effects of a disaster experienced in adolescence: I. The incidence and course of PTSD. *Journal of Child Psychology and Psychiatry, 41,* 503–511.

CHAPTER 2

Psychosocial Consequences of Disaster

A Review of Past Research

FRAN H. NORRIS
and CARRIE L. ELROD

The question of whether disasters influence mental health has been studied extensively. In this chapter, we provide a general overview of this body of research. We describe the various psychosocial consequences of disasters, the overall magnitude and duration of effects, and risk factors for adverse outcomes. We also summarize the methods that have been used in these studies and draw tentative conclusions about methodological trends. Our hope is that, by having better access to what is already known, future investigators will plan methodologically and conceptually stronger studies than have many investigators in the past.

DESCRIPTION OF PAST RESEARCH

In 2002, Norris and colleagues published a two-part empirical review of the disaster literature that presented results for 160 samples that experienced 102 distinct events and were coded as to sample type, disaster type, disaster location, outcomes observed, and overall severity of effects (Norris,

20

Route Item

5/11/2017 1:42:06 PM

ROUTE ITEM
Item Barcode:

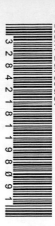

3 2 8 4 2 1 8 1 1 9 8 0 9 1

Title: Methods for disaster mental health research / edited by Fran H. Norris ... [et al.].

TO:
Library: University of Illinois at Urbana-Champaign Library

Location: UIUC ENGINEERING DESK
Address: ILDS: UIU
1301 W. Springfield Avenue
MC-274
Urbana, IL 61801

Friedman, & Watson, 2002; Norris, Friedman, Watson, et al., 2002). We updated this review for the purposes of this chapter. The studies included within our updated review were quantitative in approach and published in English between 1981 and 2004.[1] As discussed by McFarlane and Norris (Chapter 1, this volume), what exactly constitutes a disaster is not always clear at the boundaries. The focus of this review was on acute, collectively experienced events with sudden onset, thereby excluding research on chronic hazards and dislocation and terrorism that occurs within the context of ongoing political conflicts. Research that relied solely on archival or "social indicator" data or that focused solely on distant, indirect, or anticipated experiences was also excluded. For example, although we included several studies that examined the effects of the September 11, 2001, terrorist attacks on samples in New York and Washington, D.C., we excluded several studies that looked at the effects of terrorism on the nation as a whole or on samples outside of New York or Washington, DC. Because they were too few in number to review validly, studies of preschool-age children and bioterrorism were also excluded.

All together, the studies included in the updated review provided sample-level results pertaining to psychosocial outcomes for 225 distinct samples and 132 distinct events. Twenty-four percent of the samples experienced disasters that occurred before 1988. Events included (but were not limited to) the dam collapse in Buffalo Creek, West Virginia, the Three Mile Island nuclear accident, the Ash Wednesday bushfires in Australia, and the 1985 Mexico City earthquake. Twenty-two percent of the samples experienced events between 1988 and 1991. Illustrative events in this era included the devastating earthquake in Spitak Armenia, the Piper Alpha explosion, the sinking of the *Jupiter* cruise ship, and Hurricane Hugo. Twenty-eight percent of the samples experienced events between 1992 and 1995. Fourteen of the samples experienced Hurricane Andrew, which as of this writing remains the most studied event in the database. Other illustrative events of this era included the Mississippi River flood, the Hansin–Awaji earthquake in Kobe, Japan, and the Oklahoma City bombing. Twenty-five percent of the samples experienced events after 1995, such as the Marmara earthquake in Turkey. With 9 samples, the Chi Chi earthquake was the most thoroughly studied event in a developing country (Taiwan). To date, the September 11th terrorist attacks have contributed 11 samples to the database, a number that is likely to increase. See Galea, Appendix 1, this volume, for brief descriptions of the studied disasters.

---

[1]Readers are referred to www.redmh.org for some details excluded from this chapter, including statistical tests and the complete bibliography of the 225 samples. Alternatively, readers may contact Fran Norris for this information.

Disaster Types, Sample Types, and Disaster Locations

To date, the effects of natural disasters, such as earthquakes, hurricanes, floods, and wildfires, have been studied most often, accounting for 55% of the studies we reviewed. Nonetheless, a substantial number of technological accidents (28%) and episodes of mass violence (17%), such as terrorist attacks and shooting sprees, have been studied as well. Adult survivors predominate (70%), with school-age youths (16%) and rescue/recovery workers (15%) accounting for smaller percentages of the research. The samples are impressively diverse, coming from 34 separate countries or territories. The majority were studied in the United States or its territories (52%) or in other developed countries, such as the United Kingdom, Australia, western Europe, or Japan (28%). Disasters in the developing world, such as the former Soviet Union, Asia other than Japan, and the Americas, other than the United States or Canada, have been understudied, but there are signs of progress. Figure 2.1 shows the cumulative number of studies over time. In the most recent event era (1996 forward), 47% of the samples were drawn from developing countries, compared to only 11% of the samples in earlier

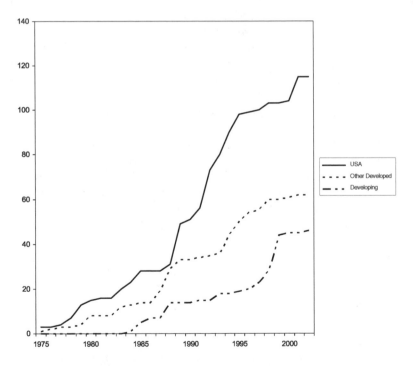

FIGURE 2.1. Cumulative frequencies (*n*'s) of samples in the database over time by disaster location (country type).

eras. Two earthquakes in Turkey and Taiwan were studied extensively (see uptick in 1999), creating some uncertainty about whether this finding represents a blip or the beginning of a trend.

Study Designs and Sampling Procedures

Most (72%) of the samples included in this review were assessed once after the disaster, and the remaining 28% were assessed two or more times. As shown in Table 2.1, longitudinal designs were less common in studies of disasters in developing countries than in studies of disasters in developed countries.

Researchers have provided a substantial amount of data about short-term disaster effects. Although these samples were first assessed at any time from immediately to 7 years postdisaster, 61% were assessed within 6 months, 28% within 2 months. In contrast, data about very long-term effects of disasters appear to be rare. Samples participating in longitudinal studies were interviewed as late as 17 years postdisaster (Green et al., 1990), but half (48% of the longitudinal samples) gave their last interview within 1 year postevent. For all panel studies, Figure 2.2 shows the month in which the study began and the month in which the study ended. (The latter was truncated at 10 years.) The data are clearly concentrated in the first 2 years.

Because disasters are typically unpredictable, it is rare for investigators to have access to true predisaster data, although it is not uncommon for such data to be collected retrospectively. In our review, we identified only 10 studies (4.4%) that had true predisaster measures (Alexander & Wells, 1991; Asarnow et al., 1999; Bravo, Rubio-Stipec, Canino, Woodbury, & Ribera, 1990; Knight, Gatz, Heller, & Bengston, 2000; Lutgendorf et al., 1995; Nolen-Hoeksema & Morrow, 1991; Norris, Phifer, & Kaniasty, 1994; Robins et al., 1986; Ullman & Newcomb, 1999; Warheit, Zimmerman, Khoury, Vega, & Gil, 1996).

Various sampling strategies have been used in past research. Most representative were samples drawn by using a census approach (27%), where investigators attempted to include all persons who experienced the event, or by means of probability sampling (19%). Some samples were drawn by using purposive or "quasi-random" sampling techniques (17%). Least representative were samples composed of individuals recruited for reasons of convenience (31%) or composed of hospitalized individuals, patients, or litigants referred for clinical evaluation (6%). Convenience sampling was the mode.

Sampling strategy covaried strongly with sample type (see Table 2.1). Purposive sampling was disproportionately common in studies of youths, because it best described methods used in many school-based studies. Ran-

TABLE 2.1. Methodological Variables by Substantive Variables in the Research

Variable Value	Sample type			Disaster location			Disaster type			Row % severe or very severe
	Child survivor (n = 37)	Adult survivor (n = 157)	Rescue/recovery (n = 33)	USA (n = 116)	Other developed (n = 63)	Developing country (n = 46)	Natural disaster (n = 124)	Technological accident (n = 62)	Mass violence (n = 39)	
Design 1										
1 post time-point	77.1	74.0	63.6	69.0	71.4	84.8	76.4	65.6	73.7	40.5
2+ post time-points	22.9	26.0	36.4	31.0	28.6	15.2	23.6	34.4	26.3	40.7
Design 2										
After only	94.3	95.5	97.0	92.2	98.4	100.0	92.7	98.4	100.0	41.9
Pre–post	5.7	4.5	3.0	7.8	1.6	0.0	7.3	1.6	0.0	0.0
Timing of first assessment										
Within 2 months	17.1	27.7	39.4	31.9	23.0	23.9	27.6	29.5	25.6	33.3
3–6 months	40.0	31.0	36.4	32.8	32.8	34.8	32.5	29.5	41.0	43.8
7–12 months	25.7	25.2	9.1	24.1	21.3	21.7	23.6	21.3	23.1	42.0
>12 months	17.1	16.1	15.2	11.2	23.0	19.6	16.3	19.7	10.3	40.0
Sampling method										
Clinical	2.9	7.7	3.0	3.4	11.3	6.5	0.8	11.3	15.4	85.7
Convenience	25.7	35.9	18.2	32.8	27.4	34.8	40.7	17.7	25.6	31.0
Purposive	37.1	14.1	6.1	14.7	8.1	32.6	22.8	4.8	15.4	54.1
Random	8.6	24.4	3.0	25.9	6.5	17.4	25.2	8.1	15.4	23.8
Census	25.7	17.9	69.7	23.3	46.8	8.7	10.6	58.1	28.2	45.0
Sample size										
1–100	25.7	32.5	51.5	31.9	49.2	19.6	24.2	46.8	46.2	44.0
101–400	45.7	43.9	36.4	44.0	38.1	47.8	50.8	41.9	20.5	39.4
401–1000	8.6	16.6	9.1	13.8	7.9	23.9	17.7	6.5	15.4	46.9
>1000	20.0	7.0	3.0	10.3	4.8	8.7	7.3	4.8	17.9	15.8

Note. Column percentages, except where noted.

24

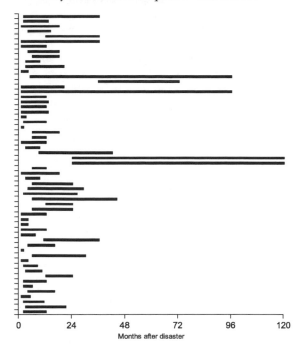

FIGURE 2.2. Beginning and end points of data collection in past panel studies of disaster. Values on the horizontal axis are months since disaster, truncated at 10 years. Each bar represents one panel study.

dom sampling was most common in studies of adult survivors, because population surveys primarily recruit community-dwelling adults. A large proportion of rescue workers but relatively small proportions of survivors were studied using the census method. In these studies, all workers of a given profession (e.g., body handlers) who worked a particular event were recruited. It was not always clear whether the sample truly represented a census or was selected for reasons of convenience. This point should be made more clearly in descriptions of samples in future research.

When possible, larger N's are generally preferred because smaller N's yield error and low power and limit ability to examine important subgroups. The size of these samples varied from very small (11) to very large (5,687). The median size was 150. Small samples (≤ 100) were disproportionately common in studies of rescue/recovery workers, and large samples ($N > 1,000$) were disproportionately common in studies of youths, probably because of the use of school-based studies (see Table 2.1). Small samples were more common in studies of technological accidents than in studies of other disaster types.

There was little evidence that the field is making methodological progress. Recent investigations are beginning earlier, on average, than did earlier studies, but they are not necessarily making use of preferred designs or sampling procedures. In fact, the proportion of studies with two or more postdisaster assessments has been decreasing, as has the proportion of samples that are high in representativeness. Recent studies did not differ from earlier studies in sample size. The correlation between sample N and event year approached 0.

MENTAL HEALTH EFFECTS OF DISASTERS

Psychosocial Consequences

Effects of the disaster on at least some aspect of mental or behavioral health were identified in most of the studies we reviewed. The studies are too numerous to mention each one, but we provide some examples of each point. Undoubtedly, the condition most often assessed and observed in these samples was posttraumatic stress disorder (PTSD; e.g., Başoğlu, Kiliç, Şalcioğlu & Livanou, 2004; Fullerton, Ursano, & Wang, 2004; Galea et al., 2002; Norris, Murphy, Baker, & Perilla, 2004; see Galea, Nandi, & Vlahov, 2005, for a review). A common finding was for intrusion and arousal to be highly prevalent and avoidance less so (e.g., Catapano et al., 2001; McMillen, North, & Smith, 2000; Maes et al., 1998). Dissociative responses (Koopman, Classen, & Spiegel, 1996) and acute stress disorder (e.g., Grieger et al., 2000; Waelde, Koopman, Rierdan, & Spiegel, 2001) also have been observed in the immediate aftermath of disasters.

Depression and anxiety are also commonly observed psychological problems in this research (e.g., Bokszczanin, 2002; Bromet, Parkinson, Schulberg, & Gondek, 1982; Norris et al., 2004; Palinkas, Russell, Downs, & Petterson, 1993; Shore, Tatum, & Vollmer, 1986; Thiel de Bocanegra & Brickman, 2004). Death anxiety, phobias, and panic disorder have been assessed and observed only occasionally in samples of disaster victims (e.g., Armenian et al., 2000; Bolton, O'Ryan, Udwin, Boyle, & Yule, 2000), although there is growing evidence that peri-event panic attacks are highly predictive of subsequent consequences (e.g., Galea et al., 2002).

Many studies have observed an elevation of various stress-related psychological and psychosomatic symptoms rather than (or in addition to) a particular syndrome, such as anxiety or depression (e.g., Carr et al., 1997; McFarlane, 1989). Demoralization (Dohrenwend, 1983), perceived stress (Thompson, Norris, & Hanacek, 1993), and negative affect (Smith, 1996) refer to similar states of nonspecific distress.

Physical health problems and/or somatic concerns were identified in many samples. Disaster victims score higher than norms or controls on objective measures (e.g., Holen, 1991) as well as on self-reported somatic complaints or checklists of medical conditions (e.g., Clayer, Bookless-Pratz, & Harris, 1985; Murphy, 1984). Physiological indicators of stress are often elevated, and sleep quality is poor (e.g., Baum, Gatchel, & Schaeffer, 1983; Ironson et al., 1997; Krakow et al., 2004). Less common than other outcomes but observed in a few samples was an increase in the use of alcohol, drugs, or cigarettes (e.g., Grieger, Fullerton, & Ursano, 2003; Vlahov et al., 2003). Alcohol consumption may increase the most in persons who were already problem drinkers or who developed other psychological disorders (North et al., 1999). Disaster exposure may increase the likelihood of relapse (clinical worsening of symptoms) in previously disabled populations (Lutgendorf et al., 1995).

Chronic problems in living (secondary stressors) have been assessed less often, but where they have been assessed, they typically have been observed. In the months that follow a disaster, disaster victims are more likely than nonvictims to experience interpersonal, familial, financial, and ecological changes and stress (e.g., Bowler, Mergler, Huel, & Cone, 1994; Murphy, 1984; Norris, Perilla, Riad, Kaniasty, & Lavizzo, 1999). These outcomes sometimes have been conceptualized and analyzed as mediators, that is, as factors that intervene between acute exposure and chronic psychological effects (Norris & Uhl, 1993).

Resources are themselves vulnerable to disaster-related stress, a phenomenon that severely limits the protection they can afford. Influenced strongly by the theory of conservation of resources (Hobfoll, 1988), several studies have documented declines in psychosocial resources in the aftermath of disasters (Arata, Picou, Johnson, & McNally, 2000; Benight et al., 1999; Bland et al., 1997; Freedy, Shaw, Jarrell, & Masters, 1992; Ironson et al., 1997). In tests of their "social support deterioration model," Kaniasty and Norris (1993; Norris, Baker, Murphy, & Kaniasty, 2005; Norris & Kaniasty, 1996) have shown more specifically that disaster victims experience declines in social embeddedness and perceived social support.

Magnitude of Effects

Of course, not all disasters are equally serious from a public health perspective. A few samples in this review (9%) showed only minimal or highly transient effects. The majority of the samples (50%) showed moderate effects, indicative of prolonged stress but little psychopathology. In these samples, depending upon the study's design, there were significant differences between exposed participants and some comparison group, changes between predisaster and postdisaster mental health measures, or significant correlations between exposure measures and mental health measures. The remaining samples showed severe (24%) or very severe (17%) effects, indicative of a high (25–49%) or very high (≥ 50%) prevalence of clinically significant distress (determined on the basis of percentages scoring above established cutoff points on standardized scales) or criterion-level psychological disorder (determined on the basis of diagnostic instruments).

Influence of Substantive Variables on Magnitude of Effects

The ability of sample-level variables to predict the overall severity of effects observed in the sample was tested in a regression analysis. The predictors included both substantive variables (sample type, disaster type, disaster location) and methodological variables (design, sample size, sampling strategy). Sample type was coded as two dummy variables, Youths and Rescue Workers, with Adult Survivors serving as the reference category. Location of disaster was likewise coded as two dummy variables, Other Developed Country and Developing Country, with the United States serving as the reference category. Type of disaster was also coded as two dummy variables, Technological Accident and Mass Violence, with Natural Disaster as the reference category. The advantage of this method is that all effects were independent of the effects of the other variables in the equation.

In the regression analyses, both sets of predictors influenced the effects observed. Child samples had been most likely to show severe effects in the original review (Norris, Friedman, Watson, et al., 2002). In the 2005 update, however, samples composed of youth were no more likely to fall into the severe range of effects than samples composed of adult survivors. Because there are fewer child samples, overall, their results may continue to fluctuate as new studies are conducted. In both the original and updated review, samples were far less likely to show severe effects if they were composed of rescue and recovery workers rather than survivors, but this result should also be interpreted with caution. These rescue and recovery workers seldom experienced direct losses or extensive bereavement. The heterogeneity of the responder samples was problematic, and as research on this topic grows, it would be advisable to make finer distinctions between responder groups exposed to physical danger (e.g., firefighters), horror, and the dead (e.g., body handlers, medical personnel), and vicarious trauma (e.g., counselors). These various caveats notwithstanding, it is also possible that we could learn much about the factors that foster resilience in these groups that seem to fare better than objective circumstances suggest they should (e.g., Alexander & Wells, 1991; McCarroll, Fullerton, Ursano, & Hermsen, 1996).

Samples that experienced technological disasters were not significantly more distressed, on average, than were samples that experienced natural disasters. With other characteristics held constant, however, it did appear that severe effects were most likely to occur in samples that had experienced mass violence. Intentional disasters may be especially difficult for victims to comprehend or assimilate. Shooting sprees (e.g., North, Smith, & Spitznagel, 1994) and terrorist attacks (e.g., North et al., 1999) tend to be indiscriminate and random, creating acute helplessness and anxiety.

Relative to the United States, samples were more likely to show severe effects if they were from either developing or other developed countries, but the effect of location in a developing country was particularly large. This finding may indicate that, outside of the United States, only the most severe events tend to be studied, or it may reflect the fact that disasters tend to be more severe when they occur in the developing world. Many of the samples from developing countries survived disasters where death tolls were measured in thousands or even tens of thousands, such as the horrendous Armenian and Marmara earthquakes and Hurricane Mitch. The difference may also attest to the ability of government services and other resources to make a difference in the lives of disaster victims.

Influence of Methodological Variables on Magnitude of Effects

It was very clear in our analyses that effects observed at the sample level were not solely dependent upon substantive variables, such as the sample type, disaster type, or disaster location, but were also influenced by the methodology used. Studies using pre–post designs were less likely to find severe or very severe effects than were studies using after-only designs. This finding may indicate, on the one hand, that controlling for predisaster symptoms makes for a more conservative test that lessens confounding of postdisaster mental health with predisaster mental health. This finding is consistent with Rubonis and Bickman's (1991) interpretation of their findings from a meta-analysis of 52 controlled studies. On the other hand, there were a few examples in this literature of samples that were only minimally exposed but studied precisely because there were predisaster data available for the research.

Sampling method and sample size also predicted the severity of observed effects. Severe effects were disproportionately common in clinical samples and disproportionately uncommon in both convenience samples and random samples (see Table 2.1). Only 16% of very large samples showed severe or very severe effects, compared to 43% of samples with $N \leq 1,000$. With sample size controlled, the effects of random sampling disappeared, which suggests that it is not the randomness of participants' selection per se that reduced the severity of observed effects but rather that random selection is typically used for large sample surveys. As Galea et al. (2005) pointed out, general populations should not be expected to show the severity of impact that victim groups do. A sizable proportion of persons making up most general population samples were only indirectly exposed to the focal event. Not all large samples were probability samples. Many of the largest samples were purposive samples, drawn from schools. These samples also often include substantial numbers of students with indirect forms of exposure to the disaster.

Of the various methodology findings, the most intriguing was the weaker effects shown by convenience samples. This finding contradicts Rubonis and Bickman's (1991) earlier result but is based upon a much larger number of studies, including many that would not have met their criteria for inclusion. Moreover, in Rubonis and Bickman's analysis, "nonrepresentative" samples included clinical/litigant as well as convenience samples. Although the assumption may be that convenience samples are composed of disproportionately exposed or distressed persons, in reality this is not always the case. In fact, sometimes samples are chosen not because they are the most important but solely because they are accessible. These samples may do a disservice to the research as a whole.

Duration of Effects

Forty-six studies were most relevant for discerning the course of postdisaster symptoms because the same individuals were assessed with the same measures at each wave, and effects were observed at some point during the study. In general, the first year postdisaster was the time of peak symptoms and effects. Seventy percent of these samples improved as time passed. Sometimes symptoms declined in a linear fashion, but sometimes they declined at first, then stabilized; or stabilized for a while, then began a new downward trend.

In many studies, levels of symptoms in the early phases of disaster recovery were good predictors of symptom levels in later phases of recovery (e.g., Fullerton et al., 1999; La Greca, Silverman, Vennberg, & Prinstein, 1996; McFarlane, 1987, 1989; Nader, Pynous, Fairbanks, & Frederick, 1990; Norris et al., 1999; Waelde et al., 2001). Where examined, delayed onsets of disorders were rare (e.g., North, Smith, & Spitznagel, 1997; Yule et al., 2000), although there were exceptions to this rule (Sungar & Kaya, 2001).

RISK AND PROTECTIVE FACTORS

It is well established that individuals vary markedly in their outcomes even when they have experienced the same event. A variety of factors have been found to influence the likelihood that an individual within a community will develop serious or lasting psychological problems in the wake of disasters. Again, the studies are too numerous to mention each one, but we provide some examples of each point. Also, it should be noted that there is much room for advancement here, especially in terms of interrelations of risk factors and timing of their effects.

Severity of Exposure

When the study's design allowed consideration of variations in participants' experiences in the disaster, severity of exposure typically was operationalized and included in the analysis in some way. A few investigators counted the number of stressors as an index of severity of exposure (Palinkas et al., 1993; Thompson et al., 1993) and generally found that, as the number of stressors increased, the participant's symptoms increased. Other investigators created ordinal measures that reflected their assumptions about the relative severity and comparability of different aspects of exposure (Bravo et al., 1990; Shore et al., 1986), and these measures also generally predicted psychological outcomes. Specific stressors that have been found to affect mental health include bereavement (Armenian et al., 2000; Gleser, Green, & Winget, 1981; Fullerton et al., 1999; Murphy, 1984), injury to self or family member (Catapano et al., 2001; Udwin, Boyle, Yule, Bolton, & O'Ryan, 2000), life threat (Creamer, Burgess, Buckingham, & Pattison, 1993; Dew & Bromet, 1993; Thompson et al., 1993), panic during the disaster (Galea et al., 2002; McFarlane, 1989), property damage or financial loss (Clayer et al., 1985; Thiel de Bocanegra & Brickman, 2004; Waelde et al., 2001), and relocation (Bland et al., 1997; Bromet et al., 2000; Norris et al., 2001).

There is relatively little research on collective loss or trauma, although it has long been held to be a defining feature of disasters. Occasionally, severity of exposure has been assessed at the neighborhood or community level. Three approaches to ecological assessment were demonstrated in this literature: (1) participants have been asked to describe conditions in their neighborhoods or communities (e.g., Hanson, Kilpatrick, Freedy, & Saunders, 1995); (2) data have been aggregated "up" from the individual to the neighborhood or community level (e.g., Perilla, Norris, & Lavizzo, 2002); and (3) archival data have been collected that reflect collective loss independent of personal loss (e.g., Norris et al., 1994). In general, such measures tend to have modest effects; yet, they often do explain variance in outcomes over and above those of individual-level measures. Community and school surveys conducted in the aftermath of terrorism provide excellent reminders that disasters impact upon whole communities, not just selected individuals (e.g., Galea et al., 2002; Pfefferbaum et al., 2001; Pfefferbaum et al., 2003). In our opinion, capturing the collective aspects of disaster exposure (and resulting complexities) is an important goal for future research.

Gender

With few exceptions, studies that have examined gender differences have almost always found female survivors to be more adversely affected. After many disasters, women were twice as likely to develop posttraumatic stress disorder (PTSD) as men (e.g., Green et al., 1990; North et al., 1999; Steinglass & Gerrity, 1990). Effects of gender are stronger in some cultures or contexts than in others (Norris, Perilla, Ibañez, & Murphy, 2001; Webster, McDonald, Lewin, & Carr, 1995).

Effects of Age in Adulthood

In contrast to conventional wisdom, only rarely have older persons been found to be at greater risk than other adults, and, in fact, middle-aged adults are often the most adversely affected by disasters (Gleser et al., 1981; Phifer, 1990; Shore et al., 1986). Explanations of these differences have sometimes focused on the maturity and experience that come with age (Norris & Murrell, 1988) and sometimes on the burdens of the middle-aged (Thompson et al., 1993). Norris, Kaniasty, et al. (2002) presented a caveat with regard to these findings in their cross-cultural study of age effects among disaster victims in the United States, Mexico, and Poland. In this study, there was no one consistent effect of age; rather, it depended upon the social, economic, cultural, and historical context of the disaster-stricken setting.

Ethnicity

Despite a few exceptions, most disaster studies that have examined the effects of ethnicity on outcomes have found that specific minority ethnic groups fare worse than persons who are of majority group status (e.g., Galea et al., 2002; Green et al., 1990; March, Amaya-Jackson, Terry, & Costanzo, 1997; Palinkas et al., 1993; Perilla et al., 2002; Webster et al., 1995). A few noncomparative studies have similarly shown that post-disaster stress was quite high in particular ethnic communities (e.g., Thiel de Bocanegra & Brickman, 2004). Ethnicity is sometimes related to other risk/protective factors, such as socioeconomic status, severity of exposure, receipt of support, and sense of personal control (Kaniasty & Norris, 1995; Palinkas et al., 1993; Perilla et al., 2002).

Socioeconomic Status

Relatively few studies have focused explicitly on the effects of socioeconomic status (SES) indicators, such as education, income, literacy, or occupational prestige, on postdisaster mental health. Where examined, lower SES was typically associated with poorer postdisaster outcomes (e.g., Catapano et al., 2001; Hanson et al., 1995; Norris et al., 2005; Vila et al., 2001). Phifer (1990) and Ginexi, Weihs, and Simmens (2000) tested interactive effects and found that the adverse effects of severity of exposure grew stronger as SES decreased.

Family Factors

Family factors are important in a variety of complex and systemic ways in the aftermath of disasters. Marital stress has been found to increase after disasters (Norris & Uhl, 1993). Husbands' symptom severity predicts their wives', and vice versa (Gleser et al., 1981; Vila et al., 2001), even with exposure and other demographics controlled. Being a parent also adds to the stressfulness of disaster recovery (Bromet et al., 1982; Havenaar et al., 1997; Solomon, Bravo, Rubio-Stipec, & Canino, 1993). In the face of uncertain health threats, mothers may become very concerned over their children's health (Bromet et al., 2000). Parental distress is a strong predictor of their children's distress (e.g., McFarlane, 1987; Rustemli & Karanci, 1996; Vila et al., 2001; Wasserstein & La Greca, 1998).

Predisaster Functioning

Whether they are assessed retrospectively or before the disaster, predisaster psychological symptoms are almost always among the best predictors of postdisaster symptoms. For example, North et al. (1999) found that victims of the Oklahoma City bombing with predisaster disorder were more likely to experience PTSD specifically related to the bombing, with a rate of 46%, than were victims with no prior disorder, for whom the rate of bombing-related PTSD was 26%. Testing interactive effects, Phifer (1990) found that respondents with higher preflood depression were more strongly affected by a flood than respondents with lower preflood depression. Prior clinical cases exposed to disasters are more likely to experience a relapse than cases not so exposed (Shore et al., 1986).

Psychological Coping and Resources

The data on coping are sometimes confusing but do consistently suggest that avoidance coping is problematic, as is the assignment of blame (Asarnow et al., 1999; Cleary & Houts, 1984; La Greca et al., 1996; Smith, 1996). Most individuals use many different types of coping simultaneously, making it difficult to isolate their unique effects. The inherent confounding (distress leads to increased coping) makes it very difficult to capture the reciprocal effect (coping leads to reduced distress), especially in cross-sectional designs. In a prospective analysis, North, Spitznagel, and Smith (2001) found three types of coping (active outreach, informed pragmatism, reconciliation) to be associated with decreased risk for psychiatric disorders. Coping self-efficacy—the perception that one is capable of managing the specific demands related to the disaster—has been strongly predictive of good outcomes (e.g., Benight & Harper, 2002; Benight et al, 1999). Lower distress also has been linked to higher perceived control, self-esteem, trait hopefulness, future temporal orientation, optimism, and hardiness (Bartone, Ursano, Wright, & Ingraham, 1989; Dougall, Hyman, Hayward, McFeeley, & Baum, 2001; Holman & Silver, 1998; Murphy, 1988; Norris et al., 1999).

Social Support

Social support researchers often differentiate among social embeddedness, received social support, and perceived social support. Social embeddedness, the structural component of social support describing the size, activeness, and closeness of the network, has been found to protect disaster victims from psychological distress (e.g., Cleary & Houts, 1984; Udwin et al., 2000), as has received support, the actual help received from others (e.g., Bolin, 1982; Joseph, Yule, Williams, & Andrews, 1992). Norris and Kaniasty (1996) found that the effects of received support on distress were mediated by perceived support, which is defined as the general sense of belongingness and belief in the availability of support, rather than actual receipt. The ability of perceived social support to protect disaster victims' health and mental health has been demonstrated repeatedly (e.g., Bartone et al., 1989; Bromet et al., 1982; Creamer et al., 1993; Dougall et al., 2001; La Greca et al., 1996; Weiss, Marmar, Metzler, & Ronfeldt, 1995).

SUMMARY AND CONCLUSIONS

A substantial amount of research pertinent to understanding the effects of disasters on mental health has been published over the past 25 years. Disaster victims' experiences and outcomes have been studied using a variety of designs, time frames, assessment strategies, and sampling methods. The research is impressively diverse, including children and adults from 34 countries or territories who experienced almost every imaginable type of disaster. Individuals' experiences ranged from little more than inconvenience to life-threatening danger, severe injuries, multiple bereavements, and the total destruction of their communities. Accordingly, it is not surprising that psychological outcomes varied across samples from a predominance of transient stress reactions to prevalent and persistent psycho-pathology.

Taken together, the data show that disasters do have implications for mental health for a significant proportion of the communities that experience them. Severe effects were especially likely when the disasters involved intentional harm or when they occurred in developing countries. Published studies identified specific psychological problems, such as anxiety, depression, and most notably PTSD, nonspecific psychological distress, varying health problems, chronic problems in living (or secondary stressors), and resource loss. The breadth of the outcomes observed indicated that researchers should not focus too narrowly on any one aspect of mental health in either epidemiological or intervention research. Although community recovery was the norm, numerous exceptions point to the need for longer-term studies after especially severe events.

A variety of factors have been found to influence the likelihood that an individual within a community will develop serious or lasting psychological problems in the wake of disasters. More severe exposure, female gender, middle age, ethnic minority status, family strains, prior psychiatric problems, secondary stressors, and weak or deteriorating psychosocial resources most consistently increased the likelihood of adverse outcomes. Undoubtedly these factors work together in ways more complex than captured in the research to date, and, in fact, interactive effects of these risk factors often emerged when such effects were tested. The effects of certain variables are mediated by other variables; for example, acute stressors increase the likelihood of chronic stressors that in turn increase the likelihood of psychological distress. Furthermore, some of these effects may be confounded with others; for example, findings that middle-aged adults, parents, and married women are disproportionately distressed all may be capturing the same processes: that caring for others is a source of stress (as well as a source of comfort) in the aftermath of disasters. We still know relatively little about how ethnicity and culture shape the influence of other variables. The state of the art is such that we cannot provide a fully integrated understanding of how all of these factors work together to increase or decrease vulnerability, making this an important arena for future research.

The review pointed to a number of methodological shortcomings in the research overall that we hope will be improved upon by future investigators. The quality of disaster research has not kept pace with the quantity of disaster research. The use of longitudinal designs and representative samples has decreased over time, although the rapidity of first assessment has increased. Rapid assessment should facilitate a better understanding of the acute postdisaster period and aid early identification of persons at long-term risk. However, we should be cautious not to trade rapidity for quality; in this review, samples that were assessed rap-

idly (within 2 months) were disproportionately likely to have been selected for reasons of convenience.

In closing, we will note our opinion that there is little need for additional correlational studies that merely replicate the purposes, methods,
and findings of past research. When there is much previous research on a
topic, it becomes more difficult to justify exploratory or "quick and dirty"
research. The field is now sufficiently mature to require investigators to derive novel and theoretically sound questions (Benight, McFarlane, &
Norris, Chapter 4, this volume), exercise good scholarship (Lerner, Appendix 2, this volume), choose the strongest possible methodologies (North &
Norris, Chapter 3, this volume), and collect their data according to the
highest ethnical standards (Fleischman, Collogan, & Tuma, Chapter 5, this
volume).

ACKNOWLEDGMENTS

Preparation of this article was supported by Grant No. R25 MH068298 from the
National Institute of Mental Health awarded to Fran H. Norris. The Department of
Veterans Affairs also provided support. Appreciation is extended to Peggy Wil-
loughby for her assistance in updating the literature review.

REFERENCES

Alexander, D., & Wells, A. (1991). Reactions of police officers to body-handling after a
major disaster: A before and after comparison. *British Journal of Psychiatry, 159,*
547–555.
Arata, C., Picou, J., Johnson, G., & McNally, T. (2000). Coping with technological disaster: An application of the conservation of resources model to *Exxon Valdez* oil spill.
Journal of Traumatic Stress, 11, 23–39.
Armenian, H., Morikawa, M., Melkonian, A., Hovanesian, A., Haroutunian, N., Saigh, P.,
et al. (2000). Loss as a determinant of PTSD in a cohort of adult survivors of the 1988
earthquake in Armenia: Implications for policy. *Acta Psychiatrica Scandinavica, 102,*
58–64.
Asarnow, J., Glynn, S., Pynoos, R., Nahum, J., Guthrie, D., Cantwell, D., et al. (1999).
When the earth stops shaking: Earthquake sequelae among children diagnosed for
pre-earthquake psychopathology. *Journal of the American Academy of Child and
Adolescent Psychiatry, 38,* 1016–1023.
Bartone, P., Ursano, R., Wright, K., & Ingraham, L. (1989). The impact of a military air disaster on the health of assistance workers: A prospective study. *Journal of Nervous
and Mental Disease, 177,* 317–328.
Başoğlu, M., Kiliç, C., Şalcioğlu, E., & Livanou, M. (2004). Prevalence of posttraumatic
stress disorder and comorbid depression in earthquake survivors in Turkey: An epidemiological study. *Journal of Traumatic Stress, 17,* 133–141.
Baum, A., Gatchel, R., & Schaeffer, M. (1983). Emotional, behavioral and physiological

effects at Three Mile Island. *Journal of Consulting and Clinical Psychology, 51*, 565–572.

Benight, C. C., & Harper, M. L. (2002). Coping self-efficacy perceptions as a mediator between acute stress response and long-term distress following natural disasters. *Journal of Traumatic Stress, 15*, 177–186.

Benight, C., Ironson, G., Klebe, K., Carver, C., Wynings, C., Burnett, K., et al. (1999). Conservation of resources and coping self-efficacy predicting distress following a natural disaster: A causal model analysis where the environment meets the mind. *Anxiety, Stress, and Coping, 12*, 107–126.

Bland, S., O'Leary, E., Farinaro, E., Jossa, F., Krogh, V., Violanti, J., et al. (1997). Social network disturbances and psychological distress following earthquake evacuation. *Journal of Nervous and Mental Disease, 185*, 188–194.

Bokszczanin, A. (2002). Long-term negative psychological effects of a flood on adolescents. *Polish Psychological Bulletin, 33*, 55–61.

Bolin, R. (1982). *Long-term family recovery from disaster.* Boulder, CO: Institute of Behavioral Science, University of Colorado.

Bolton, D., O'Ryan, D., Udwin, O., Boyle, S., & Yule, W. (2000). The long-term psychological effects of a disaster experienced in adolescence: II. General psychopathology. *Journal of Child Psychology and Psychiatry, 41*, 513–523.

Bowler, R., Mergler, D., Huel, G., & Cone, J. E. (1994). Psychological, psychosocial and psychophysiological sequelae in a community affected by a railroad chemical disaster. *Journal of Traumatic Stress, 7*, 601–624.

Bravo, M., Rubio-Stipec, M., Canino, G., Woodbury, M., & Ribera, J. (1990). The psychological sequelae of disaster stress prospectively and retrospectively evaluated. *American Journal of Community Psychology, 18*, 661–680.

Bromet, E., Parkinson, D., Schulberg, H., & Gondek, P. (1982). Mental health of residents near the Three Mile Island reactor: A comparative study of selected groups. *Journal of Preventive Psychiatry, 1*, 225–276.

Bromet, E., Goldgaber, D., Carlson, G., Panina, N., Golovakha, E., Gluzman, S., et al. (2000). Children's well-being 11 years after the Chornobyl catatrophe. *Archives of General Psychiatry, 57*, 563–571.

Carr, V., Lewin, T., Webster, R., Kenardy, J., Hazell, P., & Carter, G. (1997). Psychosocial sequelae of the 1989 Newcastle earthquake: II. Exposure and morbidity profiles during the first 2 years post-disaster. *Psychological Medicine, 27*, 167–178.

Catapano, F., Malafronte, R., Lepre, F., Cozzolino, P., Armone, R., Lorenzo, E., et al. (2001). Psychological consequences of the 1998 landslide in Sarno, Italy: A community study. *Acta Psychiatrica Scandinavica, 104*, 438–442.

Clayer, J., Bookless-Pratz, C., & Harris, R. (1985). Some health consequences of a natural disaster. *The Medical Journal of Australia, 143*, 182–184.

Cleary, P., & Houts, P. (1984). The psychological impact of the Three Mile Island incident. *Journal of Human Stress, 10*, 28–34.

Creamer, M., Burgess, P., Buckingham, W., & Pattison, P. (1993). Posttrauma reactions following a multiple shooting: A retrospective study and methodological inquiry. In J. Wilson & B. Raphael (Eds.). *International Handbook of Traumatic Stress Syndromes* (pp. 201–212). New York: Plenum.

Dew, M., & Bromet, E. (1993). Predictors of temporal patterns of psychiatric distress during 10 years following the nuclear accident at Three Mile Island. *Social Psychiatry and Psychiatric Epidemiology, 28*, 49–55.

Dohrenwend, B. P. (1983). Psychological implications of nuclear accidents: The case of

Three Mile Island. *Bulletin of the New York Academy of Medicine, 59,* 1060–1076.

Dougall, A., Hyman, K., Hayward, M., McFeeley, S., & Baum, A. (2001). Optimism and traumatic stress: The importance of social support and coping. *Journal of Applied Social Psychology, 31,* 223–245.

Freedy, J., Shaw, D., Jarrell, M., & Masters, C. (1992). Towards an understanding of the psychological impact of natural disasters: An application of the conservation resources stress model. *Journal of Traumatic Stress, 5,* 441–454.

Fullerton, C., Ursano, R., Tzu-Cheg, K., & Bharitya, V. (1999). Disaster-related bereavement: Acute symptoms and subsequent depression. *Aviation, Space and Environmental Medicine, 70,* 902–909.

Fullerton, C. S., Ursano, R. J., & Wang, L. (2004). Acute stress disorder, posttraumatic stress disorder, and depression in disaster or rescue workers. *American Journal of Psychiatry, 161,* 1370–1376.

Galea, S., Ahern, J., Resnick, H., Kilpatrick, D., Bucuvalas, M., Gold, J., et al. (2002). Psychological sequelae of the September 11 terrorist attacks in New York City. *The New England Journal of Medicine, 346,* 982–987.

Galea, S., Nandi, A., & Vlahov, D. (2005). The epidemiology of post-traumatic stress disorder after disaster. *Epidemiologic Reviews, 27,* 1–14.

Ginexi, E., Weihs, K., & Simmens, S. (2000). Natural disaster and depression: A prospective investigation of the reactions to the 1993 Midwest floods. *American Journal of Community Psychology, 28,* 495–518.

Gleser, G., Green, B., & Winget, C. (1981). *Prolonged psychological effects of disaster: A study of Buffalo Creek.* New York: Academic Press.

Green, B., Lindy, J., Grace, M., Gleser, G., Leonard, A., Korol, M., et al. (1990). Buffalo Creek Survivors in the second decade: Stability of stress symptoms. *American Journal of Orthopsychiatry, 60,* 43–54.

Grieger, T. A., Fullerton, C. S., & Ursano, R. J. (2003). Posttraumatic stress disorder, alcohol use, and perceived safety after the terrorist attack on the Pentagon. *Psychiatric Services, 54,* 1380–1382.

Grieger, T., Staab, J., Cardena, E., McCarroll, J., Brandt, G., Fullerton, C., et al. (2000). Acute stress disorder and subsequent posttraumatic stress disorder in a group of exposed disaster workers. *Depression and Anxiety, 11,* 183–184.

Hanson, R., Kilpatrick, D., Freedy, J., & Saunders, B. (1995). Los Angeles County after the 1992 civil disturbances: Degree of exposure and impact on mental health. *Journal of Consulting and Clinical Psychology, 63,* 987–996.

Havenaar, J., Rumyantzeva, G., van den Brink, W., Poelijoe, N., van den Bout, J., van Engeland, H., et al. (1997). Long-term mental health effects of the Chornobyl disaster: An epidemiologic survey in two former Soviet regions. *American Journal of Psychiatry, 154,* 1605–1607.

Hobfoll, S. (1988). *The ecology of stress.* New York: Hemisphere.

Holen, A. (1991). A longitudinal study of the occurrence and persistence of post-traumatic health problems in disaster survivors. *Stress Medicine, 7,* 11–17.

Holman, E., & Silver, R. (1998). Getting "stuck" in the past: Temporal orientation and coping with trauma. *Journal of Personality and Social Psychology, 74,* 1146–1163.

Ironson, G., Wynings, C., Schneiderman, N., Baum, A., Rodriguez, M., Greenwood, D., et al. (1997). Posttraumatic stress symptoms, intrusive thoughts, loss, and immune function after Hurricane Andrew. *Psychosomatic Medicine, 59,* 128–141.

Joseph, S., Yule, W., Williams, R., & Andrews, B. (1993). Crisis support in the aftermath of disaster: A longitudinal perspective, *British Journal of Clinical Psychology, 32*, 177–185.

Kaniasty, K., & Norris, F. (1993). A test of the support deterioration model in the context of natural disaster. *Journal of Personality and Social Psychology, 64*, 395–408.

Kaniasty, K., & Norris, F. (1995). In search of altruistic community: Patterns of social support mobilization following Hurricane Hugo. *American Journal of Community Psychology, 23*, 447–477.

Knight, B., Gatz, M., Heller, K., & Bengtson, V. L. (2000). Age and emotional response to the Northridge earthquake: A longitudinal analysis. *Psychology and Aging, 15*, 627–634.

Koopman, C., Classen, C., & Spiegel, D. (1996). Dissociative responses in the immediate aftermath of the Oakland/Berkeley firestorm. *Journal of Traumatic Stress, 9*, 521–540.

Krakow, B., Haynes, P. L., Warner, T. D., Santana, E. M., Melendrez, D., Johnston, L., et al. (2004). Nightmares, insomnia, and sleep-disordered breathing in fire evacuees seeking treatment for posttraumatic sleep disturbance. *Journal of Traumatic Stress, 17*, 257–268.

La Greca, A., Silverman, W., Vernberg, E., & Prinstein, M. (1996). Symptoms of posttraumatic stress in children after Hurricane Andrew: A prospective study. *Journal of Consulting and Clinical Psychology, 64*, 712–723.

Lutgendorf, S., Antoni, M., Ironson, G., Fletcher, M., Penedo, F., Baum, A., et al. (1995). Physical symptoms of chronic fatigue syndrome are exacerbated by the stress of Hurricane Andrew. *Psychosomatic Medicine, 57*, 310–323.

Maes, M., Delmeire, L., Schotte, C., Janca, A., Creten, T., Mylle, J., et al. (1998). Epidemiological and phenomenological aspects of post-traumatic stress disorder: DSM-III-R diagnosis and diagnostic criteria not validated. *Psychiatry Research, 81*, 179–193.

March, J., Amaya-Jackson, L., Terry, R., & Costanzo, P. (1997). Posttraumatic symptomatology in children and adolescents after an industrial fire. *Journal of the American Academy of Child and Adolescent Psychiatry, 36*, 1080–1088.

McCarroll, J., Fullerton, C., Ursano, R., & Hermsen, J. (1996). Posttraumatic stress symptoms following forensic dental identification: Mt. Carmel, Waco, Texas. *American Journal of Psychiatry, 153*, 778–782.

McFarlane, A. (1987). Posttraumatic phenomena in a longitudinal study of children following a natural disaster. *Journal of the American Academy of Child and Adolescent Psychiatry, 26*, 764–769.

McFarlane, A. (1989). The aetiology of post-traumatic morbidity: Predisposing, precipitating and perpetuating factors. *British Journal of Psychiatry, 154*, 221–228.

McMillen, J., North, C., & Smith, E. (2000). What parts of PTSD are normal: Intrusion, avoidance, or arousal? Data from the Northridge, California, earthquake. *Journal of Traumatic Stress, 13*, 57–75.

Murphy, S. (1984). Stress levels and health status of victims of a natural disaster. *Research in Nursing and Health, 7*, 205–215.

Murphy, S. (1988). Mediating effects of intrapersonal and social support on mental health 1 and 3 years after a natural disaster. *Journal of Traumatic Stress, 1*, 155–172.

Nader, K., Pynoos, R., Fairbanks, L., & Frederick, C. (1990). Children's PTSD reactions one year after a sniper attack in their school. *American Journal of Psychiatry, 147*, 1526–1530.

Nolen-Hoeksema, S., & Morrow, J. (1991). A prospective study of depression and posttraumatic stress symptoms after a natural disaster. *Journal of Personality and Social Psychology, 61,* 115–121.

Norris, F., Baker, C., Murphy, A., & Kaniasty, K. (2005). Social support deterioration after Mexico's 1999 flood: Effects of disaster severity, gender, and time. *American Journal of Community Psychology, 36,* 15–28.

Norris, F., Friedman, M., Watson, P., Byrne, C., Diaz, E., & Kaniasty, K. (2002). 60,000 disaster victims speak, Part I: An empirical review of the empirical literature, 1981–2001. *Psychiatry, 65,* 207–239.

Norris, F., Friedman, M., & Watson, P. (2002). 60,000 disaster victims speak: Part II. Summary and implications of the disaster mental health research. *Psychiatry, 65,* 240–260.

Norris, F., & Kaniasty, K. (1996). Received and perceived social support in times of stress: A test of the social support deterioration deterrence model. *Journal of Personality and Social Psychology, 71,* 498–511.

Norris, F., Kaniasty, K., Conrad, M., Inman, G., & Murphy, A. (2002). Placing age differences in cultural context: A comparison of the effects of age on PTSD after disasters in the U.S., Mexico, and Poland. *Journal of Clinical Geropsychiatry, 8,* 153–173.

Norris, F., Murphy, A., Baker, C., & Perilla, J. (2004). Postdisaster PTSD over four waves of a panel study of Mexico's 1999 flood. *Journal of Traumatic Stress, 17,* 283–292.

Norris, F., & Murrell, S. (1988). Prior experience as a moderator of disaster impact on anxiety symptoms in older adults. *American Journal of Community Psychology, 16,* 665–683.

Norris, F., Perilla, J., Riad, J., Kaniasty, K., & Lavizzo, E. (1999). Stability and change in stress, resources, and psychological distress following natural disaster: Findings from Hurricane Andrew. *Anxiety, Stress, and Coping, 12,* 363–396.

Norris, F., Perilla, J., Ibañez, G., & Murphy, A. D. (2001). Sex differences in symptoms of posttraumatic stress: Does culture play a role? *Journal of Traumatic Stress, 14,* 7–28.

Norris, F., Phifer, J., & Kaniasty, K. (1994). Individual and community reactions to the Kentucky floods: Findings from a longitudinal study of older adults. In R. Ursano, B. McCaughey, & C. Fullerton (Eds.), *Individual and Community Responses to Trauma and Disaster.* Cambridge, UK: Cambridge University Press.

Norris, F., & Uhl, G. (1993). Chronic stress as a mediator of acute stress: The case of Hurricane Hugo. *Journal of Applied Social Psychology, 23,* 1263–1284.

North, C., Nixon, S., Shariat, S., Mallonee, S., McMillen, J., Spitznagel, E., et al. (1999). Psychiatric disorders among survivors of the Oklahoma City bombing. *Journal of the American Medical Association, 282,* 755–762.

North, C., Smith, E., & Spitznagel, E. (1994). Posttraumatic stress disorder in survivors of a mass shooting. *American Journal of Psychiatry, 151,* 82–88.

North, C., Smith, E., & Spitznagel, E. (1997). One-year follow-up of survivors of a mass shooting. *American Journal of Psychiatry, 154,* 1696–1702.

North, C., Spitznagel, E., & Smith, E. (2001). A prospective study of coping after exposure to a mass murder episode. *Annals of Clinical Psychiatry, 13,* 81–87.

Palinkas, L., Downs, M., Petterson, J., & Russell, J. (1993). Social, cultural, and psychological impacts of the *Exxon Valdez* oil spill. *Human Organization, 52,* 1–13.

Palinkas, L., Russell, J., Downs, M., & Petterson, J. (1992). Ethnic differences in stress, coping, and depressive symptoms after the *Exxon Valdez* oil spill. *Journal of Nervous and Mental Disease, 180,* 287–295.

Perilla, J., Norris, F., & Lavizzo, E. (2002). Ethnicity, culture, and disaster response: Identifying and explaining ethnic differences in PTSD six months after Hurricane Andrew. *Journal of Social and Clinical Psychology, 21,* 20–45.

Pfefferbaum, B., North, C. S., Doughty, D. E., Gurwitch, R. H., Fullerton, C. S., & Kyula, J. (2003). Posttraumatic stress and functional impairment in Kenyan children following the 1998 American Embassy bombing. *American Journal of Orthopsychiatry, 73,* 133–140.

Pfefferbaum, B., Seale, T., McDonald, N., Brandt, E., Rainwater, S., Maynard, B., et al. (2001). Posttraumatic stress two years after the Oklahoma City bombing in youths geographically distant from the explosion. *Psychiatry, 63,* 358–370.

Phifer, J. (1990). Psychological distress and somatic symptoms after natural disaster: Differential vulnerability among older adults. *Psychology and Aging, 5,* 412–420.

Robins, L., Fischbach, R., Smith, E., Cottler, L., Solomon, S., & Goldring, E. (1986). Impact of disaster on previously assessed mental health. In J. Shore (Ed.), *Disaster stress studies: New methods and findings* (pp. 22–48). Washington, DC: American Psychiatric Press.

Rubonis, A., & Bickman, L. (1991). Psychological impairment in the wake of disaster: The disaster–psychopathology relationship. *Psychological Bulletin, 109,* 384–399.

Rustemli, A., & Karanci, A. N. (1996). Distress reactions and earthquake-related cognitions of parents and their adolescent children in a victimized population. *Journal of Social Behavior and Personality, 11,* 767–780.

Shore, J., Tatum, E., & Vollmer, W. (1986). Psychiatric reactions to disaster: The Mount St. Helens experience. *American Journal of Psychiatry, 143,* 590–595.

Smith, B. (1996). Coping as a predictor of outcomes following the 1993 Midwest flood. *Journal of Social Behavior and Personality, 11,* 225–239.

Solomon, S., Bravo, M., Rubio-Stipec, M., & Canino, G. (1993). Effect of family role on response to disaster. *Journal of Traumatic Stress, 6,* 255–269.

Steinglass, P., & Gerrity, E. (1990). Natural disaster and post-traumatic stress disorder: Short term versus long-term recovery in two disaster-affected communities. *Journal of Applied Social Psychology, 20,* 1746–1765.

Sungar, M., & Kaya, B. (2001). The onset and longitudinal course of a man-made posttraumatic morbidity: Survivors of the Sivas disaster. *International Journal of Psychiatry in Clinical Practice, 5,* 195–202.

Thiel de Bocanegra, H., & Brickman, E. (2004). Mental health impact of the World Trade Center attacks on displaced Chinese workers. *Journal of Traumatic Stress, 17,* 55–62.

Thompson, M., Norris, F., & Hanacek, B. (1993). Age differences in the psychological consequences of Hurricane Hugo. *Psychology and Aging, 8,* 606–616.

Udwin, O., Boyle, S., Yule, W., Bolton, D., & O'Ryan, D. (2000). Risk factors for long-term psychological effects of a disaster experienced in adolescence: Predictors of PTSD. *Journal of Child Psychology and Psychiatry and Allied Disciplines, 41,* 969–979.

Ullman, J., & Newcomb, M. (1999). I felt the earth move: A prospective study of the 1994 Northridge Earthquake. In P. Cohen, C. Slomkowski, & L. Robins (Eds.), *Historical and geographical influences on psychopathology* (pp. 217–246). Mahwah, NJ: Erlbaum.

Vila, G., Witkowski, P., Tondini, M., Perez-Diaz, F., Mouren-Simeoni, M., & Jouvent, R. (2001). A study of posttraumatic disorders in children who experienced an industrial disaster in the Briey region. *European Child and Adolescent Psychiatry, 10,* 10–18.

Vlahov, D., Galea, S., Resnick, H., Ahern, J., Boscarino, J., Bucavalas, M., et al. (2002). Increased use of cigarettes, alcohol, and marijuana among Manhattan, New York, residents after the September 11th terrorist attacks. *American Journal of Epidemiology, 155*, 988–996.

Waelde, L., Koopman, C., Rierdan, J., & Spiegel, D. (2001). Symptoms of acute stress disorder and posttraumatic stress disorder following exposure to disastrous flooding. *Journal of Trauma and Dissociation, 2*, 37–52.

Warheit, G., Zimmerman, R., Khoury, E., Vega, W., & Gil, A. (1996). Disaster related stresses, depressive signs and symptoms, and suicidal ideation among a multi-racial/ethnic sample of adolescents: A longitudinal analysis. *Journal of Child Psychology and Psychiatry, 37*, 435–444.

Wasserstein, S., & La Greca, A. (1998). Hurricane Andrew: Parent conflict as a moderator of children's adjustment. *Hispanic Journal of Behavioral Science, 20*, 212–224.

Webster, R., McDonald, R., Lewin, T., & Carr, V. (1995). Effects of a natural disaster on immigrants and host population. *Journal of Nervous and Mental Disease, 183*, 390–397.

Weiss, D., Marmar, C., Metzler, T., & Ronfeldt, H. (1995). Predicting symptomatic distress in emergency services personnel. *Journal of Consulting and Clinical Psychology, 63*, 361–368.

Yule, W., Bolton, D., Udwin, O., Boyle, S., O'Ryan, D., & Nurrish, J. (2000). The long-term psychological effects of a disaster experienced in adolescence: I. The incidence and course of PTSD. *Journal of Child Psychology and Psychiatry, 41*, 503–511.

PART II

Research Fundamentals

CHAPTER 3

Choosing Research Methods to Match Research Goals in Studies of Disaster or Terrorism

Carol S. North and Fran H. Norris

Ten different researchers investigating the same disaster might come up with 10 very different studies with important, nonoverlapping findings. This chapter is concerned with choosing the design and methods that can best answer the researcher's questions. If the methods are not appropriate for the research questions, the researcher might learn some interesting things, but what is learned might be very different from what he or she is trying to study. To organize the challenging process of designing a study, investigators can begin by asking themselves five questions relating to the *why*, *who*, *what*, *when*, and *how* of the research. In some ways, the "why" is both the beginning and end of the process because it shapes the questions that are asked and the interpretation of data that are collected. The "who" entails deciding what group of people should be studied, such as patients in a clinic, the general population, or rescue workers. The "what" is the construct or constructs to be measured, including posttraumatic stress disorder (PTSD) and other psychiatric disorders, distress, stress, and social support or other resources. The "when" refers to the time frame, the point or points in time at which the constructs should be assessed. The "how" pertains to logistical considerations and to the methods used to collect the data. In the remainder of this chapter, we discuss each of these questions—why, who,

45

what, when, and how—sequentially. In some ways, this chapter provides a "roadmap" to the rest of this book, and the reader is often referred to other chapters for details on questions, methods, ethical considerations, and special challenges.

WHY

Why is the research being conducted? What does the investigator hope to learn? As in behavioral science generally, the goals of disaster research are to describe, explain, predict, and influence behavior, broadly defined to include thoughts, feelings, and actions. These goals are not necessarily mutually exclusive; that is, one study might achieve multiple scientific goals, but each goal should be considered separately for the purpose of research planning. Table 3.1 provides an overview of the goals and appropriate methods. Regardless of goal, any justification for why a new study should take place must begin with a solid understanding of past research. Lerner (Appendix 2, this volume) provides a useful overview of how to search the literature on disasters and traumatic stress effectively.

Description

Describing Phenomena

The two main categories of descriptive research differ vastly in terms of methodology depending upon whether the researcher aims to describe phenomena or populations. Researchers sometimes aim for "deep description," a richly detailed account of a phenomenon, such as a particular community's experience in a disaster. This purpose usually leads one to the realm of qualitative methods. As Palinkas (Chapter 10, this volume) discusses, these methods provide a depth of understanding of an issue or topic that complements the breadth of understanding afforded by quantitative and epidemiological methods. Qualitative descriptive studies often have an exploratory purpose. Exploratory studies are especially important when there is little prior research about a culture, context, construct, or some combination of these variables. Ideally, these studies lead to hypotheses and confirmatory studies down the road.

Describing Populations

Disaster mental health research often aims to describe the prevalence or incidence of psychological disorders in populations afflicted by the disas-

TABLE 3.1. Research Methods by Research Goals

Goal	Requirements and/or approach	See also
Describe phenomenon or community	Qualitative methods	Palinkas (Chapter 10)
Describe population (prevalence/incidence/ risk factors)	Epidemiological methods; highly representative samples	Bromet & Havenaar (Chapter 6) Galea et al. (Chapter 7) Schlenger & Silver (Chapter 8)
Describe mental health services/ consumers/needs	Mental heath services/ evaluation research	Rosen & Young (Chapter 12) Galea & Norris (Chapter 11)
Describe/estimate effects of disaster on community or victims	Comparison data, either pre–post or two or more groups who differ only in exposure	Bromet & Havenaar (Chapter 6)
Explain effects; identify mechanisms by which exposure influences mental health	Highly valid and reliable measures; multivariate statistical strategies; adequate representation of severely exposed and impaired persons; sound conceptualization	Benight et al. (Chapter 4)
Predict long-term outcomes or course of postdisaster distress	Longitudinal designs	Benight et al. (Chapter 4) Bromet & Havenaar (Chapter 6)
Influence/change outcomes	Strong interval validity (experimental or quasi-experimental design); highly valid and sensitive measures	Gibson et al. (Chapter 13) Marshall et al. (Chapter 14)
Describe/explain/predict/ influence effects in children, rescue/recovery workers, and various understudied populations	Access; trust; measures that are valid and reliable in target population	Bromet & Havenaar (Chapter 6) La Greca (Chapter 9) Steinberg et al. (Chapter 15) Fullerton et al. (Chapter 16) Palinkas (Chapter 10) Jones et al. (Chapter 17) Murphy et al. (Chapter 18)
Provide formal diagnoses	Clinician-administered or structured interviews	
Identify potential or probable cases	Validated screening tools	Galea & Norris (Chapter 11)

ter. Often this purpose is combined with the identification of risk and protective factors, the correlates of postdisaster distress or psychopathology. Typically, such research is undertaken to identify the magnitude or extent of the problem and for whom or where in the community the problem is greatest: How many people of what characteristics have how much of a problem? The extent to which study findings can be generalized from a given sample to the population is critical for research of this type. Descriptive research in nonrepresentative samples has limited value. For describing populations, researchers generally turn to the methods of epidemiology (see Bromet & Havenaar, Chapter 6, this volume; Galea et al., Chapter 7, this volume). In their purest form, descriptive studies aim to describe what *is*, and are not concerned with explaining why the problem exists or even whether the disaster is uniquely responsible for the problem.

Describing Services and Consumers

Another potential goal of disaster research is to describe postdisaster mental health services and users of services. Disaster mental health services research is concerned with describing the availability, reach, utilization, quality, and effectiveness of services in the community. This description may be critical for public mental health planners and providers both to assess extant services and to determine whether or not the available services are meeting the need. Typically, such research considers questions such as: How many people have sought mental health services due to the disaster? Is that number substantially fewer than those who may need mental health services? Are there disparities between subpopulations in the use of services? The validity of answers to questions like these depends upon the study's applicability to a clearly defined population, which could be the general population of an area or the population composed of recipients of mental health services. Therefore, the quality of sampling procedures is very important. In this volume, Galea and Norris (Chapter 11) and Rosen and Young (Chapter 12) further discuss these purposes and approaches. When descriptive in purpose, the research aims only to describe the frequency and correlates of service use. The researcher has not actively intervened, such as in conducting research that aims to influence behavior.

Describing/Estimating Effects of Disasters

Disaster studies rarely have a purely descriptive purpose because they generally aim to show that the disaster influenced the mental health of the afflicted population in some way. Therefore, even if the study professes to have only a descriptive purpose, there is an implicit concern with causality.

Causality is difficult to demonstrate in the absence of comparison data. Comparison or "control" data take two forms.

First, severely exposed groups are sometimes compared with less severely exposed or unexposed groups, and differences between them are attributed to the disaster. Earthquake research provides some good examples where investigators have compared otherwise similar communities that differed in their physical distance from the epicenter. Although comparison groups can be helpful, even the most carefully selected comparison group may have many important preexisting differences from the disaster-affected group, making interpretation of postdisaster differences perilous (North & Pfefferbaum, 2002). Often, researchers draw conclusions about the effects of the disaster not by comparing distinct populations or groups but by conducting "within-sample" analyses, for example, by showing that, as severity of exposure increases, psychological outcomes worsen. Disaster researchers generally rely on statistical controls to supplement their designs and must remain cautious about inferring causality.

A second comparative approach is to include predisaster mental health in the study design, creating a one-group pretest–posttest design. Usually predisaster mental health is assessed retrospectively after the disaster by "lifetime" diagnostic measures that date the onset and recency of symptoms. Importantly, some disaster studies using this method have found high rates of psychopathology that predated the disaster. For example, a study of 1993 Mississippi River flood victims (North, Kawasaki, Spitznagel, & Hong, 2004) found high rates of postdisaster psychopathology, but it turned out this sample of lower-income people who lived on a flood plain because the land was affordable had a high prevalence of psychiatric disorders before the floods. Studies lacking predisaster data might have attributed the prevalence of psychopathology to the floods themselves. Retrospective assessments are imperfect, despite their frequent use, but only occasionally do investigators have access to diagnostic data that are actually collected before the disaster (see Norris & Elrod, Chapter 2, this volume).

Researchers can, and often do, employ both premeasures and comparison groups to strengthen their studies. In such studies, the highly exposed group is generally expected to show more change from before to after the disaster than is the less exposed group. If so, it is reasonable to attribute the effect to the disaster. The problem with this interpretation, however, is that some other factor could be confounded with the disaster—an economic recession, for example—and might account for more alteration of people's mental health status than the disaster itself. Thus, regardless of whether the design has one or more groups with posttest only, one group with pretest and posttest, or two or more groups with pretest and posttest, researchers must always remember to think through the plausible alternatives to their conclusions.

Explanation

Other disaster studies are less concerned with describing populations or phenomena. That disasters influence mental health is conceptually the starting point, and the study is undertaken to explain why or how disasters influence mental health. These studies are concerned about the mechanisms by which stress affects health, be they social, cognitive, or physiological. Often, explanatory questions are expressed in terms of mediating or intervening variables, and these studies typically employ regression methods, such as path analysis or structural equation modeling. Because these studies are focused on testing abstract theories, they do not need to be as concerned as are descriptive studies about generalizability to specific populations, but they must be acutely concerned with construct validity and the quality of measures.

Explanatory studies should aim to ask new and interesting questions (see Benight, McFarlane, & Norris, Chapter 4, this volume). Some systematic replication is helpful in assuring the reliability of previous findings, but testing the identical model repeatedly is of limited value unless there was a theoretically sound rationale for anticipating that the latest test could falsify or expand the theory in a meaningful way.

Prediction

Some disaster studies are undertaken to determine how future outcomes are influenced by earlier conditions. This purpose overlaps with risk factor research, with the key distinction that relations are examined over time: How soon do problems emerge? How long do they last? Who is at risk for chronic problems? Are factors associated with development of psychological disorders the same as those associated with their maintenance? Time, of course, is a critical variable in disaster research that is discussed further under the question of *when*.

Influence

Relatively few postdisaster studies aim to influence behavior (i.e., thoughts, feelings, or actions), but this purpose does subsume intervention and treatment studies. These studies do not simply observe change naturalistically or passively but actively seek to create change. They bear the highest burden of proof, and their designs and measures are judged according to the strictest standards with regard to internal validity. Gibson, Hamblen, Zvolensky, and Vujanovic (Chapter 13, this volume) discuss these standards in more detail and provide useful examples. Intervention studies are generally less concerned with external validity or generalizability, although there is increasing attention to issues of dissemination and transferability (see Marshall, Amsel, Neria, & Suh, Chapter 14, this volume). Treatment and intervention researchers should make sure that they include measures that are sensitive to change and end-state functioning in addition to diagnostic categories.

WHO?

Selecting a population of interest is a fundamental issue driving other parts of the methodology, including but not limited to the sampling plan and sample size. Decisions about whom to study tend to be based on the nature/severity of exposure or characteristics of the survivors, such as ethnicity or age.

Selections Based on Nature/Severity of Exposure

Broadly speaking, populations of interest to disaster research fall into three categories of exposure: (1) communities or general populations composed of people with a variety of exposure levels, often including people who are indirectly exposed as well as directly exposed, (2) selected groups of directly, often severely, exposed disaster victims, and (3) rescue and recovery workers exposed to the disaster by the nature of their work, often in horrific ways.

Communities, Populations, and Schools

For understanding communities or populations, it is critical to consider the nature, level, and variability of participants' exposure to the disaster. Exposure is a multifaceted concept, one that is more complex than is sometimes realized. Disasters may engender an array of stressors, including threat to one's own life and physical integrity, exposure to the dead and dying, bereavement, profound loss, social and community disruption, and ongoing hardship. Effects are not necessarily confined to people who had personal losses (direct or primary victims) but may extend to people who lived in the stricken area but suffered no personal loss or damage (indirect or secondary victims). Researchers need to think through how the direct/indirect distinction will be conceptualized, measured, and analyzed in their particular context.

The issue of indirect consequences has been especially salient in the case of terrorism. Major terrorist events have demonstrated that emotional and psychosocial effects are more far-reaching than was generally recognized. These broader populations lend themselves to different research questions. Indirectly exposed groups may not provide the kind of data needed for studying the diagnosis of PTSD (discussed in more detail subsequently); however, they may yield important information on distress, attitudes, and behaviors. In chemical, biological, and radiological terrorist attacks, the affected population may not be well defined (Holloway, Norwood, Fullerton, Engel, & Ursano, 1997). Large numbers of people who were not actually exposed may perceive that they were (Salter, 2001), overwhelming the health care system (Ohbu et al., 1997). Therefore, studies of these disasters call for attention to early behaviors, symptoms, and attitudes of broader populations rather than the psychiatric disorders that have been investigated more extensively after conventional terrorist events with explosives and other kinds of disasters.

Victims and Survivors

Much of the research on postdisaster mental health has been conducted with more select groups of individuals who were presumably highly affected. After natural disasters, samples of victims/survivors are often obtained by canvassing badly affected neighborhoods or schools. These samples may be highly representative of disaster victims (an abstract notion, really) but cannot be said to represent an entire geographic area. For example, after Hurricane Andrew, Norris, Perilla, Riad, Kaniasty, and Lavizzo (1999) selected seven badly stricken neighborhoods from which to draw their in-home sample. The data could be used to examine mediators of disaster effects on mental health (an explanatory purpose) but could not be used to estimate the prevalence of psychopathology in Dade County (a descriptive purpose).

It can be difficult to study victims and survivors in some circumstances. After public transportation accidents, for example, survivors often disperse rapidly with no record of their presence. Another obstacle, encountered in airline accidents, is the lack of survivors to participate in research. Studies might instead investigate effects of the disaster on surviving relatives and friends of deceased victims.

The larger the disaster in terms of scope and magnitude, and the greater the emotional and political complexity added by factors such as terrorist elements, the greater may be the barriers to gaining access to potential study participants (North & Smith, 1994). Gatekeepers to portals of access to survivors are understandably highly protective and may shield survivors from contact with would-be researchers. Gatekeepers may be unable to differentiate serious researchers and projects with high potential to make major contributions to human knowledge from frivolous or nuisance proposals portrayed as scientific research. They may fear emotional harm to their constituency or legal liabilities. Disaster research experts have recently considered that this fear may be out of proportion to potential risks in appropriately and ethically designed and implemented research (see Fleischman, Collogan, & Tuma, Chapter 5, this volume).

Regardless, such concerns may incite the erection of protective barriers designed to block access to potential research populations. After the Oklahoma City bombing, the state's governor declared that only very selected research groups would be permitted to conduct research on the bombing survivors (Tucker, Pfefferbaum, Vincent, Boehler, & Nixon, 1998). Fears that people might be emotionally upset, "retraumatized," or otherwise mentally damaged by participation in a research study have led to institutional human studies constraints on the conduct of research (Fleischman et al., Chapter 5, this volume). Current rules set forth by the Federal Office for Human Research Protections disallowing direct contact with potential study participants to recruit them from agencies without written consent (Code of Federal Regulations, 2001) seem to be designed with the interest of protecting human subjects, but in fact may make it impossible to achieve representative samples that have been routinely obtained in the past without negative consequences. Such restrictions are proving to be a massive blow to the broader field of epidemiology as well as epidemiological disaster research.

When survivors are difficult to access, researchers sometimes make questionable choices. Convenience (i.e., studying whom one has access to rather than whom one needs to study) is seldom a good basis for conducting important research. College student samples have been used to examine psychological responses to disasters and hypothetical scenarios ("What would you do if . . . ?"). However, findings may be poorly generalizeable to actual events, which might elicit entirely different responses than the students can imagine in such hypothetical scenarios. Further, student populations represent narrow demographic groups, and their exposure may not be great enough to draw conclusions about direct mental health effects of a disaster.

Occasionally researchers draw samples of severely affected persons from psychiatric or patient populations. They are a poor source of data on incidence of psychopathology or general phenomenology because of their general nonrepresentativeness, but they are appropriate for treatment studies or for studies of populations with preexisting mental illness. Of course, service recipients and providers are essential to study if the research questions pertain to the reach or quality of disaster mental health services (see Rosen & Young, Chapter 12, this volume).

Rescue/Recovery Workers

A substantial amount of the research on disaster mental health has been focused on the effects of rescue work, body recovery, and similar tasks. Often these studies do not sample, but attempt to reach all persons who performed a particular function after a disaster. Issues of cause and effect as well as generalizability are especially salient when studying rescue workers because they may differ from direct victims in important ways before the disaster, such as prevalence of alcohol abuse/dependence, experience with trauma situations on the job, and self-selection of individuals for this line of work. Fullerton, McCarroll, and Ursano (Chapter 16, this volume) provide many insights into how to conduct research with this population.

Selections Based on Age, Ethnicity, and Other Survivor Characteristics

Whether selected on the basis of their age (children, older adults), ethnicity, culture, or national origin, special populations of disaster victims require additional attention to issues of access to the population, building trust, and appropriate interviewing procedures. Care must be taken in selecting, translating, or validating measures for the select populations. These issues are discussed further by Jones, Hadder, Carvajal, Chapman, and Alexander (Chapter 17), Steinberg, Brymer, Steinberg, and Pfefferbaum (Chapter 15), and Murphy, Perilla, and Jones (Chapter 18) in the "special challenges" section of this book.

WHAT?

This question refers to decisions about the constructs of interest and how to measure them. The list of possible variables that can be studied is virtually endless, but given the focus of this book, two categories of constructs are of particular concern: mental health and correlates of mental health, such as psychosocial resources.

Mental Health

Few areas generate as much controversy as do researchers' choices of mental health measures. Researchers need to begin by asking whether formal diagnoses are required, whether the identification of probable cases is sufficient, or whether placing people on a continuum of mental health or distress is better for the questions of the study. Continuous measures are often the best choice for explanatory research, but they can be problematic for descriptive studies that aim to estimate prevalence or incidence of disorders. Trade-offs need to be considered.

  Diagnostic assessment using accepted criteria for psychiatric disorders can be demanding and laborious. In relatively small samples where a high prevalence of disorder is anticipated, it may be practical to provide all members with a full diagnostic assessment. Diagnoses are best assessed by using clinician-administered measures, followed by structured diagnostic interviews designed for lay interviewers. Often, however, the time and resources required to fully assess psychiatric diagnoses are prohibitive. Symptom checklists are much easier to apply, especially in difficult settings or to large populations, but one must be circumspect in drawing conclusions about symptoms, which may point to general distress rather than specific psychiatric illness.

Screening tools can offer a reasonable solution to approaching large populations with anticipated disease prevalence rates that are not high enough to warrant blanket application of a time-consuming full diagnostic measure. Brief tools with adequate sensitivity can identify those with greater risk for disorders. If the instrument's specificity is also high enough, its administration may yield a small enough subsample to target for full diagnostic assessment and intervention appropriate to the diagnostic category. Screening tools are not diagnostic instruments and should not be used for diagnosis of any given individual. Individuals who screen positive for increased risk of a disorder on one of these instruments still require a full diagnostic interview for confirmation. Screening tools do not provide precise prevalence rates of disorders after disasters. Large studies that have relied on self-report measures often qualify their findings by drawing conclusions about "probable cases."

The mental health outcome that has been studied most extensively in the aftermath of disasters is PTSD (see Norris & Elrod, Chapter 2, this volume). In directly exposed populations, the incidence of PTSD is higher than that of other psychiatric disorders. Major depression is frequently present or comorbid with PTSD after disasters. Other anxiety disorders such as panic disorder and generalized anxiety disorder may also arise, but less commonly. Although previous studies have described reported changes in substance use patterns in relation to disasters (e.g., Vlahov et al., 2002), there is no evidence to suggest that such reported behavioral changes regularly translate into substance abuse/dependence that was not already preexisting (e.g., North et al., 1999; North & Pfefferbaum, 2002). Schizophrenia, bipolar disorder, somatization disorder, and personality disorder are not among the disorders described as arising regularly after disasters.

Research focusing on PTSD is complicated by its unusual defining feature that includes causality as part of its definition, that is, the requirement of personal exposure or eyewitness to a specific type of traumatic event (one that threatens life or limb) of self or close loved ones. A diagnosis of PTSD presupposes sufficient exposure to a qualifying traumatic event conforming to this definition. Studies of unexposed samples must, by definition, ignore the exposure criterion, instead focusing on the symptom criteria as assessed by measures of intrusion, arousal, and avoidance and numbing symptoms. Interpretation of these symptoms outside the context of exposure requires considerable care.

Correlates of Mental Health

Physical health, health behavior, and a variety of psychosocial variables are of interest to many stress researchers. Although researchers sometimes study physical symptoms or conditions as outcomes of trauma in their own right (Schnurr & Green, 2004), researchers may be specifically interested in medically unexplained symptoms, referred to as somatization. Somatization refers to complaints lacking or in excess of medically explainable pathology or symptoms that are medically or physiologically untenable (North & Guze, 1998). Differentiation of medically explainable from medically unexplained symptoms is not easy and requires review of outside data with medical judgment to fully assess the medical explanation of symptoms.

A variety of psychosocial measures may also be of interest: attitudes such as trust in authorities after terrorist attacks, perceptions of personal safety and fear of future events, and changes in ability to function. Many research goals also require the inclusion of hypothesized protective factors, such as social support, self-efficacy, locus of control, or personality. Regardless of what aspect of disaster is studied, disasters occur within the fabric of people's lives. Therefore, it is vital to find out what was going on with people at the time and what their history is, such as patterns of alcoholism before the disaster, ongoing marital problems, financial problems, prolonged illness and death of an aging parent, context of litigation, or termination of employment. All of these factors could be expected to contribute significantly to the individual's outcome (North, 2004).

Each of these variables (health, social support, concurrent stress, past history) is represented by its own body of work and sets of measures that differ in length, format, and psychometrics. Selection of measures for study questionnaires is sometimes a haphazard or idiosyncratic process, especially when researchers are trying to respond to events rapidly, but the more one knows about a topic, the more one is likely to appreciate nuances in the construct and measures. Social support, for example, can be conceptualized and measured as received support, perceived support, or social embeddedness, and the findings may be very different depending upon this choice (Kaniasty & Norris, 1997). One of the true advantages of proactive disaster research (i.e., a strategy in which one chooses the questions and approaches before a disaster) is the ability it affords to consider the meaning and measurement of each study variable carefully. Whether the approach is proactive or reactive, the breadth of knowledge required to create an expert questionnaire argues for collaboration in disaster research.

WHEN?

Two key "when" questions must be answered when planning a study: How soon must (or can) the study begin, and how long must (or can) it last? Disasters and their sequelae unfold in a sequential time course with defined phases. Human responses evolve through these different phases, and thus observation at different points in time yield very different pictures. Ideally, participants are assessed at more than one time point, using a longitudinal design so that the influence of time can be taken into account. This is especially important if the "why" is prediction, and questions concern onset, course, duration, and recovery. Only one-third of the studies on disasters have been longitudinal in design, which is one of the shortcomings of the research as a whole (Norris & Elrod, Chapter 2, this volume).

When to Begin?

Beginning disaster research too soon can actually be problematic. Immediately after disaster impact, people are focused on their physical safety and assimilating the unthinkable into their worldview. People are preoccupied with removing themselves from danger, obtaining treatment for injuries, and locating loved ones. Adrenaline is pumping; initial shock and disbelief give way to profound emotions including fear, anger, and grief. Moreover, in the first hours and days after a disaster, virtually all directly exposed individuals are very upset and experience posttraumatic symptoms (North et al., 1999). Postdisaster psychiatric disorders have not had time to fully develop before 2–4 weeks (2 weeks to diagnose major depression and 4 to diagnose PTSD, by DSM-IV definition). These time requirements, incidentally, are intended to avoid inadvertent inclusion of individuals who are so upset in the early period after disaster that their upset may briefly appear indistinguishable from PTSD or depression but are demonstrated by the passage of time not to develop an enduring illness.

During this same time period, people may also be preoccupied with efforts to bury their deceased loved ones, secure shelter, repair damages, and seek resources and compensation. At this time, those so affected by the disaster may find research endeavors to be intrusive and insensitive. Research conducted during this period may be sensitive to these issues by using simple measures creating a light participant burden, although with some sacrifice of methodological integrity.

Despite these challenges, there are a number of good reasons for beginning fieldwork within a few weeks postdisaster. For one thing, data on initial responses are more accurate when collected with minimal delay. Previous research in other areas of psychiatric epidemiology has demonstrated that even normal populations show discrepancy in reporting psychiatric information in repeated interviews. A well-documented phenomenon in longitudinal follow-up studies is decay in diagnoses derived from reported symptoms from one interview to another over time (North et al., 2004; Rubio-Stipic et al., 1992; Shillington, Cottler, Mager, & Compton, 1995). A certain proportion of individuals who report symptoms meeting criteria for PTSD in the early months after a disaster may fail to disclose the same symptoms retrospectively at follow-up 1 or more years later that had qualified them for the diagnosis at the earlier interview. Studies carried out some time after the disaster may fail to identify some people who had PTSD that would have been detected at an earlier time.

A second good reason for beginning the research soon after the disaster is the ability to answer the predictive questions outlined earlier. Rapid-response research is often (perhaps ideally) combined with a longitudinal design. Interesting information on early predictors of PTSD and other adverse outcomes has emerged from rapid-response studies (e.g., Koopman, Classen, & Spiegel, 1996), although it is often limited by the constraints on the assessment tools that would preclude full diagnostic assessment.

Of course, a number of very good studies did not begin until a year or more after the disaster. What these studies sacrificed in terms of information about the acute impact period was often compensated for by the quality of their measures and the information they provided about the disaster's lingering or long-term effects. There is no single right time to begin a study, but the timing must match the questions (and sometimes the reverse).

When to End?

Longitudinal studies need to plan an end point as well as a beginning point. The proper point at which to end a study is far from universally agreed upon, and it is probably driven more by feasibility than theoretical concerns. It depends upon the severity of the disaster, the extent of ongoing disruption, and the residential stability and cooperativeness of the sample. Nonetheless, a reasonable rule of thumb would be to select, at a minimum, time points that represent the acute period (2–6 months), intermediate period (12–18 months) and long-term period (2–3 years). Only rarely have events been studied long afterward (see Norris & Elrod, Chapter 2, this volume), and there is probably a need for more of these studies after exceptionally serious disasters.

HOW?

The "hows" of disaster research require a blend of expertise on ethics, logistics, and research methods and are the focus of much of this book. Regardless of why the study is being conducted, who is being studied, or what is being assessed and when, disaster research is complicated by the chaos of the setting. Because disasters cannot be precisely predicted, studies of them must be designed and implemented in a short period of time after the event, a period that may be quite chaotic to research teams local to the affected community. Disaster research may be something these teams never previously thought about, and they need to bring themselves "up to speed" quite quickly. In such cases, finding mentors and experienced researchers with whom to collaborate is often the first and most important pragmatic consideration (Galea et al., 2002). Researchers outside the affected community have their own logistical barriers of geographical distance and lack of preexisting interpersonal networks to overcome. Resources for new research studies are traditionally not quickly obtained from federal funding agencies, further limiting the scope and complexity that may be achieved. Researchers may prepare in advance by developing a generic research design that can be applied flexibly to specific disaster settings. Funding can be obtained within a few months through NIMH Rapid Assessment Post-Impact of Disaster (RAPID) grants, and even in advance in some cases (Smith, 1996).

CONCLUSIONS

This chapter has explored the art of matching methodological choices to the study's goals, as summarized in Table 3.1. The critical decisions and issues involve finding the right population to fit the research question, choosing the right measure to fit the entity to be investigated, practicing good timing in gathering data, overcoming hurdles specific to disaster research, and interpreting the data given the limitations inherent to disaster research and its challenges. In interpreting disaster mental health data, a cardinal rule is to avoid leaping to conclusions that characteristics observed after a disaster are products of the disaster. The old adage is still true: correlation does not imply causation or causal directionality. Notwithstanding the inherent difficulties of the work, disaster research is important and exciting and, with planning, can be done well. Careful matching of methods to the research goals won't solve all the dilemmas, but it provides a very good start.

ACKNOWLEDGMENTS

Fran H. Norris's contributions to this chapter were supported in part by Grant No. R25 MH068298 from the National Institute of Mental Health.

REFERENCES

Code of Federal Regulations, Title 45, Public Welfare, Part 46, Protection of Human Subjects, Section 103. (2001). Department of Health and Human Services, National Institutes of Health, Office for Protection from Research Risks, last updated 12/13/01; last accessed 9/4/04; www.hhs.gov/ohrp/humansubjects/guidance/45cfr46.htm.

Galea, S., Vlahov, D., Resnick, H., Kilpatrick, D., Bucuvalas, M., Morgan, M., et al. (2002). An investigation of the September 11, 2001 attacks on NYC: Developing and implementing research in the acute postdisaster period. *CNS Spectrums, 7,* 585–597.

Holloway, H. C., Norwood, A. E., Fullerton, C. S., Engel, C. C., & Ursano, R. J. (1997). The threat of biological weapons. Prophylaxis and mitigation of psychological and social consequences. *Journal of the American Medical Association, 278,* 425–427.

Kaniasty, K., & Norris, F. (1997). Social support dynamics in adjustment to disasters. In B. Sarason & S. Duck (Eds.), *Personal relationships: Implications for clinical and community psychology* (pp. 595–620). New York: Wiley.

Koopman, C., Classen, C., & Spiegel, D. (1994). Predictors of posttraumatic stress symptoms among survivors of the Oakland/Berkeley, Calif., firestorm. *American Journal of Psychiatry, 151,* 888–894.

Norris, F., Perilla, J., Riad, J., Kaniasty, K., & Lavizzo, E. (1999). Stability and change in resources, stress, and psychological distress following natural disaster: Findings from Hurricane Andrew. *Anxiety, Stress, and Coping: An International Journal, 12,* 363–396.

North, C. S. (2004). Psychiatric effects of disasters and terrorism: Empirical basis from study of the Oklahoma City bombing. In J. M. Gorman (Ed.), *Fear and anxiety: The Benefits of translational research* (pp. 105–17). Washington DC: American Psychiatric Publishing.

North, C. S., & Guze, S. B. (1998). Somatoform disorders. In S. B. Guze's (Ed.), *Adult psychiatry* (pp. 269–283). St. Louis, MO: Washington University.

North, C. S., Kawasaki, A., Spitznagel, E. L., & Hong, B. A. (2004). The course of PTSD, major depression, substance abuse, and somatization after a natural disaster. *Journal of Nervous and Mental Disease, 192,* 823–829.

North, C. S., Nixon, S. J., Shariat, S., Mallonee, S., McMillen, J. C., Spitznagel, E. L., et al. (1999). Psychiatric disorders among survivors of the Oklahoma City bombing. *Journal of the American Medical Association, 282,* 755–762.

North, C. S., & Pfefferbaum, B. (2002). Research on the mental health effects of terrorism. *Journal of the American Medical Association, 288,* 633–636.

North, C. S., Pfefferbaum, B., Tivis, L., Kawasaki, A., Reddy, C., & Spitznagel, E. L. (2004). The course of posttraumatic stress disorder in a follow-up study of survivors of the Oklahoma City bombing. *Annals of Clinical Psychiatry, 16,* 209–215.

North, C. S., Pfefferbaum, B., & Tucker, P. (2002). Ethical and methodological issues in academic mental health research in populations affected by disasters: The Oklahoma City experience relevant to September 11, 2001. *CNS Spectrums, 7,* 580–584.

North, C. S., & Smith, E. M. (1994). Quick response disaster study: Sampling methods and practical issues in the field. In T. W. Miller's (Ed.), *Stressful life events II* (pp. 295–320). New York: International Universities Press.

North, C. S., Tivis, L., McMillen, J. C., Pfefferbaum, B., Spitznagel, E. L., Cox, J., et al. (2002). Psychiatric disorders in rescue workers after the Oklahoma City bombing. *American Journal of Psychiatry, 159,* 857–859.

Ohbu, S., Yamashina, A., Takasu, N., Yamaguchi, T., Murai, T., Nakano, K., et al. (1997). Sarin poisoning on Tokyo subway. *Southern Medical Journal, 90,* 587–593.

Rubio-Stipec, M., Freeman, D., Robins, L., Shrout, P., Canino, G., & Bravo, M. (1992). Response error and the estimation of lifetime prevalence and incidence of alcoholism: Experience in a community survey. *International Journal of Methods in Psychiatry Research, 2,* 217–224.

Salter, C. A. (2001). Psychological effects of nuclear and radiological warfare. *Military Medicine, 166,* 17–18.

Schnurr, P. P., & Green, B. L. (Eds.). (2004). *Trauma and health: Physical health consequences of exposure to extreme stress.* Washington, DC: American Psychological Association.

Shillington, A. M., Cottler, L. B., Mager, D. E., & Compton, W. M. (1995). Self-report stability for substance use over 10 years: Data from the St. Louis Epidemiologic Catchment Study. *Drug and Alcohol Dependence, 40,* 103–109.

Smith, E. M. (1996). Coping with the challenges of field research. In E. B. Carlson (Ed.), *Trauma research methodology* (pp. 126–152). Lutherville, MD: Sidran.

Tucker, P., Pfefferbaum, B., Vincent, R., Boehler, S. D., & Nixon, W. J. (1998). Oklahoma City: Disaster challenges mental health and medical administrators. *Journal of Behavioral Health Services Research, 25,* 93–99.

Vlahov, D., Galea, S., Resnick, H., Ahern, J., Boscarino, J. A., Bucavalas, M., et al. (2002). Increased use of cigarettes, alcohol, and marijuana among Manhattan, New York, residents after the September 11th terrorist attacks. *American Journal of Epidemiology, 155,* 988–996.

CHAPTER 4

Formulating Questions about Postdisaster Mental Health

CHARLES C. BENIGHT, ALEXANDER C. MCFARLANE,
and FRAN H. NORRIS

Conducting scholarly research within the context of enormous humanitarian suffering is difficult, inspirational, and extremely complex. Although one should not negate the need to document the history of a disaster and the experiences of the affected community, it is important to look beyond the specific disaster context and consider more general questions about the responses of individuals and organizations that could be investigated. In this chapter, we focus on theories and models that may guide the formulation of useful and significant questions about the development and prevention of mental health problems in the aftermath of disaster. We do not attempt to enumerate a list of questions that a researcher might ask, but rather point the way to sources that we believe will stimulate the reader to develop his or her own original ideas. Space prevents us from reviewing how various disaster studies were informed by specific theories, but we occasionally give examples from our own research to illustrate this point.

The chapter is divided into two sections. In the first and primary section, we describe how stress theories can guide research on postdisaster health and mental health. The theories reviewed here do not constitute an exhaustive set but are offered as an introduction to conceptual approaches. We also note the need for thinking temporally regardless of theoretical approach and briefly introduce selected analytic strategies that can help disaster researchers to test theoretical models. In the second section, we describe the potential for conducting theory-guided research on points of prevention and mitigation, focusing specifically on risk management.

STRESS AND THE DEVELOPMENT OF POSTDISASTER MENTAL HEALTH PROBLEMS

Research on postdisaster mental health belongs to the broader field of stress research. Stressors are aversive circumstances that threaten the well-being of the individual, organization, or community. Contemporary models of the stress process typically consider (1) characteristics of the stressor, such as severity and duration; (2) appraisals or perceptions of the stressor; (3) the response to or aftereffects of the stressor; and (4) various conditions that influence the relations between the stressor, stress appraisal, and stress response. The modifying conditions are typically conceptualized as vulnerabilities or, conversely, resources that come into play at various stages of the stress process to influence the outcomes, such as posttraumatic stress disorder (PTSD), depression, physical health, or generalized distress. Depending upon disciplinary orientations, theorists differentially focus on personal vulnerabilities (such as preexisting disorders, previous exposure to trauma, or personality), genetic or neurobiological predispositions, social and community contexts, or a blend of these different types of susceptibilities in predicting specific outcomes. Specific theories of the stress process differ in their relative attention to the different components of the model, be they stressor characteristics, appraisals, or vulnerabilities/resources. The influence of stress-diathesis theory (i.e., the level of exposure interacting with preexisting personal vulnerabilities to produce important outcomes) is evident in some of the earliest published frameworks for disaster research (Perry & Lindell, 1978; Vitaliano, Maiuro, Bolton, & Armsden, 1987).

Risking oversimplification, we can identify physiological, cognitive, social/ecological, and cross-cultural traditions in stress research. Each provides useful frameworks for the derivation of testable hypotheses in disaster research, and these are reviewed below.

Physiological Influences on Postdisaster Health and Mental Health

The scientific study of stress is often traced to the pioneering work of Cannon (1929) and Selye (1956), who emphasized the physiological components of the stress response. Selye's general adaptation syndrome (GAS) identified three critical stages: (1) the alarm reaction, which consists of autonomic processes, such as increased heart rate and adrenaline secretion; (2) resistance, which consists of physiological responses that aim to restore equilibrium, such as sweating in response to heat; and (3) exhaustion, which occurs when homeostatic mechanisms fail and reserves are depleted. The influence of this framework on substantive research and theories was profound, extending well past specific concern with the physiology of stress.

In fact, laboratory studies of stress can lead to ideas for naturalistic tests of stress processes. For example, Eysenck (1983) drew upon animal studies demonstrating stress tolerance to propose an "inoculation hypothesis," the idea that exposure to stress increases our resistance to subsequent stress and ultimately may protect us from harm. Norris and Murrell (1988) subsequently translated Eysenck's idea to the disaster context by hypothesizing that newly exposed flood victims would experience more anxiety than would disaster victims who had previously experienced a flood. Essentially, in areas where floods occur with some frequency, the threat should be normalized and more understandable, and people should be better prepared to respond and cope effectively.

In contemporary research, the physiological tradition is exemplified in several sets of research approaches and questions. Neurobiology has been a particularly active area for research on traumatic stress. Stress-related psychiatric disorders, such as PTSD, appear to be behavioral manifestations of stress-induced changes in brain structure and function (Bremner, Southwick, & Charney, 1999). For example, neuroimaging research (Rauch et al., 1996) has demonstrated a disruption of the neural networks involving language in persons with PTSD. They also have a greater degree of activation of a region in the right parietal cortex that is involved in somatic processing. Hence there is a neurobiological basis for the difficulty disaster survivors may have in the verbal representation of their experience and its manifestation of somatic distress.

More recently, some investigators have begun to speculate upon and to study the neurobiology of resilience (Southwick, Morgan, Vythilingam, Krystal, & Charney, 2003). For example, Charney (2004) proposed an integrative model of resilience and vulnerability that encompassed neurochemical response patterns and the neural mechanisms mediating reward and motivation (e.g., optimism), fear responsiveness, and adaptive social behavior. Many potential research questions are embedded within Charney's theoretical model.

Likewise, interest has been growing in the behavioral genetics of stress-related disorders. As Koenen (2003) noted in her review of family, twin, and association studies, we are still in the early stages of research on the genetics of posttraumatic stress. She noted that it has been difficult to distinguish family/genetic influences on PTSD from family/genetic influences on trauma exposure. Although disaster victims have been studied less often than have other types of trauma victims, conducting studies of behavioral genetics in the aftermath of disasters could have advantages, because the timing and type of exposure could be relatively well controlled. Methodological advances, including imaging technologies and the completion of the Human Genome Project, promise to facilitate new scientific discoveries.

An additional area of theory and research that follows from the physiological stress tradition relates to the consequences of trauma on physical health. Disaster victims often report declines in their physical health (Norris & Elrod, Chapter 2, this volume), making this a salient area for explanatory disaster research. Schnurr and Green (2004) summarized a growing area of research that has examined the role of PTSD as a mediator (intervening variable) of the effects of trauma exposure on physical health. Researchers are not yet certain how PTSD affects health. The association may stem in part from the negative affect (anger and depression) that is associated with PTSD and in part from core features of the disorder, such as physiological reactivity, hypervigiliance, and exaggerated startle (Friedman & McEwen, 2004). Schnurr and Green (2004) presented a complex theoretical framework that provides a rich source of interesting questions that could be asked in the aftermath of disasters.

Cognitive/Behavioral Influences on Postdisaster Health and Mental Health

Diverging significantly from earlier physiological theorists, Lazarus (1966; Lazarus & Folkman, 1984) emphasized the cognitive components of the stress response and was highly influential in shaping the ways stress was conceptualized. In this theory, appraisal was the central mechanism: an individual encountering a stressor would judge both (1) the degree to which the stressor was threatening (entailing the potential for harm or loss) or challenging (entailing potential for growth), often referred to as the primary appraisal, and (2) his or her own capacity to respond, often referred to as the secondary appraisal. This theoretical perspective instigated a tremendous amount of research that distinguished between problem-focused and emotion-focused ways of coping. Coping has been studied quite often in the context of disasters, though seldom in ideal ways (Norris, Friedman, et al., 2002). Although 40 years have passed since these ideas were first introduced, cognitions continue to play an important role in stress research.

Several current trends in trauma research have emerged from the early work of cognitive behavioral theorists. Benight and Bandura (2004) recently argued for utilizing social cognitive theory in understanding trauma recovery. Through this framework human adaptation is viewed as an interplay among environmental, intraindividual, and behavioral factors, where the individual is viewed as an active contributor to the adaptive process (i.e., human beings are agentic) rather than simply responding to changing environmental conditions. In the aftermath of a major trauma, Benight and Bandura argue, perceptions of one's ability to manage environmental challenges (i.e., coping self-efficacy) serve as a critical factor in understanding effective coping and are part of an ongoing self-evaluative process that is fundamental to human functioning. Consistent support has been found for the importance of self-perceptions of coping self-efficacy in predicting psychological outcomes from a variety of disasters, including terrorist attacks (Benight et al., 2000), hurricanes (Benight et al., 1997; Benight, Ironson et al., 1999; Benight, Swift, Sanger, Smith, & Zeppelin, 1999), fires/flash flooding (Benight & Harper, 2001), and volcanic eruptions (Murphy, 1987).

This agentic approach specifies the mechanisms through which risk and protective factors (e.g., social support or preexisting psychopathology) produce their effects and provide a framework for understanding the unfolding recovery process (Bandura, 2001). For example, social support is considered to be an important protective factor in disaster research. The beneficial effects are usually attributed to a buffering function relative to the amount of support perceived by the individual. When viewed from within the agentic theoretical framework, one can begin to speculate on the intraindividual proactive mechanisms that are influenced by social support as recovery unfolds. For example, supportive actions of fellow disaster survivors model effective coping responses, provide encouragement for continued perseverance, and provide interpersonal reinforcement for healthy adaptive actions over a period of time. These positive effects of social support serve then to elevate perceptions of one's own coping self-efficacy through successive interactions (Benight & Bandura, 2004). Mediational analyses support this hypothesis and show that social support provides its benefits to the extent that it raises perceived self-efficacy to manage environmental demands (Benight, Swift, et al., 1999).

Individuals and communities have a proactive role in the recovery process, including planning and constructing environmental conditions to promote successful resolution. In addition to the findings with individual perceptions of coping capability, recent evidence has also supported the role of perceived collective efficacy (i.e., the perception of the community's ability to effectively respond to a disaster situation) as a social resource in understanding psychological outcomes from disaster (Benight, 2004). The concept of resilience, a topic of much recent interest, likewise acknowledges that most people will thrive (e.g., Bonanno, 2004) even in the face of adversity. Future research is needed that ties in the concept of resilience with the theoretically driven construct of coping self-efficacy in understanding recovery from disaster.

Ehlers and Clark (2000) have also proposed a cognitive model of trauma response that is becoming increasingly influential. They suggested that PTSD becomes persistent when individuals make excessively negative appraisals of the trauma (e.g., "catastrophizing") and exhibit a disturbance of autobiographical memory characterized by poor elaboration and contextualization, strong associative memory, and strong perceptual priming. Ehlers and Clark furthermore argued that salutary changes in these negative appraisals and memories are prevented by a series of problematic behavioral and cognitive strategies. Turning their attention to the acute period, Halligan, Michael, Clark, and Ehlers (2003) showed that certain styles of peritraumatic cognitive processing prompt the development of disorganized or problematic memories that, in turn, increase the risk for subsequent PTSD.

Janoff-Bulman's (1992) model about the reworking of basic schemas about the self and the world is one of particular interest because it allows testable hypotheses that focus on the beliefs about the nature of the world and the ability of an individual to master destiny. Social cognitive theory, described above, provides a valuable framework for understanding the human quest for finding meaning in despair (e.g., one's perceived ability to generate meaning from trauma). A related concept is posttraumatic growth, which focuses on the idea that empathy and wisdom can be attained in the face of hardship (Park, Cohen, & Murch, 1996). Such an approach comes from the capacity of an individual to make stressors comprehensible and meaningful (Antonovsky, 1987). A range of adversities have been shown to have a positive impact on self-concept, coping, and social relationships (Park et al., 1996). Lehman et al. (1993) challenged this proposition and suggested that these reports are merely positive illusions that are not grounded in measurable changes, but there is some recent research to the contrary (Smith & Cook, 2004).

Clearly the role of cognitive processing and appraisals has strongly influenced how we view the recovery process following a disaster. However, alternative perspectives that do not emphasize the importance of perception have also been offered.

Social/Ecological Influences on Postdisaster Health and Mental Health.

Other contemporary theorists have argued against the supremacy of cognitive psychology, proposing that it serves "a Western view of the world that emphasizes control, freedom, and individualized determinism" (Hobfoll, 1998, p. 21). Beginning in the 1960s and 1970s, many researchers began to give increased emphasis to the social and sociological contexts in which stressful life events occur (e.g., Dohrenwend, 1978; Gore, 1981). For example, in his review of the effects of stress on health and mental health, Cassel (1976) identified a variety of environmental factors that could protect or buffer individuals from the effects of stressors. Typically, the "buffer hypothesis" was understood as an interaction in which stress would be more strongly related to health under conditions of weak resources than under conditions of strong resources. Research over the next decade (e.g., Norris & Murrell, 1984) convincingly showed that social resources, such as social support, socioeconomic status, and access to services, had strong effects on mental health and played a variety of roles in the stress process.

With its emphasis on identifying risk and protective factors, disaster research has borrowed heavily from models that were first derived for the study of stressful life events. Early work (Holmes & Rahe, 1967) was important for articulating the problems of measurement of the impact of events. Disaster research is ripe with opportunities to investigate how various domains of disaster exposure such as property loss, personal injury, death of relatives and friends, and disruption of business and income-earning assets should be indexed and compared. Are these domains numerically additive, multiplicative, or are there threshold effects? How does a researcher differentially quantify the death of a spouse and the loss of a house? These questions have largely been ignored (Netland, 2005). Over time, the Holmes and Rahe approach succumbed to evidence showing that individual perceptions of the negativity of the stressful events were more predictive of psychological outcomes than were objective normative ratings (Sarason, Johnson, & Siegel, 1978). The measurement of exposure is even more complicated than this discussion suggests, because impact and recovery can be conceptualized at a community or population level as well as at the individual level (see Galea & Resnick, 2005, and Kaniasty & Norris, 1999, for more detailed discussions).

Presently, the ecological tradition is best exemplified in the conservation of resources (COR) theory (Hobfoll, 1989), which is based on the premise that people are biologically primed and further learn to obtain, retain, and protect that which they value (i.e., resources). Importantly, this framework conceptualized stress in terms of resource loss and shifted the field away from the notion that resources were stable, immutable properties of the person or environment. Stress occurs when resources are threatened or lost or there is a failure to gain resources following resource investment. COR theory suggests that traumatic stress results when resources are unpredictably, suddenly, and severely depleted (Hobfoll, 1991). Distress results from the intense need to replenish critical resources (e.g., food, housing, shelter) as well as psychological resources (e.g., self-esteem and mastery). The theory is dynamic in nature, suggesting that disaster recovery is predicted by the interplay between individual- and community-level efforts to reduce losses caused by the disaster and the environmental conditions that promote further losses to occur. Loss spirals result when those with greater resource depletion lose ever more critical resources as they attempt to cope.

A number of disaster studies have tested the utility of COR theory (e.g., Freedy, Saladin, Kilpatrick, Resnick, & Saunders, 1994; Smith & Freedy, 2000). To date, this research has provided strong support for the central idea that resource loss is highly predictive of psychological outcomes. But there are several corollaries and principles of the theory (i.e., that resource loss is more salient than resource gain; that people must invest resources in order to protect against resource loss; that those with greater pre-event resources are less vulnerable to resource loss; that initial loss begets future loss) that have been less thoroughly tested. Future research questions that dig more deeply into the dynamics of this theoretical approach and evaluate the interplay among different resources, such as intraindividual factors and environmental conditions, will contribute to the knowledge of disaster adaptation.

One specific model of disaster recovery that may be understood within the broader context of COR theory is the "social support deterioration model," in which declines in perceived support and social embeddedness were proposed to be critical mediators of the adverse effects of disaster exposure on mental health (see Kaniasty & Norris, 2004, for a review). The deterioration of social support may be deterred when sufficient resources are received after the event, but various social, political, and cultural dynamics interfere with the adequacy and equity of resource distribution. Although this research has focused predominantly on natural disasters, there are both evidential and conceptual reasons to anticipate that the forces of support deterioration may be as, or even more, relevant in the aftermath of human-caused disasters.

Cultural Influences on Postdisaster Health and Mental Health

The impact of culture on disaster mental health is an area that is potentially rich for the derivation of research questions and hypotheses. The possibilities are virtually endless, as the implications of almost any model or theory previously described could be tested in light of an understanding of a particular culture or tradition. Whereas our understanding of the influence of culture on postdisaster mental health is nascent, there is an older body of work on the anthropology of disaster (see Hoffman & Oliver-Smith, 2002) that can guide the derivation of testable hypotheses. This intriguing body of work has addressed culturally based conceptions of power, risk, uncertainty, and vulnerability in the aftermath of disasters, the symbolism of disasters, and concepts helpful for understanding how the local context affects and is affected by disaster relief. Likewise, there is an extensive body of work in cross-cultural psychology (Berry, Poortinga, & Pandey, 1997; Klass, 1999) that can inform research on postdisaster mental health. For example, Norris, Perilla, Ibañez, and Murphy (2001) drew upon the literature on cross-cultural value systems to hypothesize that Mexican culture would exacerbate gender differences in postdisaster PTSD, whereas African American culture would attenuate them. Similarly, Norris, Kaniasty, Conrad, Inman, and Murphy (2002) proposed that the influence of age on postdisaster outcomes would vary, depending upon the cultural and historical contexts and family life cycles predominant in the settings.

Valid cross-cultural research of postdisaster mental health depends upon reaching a solid contextualized understanding of the idioms of distress that assist in survival or that perpetuate grief and reinforce the traumatic memory. The methodological challenge is how to explore the experience of individuals using the language of common distress as well as the viability of relevant psychiatric diagnoses across cultural contexts (Norris, Perilla, & Murphy, 2001).

Temporal Influences on Postdisaster Mental Health

Regardless of one's particular theoretical perspective, time is one of the critical frames of reference in understanding the nature of reactions to disaster. Although the predominant temporal pattern is one of recovery, a minority of survivors fail to recover, and some may show a fluctuating pattern (Norris & Elrod, Chapter 2, this volume). Large-scale longitudinal studies of disasters have much to contribute to the unravelling of different patterns of symptom progression and positive adaptation. The recent trend to study hospitalized victims of traumatic injury has biased the field conceptually to looking at short windows of effect that focus excessively on the view that early symptomatic distress is the predominant predictor of disorder (Mayou, Bryant, & Duthie, 1993). Victims of accidents do not experience the disruption in the physical and social environment that is typical of disasters. The nature, frequency, and controllability of the initiating event require more investigation as determinants of differential patterns of long-term adjustment.

There is also a need for conceptual models of the factors that may modulate the immediate symptoms of an individual, in contrast to their long-term progression. A variety of conceptual frameworks for characterizing the recovery environment make it possible to generate testable hypotheses concerning longitudinal outcomes. For example, social cognitive theory provides an interactive model for understanding the interactions between ever changing environmental conditions and self-appraisals of coping capability and the impact of this interactive process on important coping outcomes (e.g., psychological distress, effective behavioral coping). Life does not stand still, and subsequent adversities and developmental challenges test the capacity of disaster survivors (McFarlane, 1987; Norris & Uhl, 1993). There is much to learn about the impact of secondary stressors on the adaptation of individuals over longer periods of observation.

Significant opportunities exist for studying the complex recovery process as it unfolds over time, highlighting the mediating and moderating factors that influence symptoms and functioning. Extremely important longitudinal studies have followed individuals exposed to a major disaster for a relatively long period of time (Green, Grace, & Vary, 1994); yet, these investigations have not focused on identifying key mechanisms of change. Instead of looking at static outcomes from one time point to the next, future research needs to identify key adaptational variables that predict functional changes or maladaptive trajectories across time.

Importantly, contemporary analytic strategies make asking these types of dynamic questions feasible. The current state of disaster research calls for multivariate models that test theoretical predictions across time. Structural equation modeling (SEM), which has been utilized in some disaster research, makes it possible to ask more complex and theoretically interesting questions concerning disaster recovery. Under certain conditions, SEM also allows for feedback loops or bidirectional influence between variables (nonrecursive model, Maruyama, 1998).

Another contemporary method that may change the types of questions that disaster researchers are able to pose is latent growth curve (LGC) modeling (Duncan, Duncan, Strycker, Li, & Alpert, 1999). LGC modeling is a useful statistical tool for understanding data that are collected repeatedly over time. What is unique about this technique is that trajectory for change over time is generated for each individual, and therefore individual differences in these trajectories can be studied. LGC modeling allows also for identification of predictors that are related to nonlinear trajectories that may be of particular interest relative to negative (PTSD development) and positive (resiliency) recovery paths. Designing a disaster recovery study with LGC modeling in mind allows the types of questions concerning theoretical constructs that predict change over time to be more complex than is typically seen in more static regression approaches. Hierarchical Linear Modeling (Bryk & Raudenbush, 1992) offers a superior strategy for analyzing data where individuals are nested in larger units, such as neighborhoods and communities.

PREVENTION AND MITIGATION
OF DISASTER STRESS

The social and behavioral sciences have much to contribute to disaster research and practice beyond increasing our understanding of stress, health, and mental health. The range of potential applied research questions is wide, encompassing aims to increase understanding of household and organizational preparedness, response to warnings, mass communications, effects of media, help seeking, volunteer behavior, positive and negative effects of disaster relief, and secondary traumatic stress and burnout among disaster workers. Part IV of this volume focuses on models and concepts that may guide research on public mental health surveillance, disaster mental health services, treatment, and dissemination of treatments. We will here briefly discuss research on risk management as one additional example of how theory and scholarship can facilitate disaster research.

Risk management is itself a broad area of theory and research, of which we consider only the selected elements of response to warnings and hazard preparedness. Disaster warnings aim to promote public safety behaviors to reduce human casualties and property losses (Lindell & Perry, 1992). Effective warnings motivate people to take protective actions. Several researchers have generated models that depict the interaction among environmental information, sociological processes, and individual factors to predict warning responses (Lindell & Perry, 1992; Tobin & Montz, 1997). Clearly an interdisciplinary problem, evacuation behavior has been studied by researchers in public health, geography, political science, economics, psychology, communications, and sociology (see Riad, Waugh, & Norris, 2001, for a review). Among the factors that have been hypothesized to influence an individual's decision to evacuate are risk perceptions (very key), clarity and sufficiency of information provided, social influences, prior experience, access to resources, and territoriality (which can create conflicting motivations because of the desire to protect one's home and property). As may be self-evident in this statement, researchers interested in such questions can turn to basic science in a number of areas for ideas and guidance, such as decision-making heuristics and social comparison theory. Research on risk assessment as it relates to terrorism, the focus of much recent work (e.g., Fischhoff, 2002; Lerner, Gonzalaz, Small, & Fischhoff, 2003; Siöberg, 2004), has drawn heavily on classic paradigms in the field of cognitive science.

Disaster and terrorism preparedness is also an area of increasing interest that can be shaped by consideration of basic social psychological theory. Norris (1997), for example, examined the conceptual similarities and differences between hazard preparedness and other forms of self-protective behavior, and subsequently extended this work (Norris, Smith, & Kaniasty,

1999) to test the hypothesis that victims of a major disaster would perceive the impact of future disasters as more controllable than would nonvictims and would therefore exhibit increased hazard preparedness. For this work, she drew upon models of self-protective behavior in health psychology (e.g., health beliefs model, models of personal change) and criminal justice (e.g., citizen crime prevention), as well as previous research on hazard preparedness.

CLOSING THOUGHTS: THEORY, SCHOLARSHIP, AND THE RESEARCH PROCESS

Disaster researchers can draw upon a variety of theories, perspectives, and past studies to develop explanatory models. We have highlighted classic as well as contemporary sources of ideas about the physiological, cognitive, social, ecological, cultural, and temporal influences on postdisaster mental health. We have advocated for the value of gaining a broad understanding of the stress process and a deep appreciation of the background knowledge that has been generated through different disciplines (sociology, psychology, psychiatry, anthropology, public health) across the years. Reading scientific writings on historically significant disasters can also provide valuable insights for future research.

Of course, finding an intriguing theory or testable hypothesis is only the beginning. The careful selection of relevant outcomes is especially important for testing theories derived from a stress framework. Some models may be especially well suited for understanding PTSD, whereas others would be more appropriate for understanding depression or resiliency. The general idioms of distress and self-definitions of functioning are major determinants of behavior and should command more attention. The researcher then faces a variety of methodological, logistical, and ethical challenges that are addressed elsewhere in this volume. Sometimes, the focus on meeting the immediate and practical needs of the community may impede the researchers' capacity to conduct applied, but nonetheless theory-based, research. One method for solving this dilemma is to develop cooperative agreements for critical research *before* a disaster occurs. A priori research agendas can be developed that meet the needs of both the advancement of knowledge and the practical needs of governmental (e.g., Federal Emergency Management Agency) and nongovernmental (e.g., Red Cross) relief agencies. Creation of solid professional relationships before an event is much more realistic and, most likely, more effective.

In summary, questions about the development and mitigation of disaster mental health problems can be answered with careful attention to theory, scholarship, measurement, dynamic analytic strategies, and professional collaborations. The impact of a disaster on an individual, on superficial reflection, can appear to be obvious. However, there are many complexities that await innovative investigation.

ACKNOWLEDGMENTS

Preparation of this chapter was supported in part by NH&MRC Program Grant No. 300403 to Alexander C. McFarlane.

REFERENCES

Antonovsky, A. (1987). *Unravelling the mystery of health: How people manage stress and stay well.* San Francisco: Bass.

Bandura, A. (2001). Social cognitive theory: An agentive perspective. *Annual Review of Psychology, 52,* 1–26.

Benight, C. C. (2004). Collective efficacy following a series of natural disasters. *Anxiety Stress and Coping, 17,* 401–420.

Benight, C. C., Antoni, M. H., Kilbourn, K., Ironson, G., Kumar, M. A., Fletcher, M. A., et al. (1997). Coping self-efficacy buffers psychological and physiological disturbances in HIV+ men following a natural disaster. *Health Psychology, 16,* 248–255.

Benight, C. C., & Bandura, A. (2004). Social cognitive theory of posttraumatic recovery: The role of perceived self-efficacy. *Behavior Research and Therapy, 42,* 1129–1148.

Benight, C. C., Freyaldenhoven, R, Hughes, J., Ruiz, J. M., Zoesche, T. A., & Lovallo, W. (2000). Coping self-efficacy and psychological distress following the Oklahoma City Bombing: A longitudinal analysis. *Journal of Applied Social Psychology, 30,* 1331–1344.

Benight, C. C., & Harper, M (2002). Coping self-efficacy as a mediator for distress following multiple natural disasters. *Journal of Traumatic Stress, 15,* 177–186.

Benight, C. C., Ironson, G., Klebe, K., Carver, C., Wynings, C., Greenwood, D., et al. (1999). Conservation of resources and coping self-efficacy predicting distress following a natural disaster: A causal model analysis where the environment meets the mind. *Anxiety, Stress, and Coping, 12,* 107–126.

Benight, C. C., Swift, E., Sanger, J., Smith, A., & Zeppelin, D. (1999). Coping self-efficacy as a prime mediator of distress following a natural disaster. *Journal of Applied Social Psychology, 29,* 2443–2464.

Berry, J., Poortinga, Y., & Pandey, J. (1997). *Handbook of cross-cultural psychology: Vol. 1 Theory and method (2nd ed.).* Boston: Allyn & Bacon.

Bonanno, G. A. (2004). Loss, trauma, and human resilience. Have we underestimated the human capacity to thrive after extremely aversive events? *American Psychologist, 59,* 20–28.

Bremner, J., Southwick, S., & Charney, D. (1999). The neurobiology of posttraumatic stress disorder: An integration of animal and human research. In P. Saigh & J. Bremner (Eds.), *Posttraumatic stress disorder: A comprehensive text* (pp. 103–143). Boston: Allyn & Bacon.

Bryk, A., & Raudenbush, S. (1992). *Hierarchical linear models: Applications and data analysis methods.* Newbury Park, CA: Sage.

Cannon, W. B. (1929). *Bodily changes in pain, hunger, fear, and rage.* Boston: Branford.

Cassel, J. (1976). The contribution of the social environment to host resistance. *American Journal of Epidemiology, 104,* 107–123.

Charney, D. S. (2004). Psychobiological mechanisms of resilience and vulnerability: Implications for successful adaptation to extreme stress. *American Journal of Psychiatry, 161,* 195–216.

Dohrenwend, B. S. (1978). Social stress and community psychology. *American Journal of Community Psychology, 6,* 1–14.

Duncan, T. E., Duncan, S. C., Strycker, L. A., Li, F., & Alpert, A. (1999). *An introduction to latent variable growth curve modeling: Concepts, issues and, applications.* Mahwah, NJ: Erlbaum.

Ehlers, A., & Clark, D. M. (2000). A cognitive model of posttraumatic stress disorder. *Behaviour Research and Therapy, 38,* 319–345.

Eysenck, H. (1983). Stress, disease, and personality: The inoculation effect. In C. L. Cooper (Ed.), *Stress research* (pp. 121–146). New York: Wiley.

Fischhoff, B. (2002). Assessing and communicating the risk of terrorism. In A. H. Teich, S. D. Nelson, & S. J. Lita (Eds.), *Science and technology in a vulnerable world* (pp. 51–64). Washington, DC: American Association for the Advancement of Science.

Freedy J. R., Saladin, M. E., Kilpatrick, D. G., Resnick, H. S., & Saunders, B. E. (1994). Understanding acute psychological distress following natural disaster. *Journal of Traumatic Stress, 7,* 257–273.

Friedman, M., & McEwen, B. (2004). Posttraumatic stress disorder, allostatic load, and medical illness. In P. Schnurr & B. Green (Eds.), *Trauma and health: Physical health consequences of exposure to extreme stress* (pp. 157–188). Washington DC: American Psychological Association.

Galea, S., & Resnick, H. (2005). Psychological consequences of mass trauma in the general population. *CNS Spectrums, 10,* 107–115.

Gore, S. (1981). Stress buffering functions of social supports: An appraisal and clarification of research models. In B. S. Dohrenwend & B. P. Dohrenwend (Eds.), *Stressful life events and their contexts* (pp. 202–222). New York: Prodist.

Green, B. L., Grace, M. C., & Vary, M. G. (1994). Children of disaster in the second decade: A 17-year follow-up of Buffalo Creek survivors. *Journal of the American Academy of Child and Adolescent Psychiatry, 33,* 71–79.

Halligan, S. L., Michael, T., Clark, D. M., & Ehlers, A. (2003). Posttraumatic stress disorder following assault: The role of cognitive processing, trauma memory, and appraisals. *Journal of Consulting and Clinical Psychology, 71,* 419–431.

Hobfall, S. (1998). *Stress, culture, and community: The psychology and philosophy of stress.* New York: Plenum.

Hobfoll, S. E. (1989). Conservation of resources. A new attempt at conceptualizing stress. *American Psychologist, 44,* 513–524.

Hobfoll, S. E. (1991). Traumatic stress: A theory based on rapid loss of resources. *Anxiety Research, 4,* 187–197.

Hoffman, S., & Oliver-Smith, A. (2002). *Catastrophe and culture: The anthropology of disaster.* Santa Fe, NM: School of American Research Press.

Holmes, T. H., & Rahe, R. H. (1967). The social readjustment rating scale. *Journal of Psychosomatic Research, 11,* 213–218.

Janoff-Bulman, R. (1992). *Shattered assumptions: Towards a new psychology of trauma.* New York: Free Press.

Kaniasty, K., & Norris, F. (1999). Individuals and communities sharing trauma: Unpacking the experience of disaster. In R. Gist & B. Lubin (Eds), *Psychosocial, ecological, and community approaches to understanding disaster* (pp. 25–62). London: Bruner/Mazel.

Kaniasty, K., & Norris, F. (2004). Social support in the aftermath of disasters, catastrophes, and acts of terrorism: Altruistic, overwhelmed, uncertain, antagonistic, and patriotic communities. In R. Ursano, A. Norwood, & C. Fullerton (Eds.), *Bioterrorism: Psychological and public health interventions*. Cambridge, UK: Cambridge University Press.

Klass, D. (1999). Developing a cross-cultural model of grief: The state of the field. *Omega: Journal of Death and Dying, 39*, 153–178.

Koenen, K. (2003). A brief introduction to genetics research in PTSD. *PTSD Research Quarterly, 14*(3), 1–7.

Lazarus, R. (1966). *Psychological stress and the coping process*. New York: McGraw-Hill.

Lazarus, R. L., & Folkman, S. (1984). *Stress, appraisal, and coping*. New York: Springer.

Lehman, D. R., Davis, C. G., Delongis, A., Wortman, C. B., Bluck, S., Mandel, D. R., et al. (1993). Positive and negative life changes following bereavement and their relations to adjustment. *Journal of Social and Clinical Psychology, 12*, 90–112.

Lerner, J., Gonzalez, R., Small, D., & Fischhoff, B. (2003). Effects of fear and anger on perceived risks of terrorism: A national field experiment. *Psychological Science, 14*, 144–150.

Lindell, M., & Perry, R. (l992) *Behavioral foundations of community emergency planning*. Washington, DC: Hemisphere.

McFarlane, A. C. (1985). The effects of stressful life events and disasters: Research and theoretical issues. *Australian and New Zealand Journal of Psychiatry, 19*, 409–421.

McFarlane, A. C. (1987). Life events and psychiatric disorder: The role of a natural disaster. *British Journal of Psychiatry, 151*, 362–367.

Maruyama, G. M. (1998). *Basics of structural equation modeling*. Thousand Oaks, CA: Sage.

Mayou, R., Bryant, B., & Duthie, R. (1993). Psychiatric consequences of road traffic accidents. *British Medical Journal, 307*, 647–651.

Murphy, S. A. (1987). Self-efficacy and social support mediators of stress on mental health following a natural disaster. *Western Journal of Nursing Research, 9*, 58–86.

Netland, M. (2005). Event list construction and treatment of exposure data in research on political violence. *Journal of Traumatic Stress, 18*, 507–517.

Norris, F. (1997). The frequency and structure of precautionary behavior in the domains of hazard preparedness, crime prevention, vehicular safety, and health maintenance. *Health Psychology, 16*, 566–575.

Norris, F., Friedman, M., Watson, P., Byrne, C., Diaz, E., & Kaniasty, K. (2002). 60,000 disaster victims speak: Part I. An empirical review of the empirical literature, 1981–2001. *Psychiatry, 65*, 207–239.

Norris, F., Kaniasty, K., Conrad, M. L., Inman, G. L., & Murphy, A. D. (2002). Placing age differences in cultural context: A comparison of the effects of age on PTSD after disasters in the United States, Mexico, and Poland. *Journal of Clinical Geropsychology, 8*, 153–173.

Norris, F., & Murrell, S. (1984). Protective functions of resources related to life events, global stress, and depression in older adults. *Journal of Health and Social Behavior, 25*, 424–437.

Norris, F., & Murrell, S. (1988). Prior experience as a moderator of disaster impact on anxiety symptoms in older adults. *American Journal of Community Psychology, 16*, 665–683.

Norris, F., Perilla, J., Ibañez G., & Murphy, A. (2001). Sex differences in symptoms of posttraumatic stress: Does culture play a role? *Journal of Traumatic Stress, 14*, 7–28.

Norris, F., Perilla, J. L., & Murphy, A. D. (2001). Postdisaster stress in the United States and Mexico: A cross-cultural test of the multicriterion conceptual model of posttraumatic stress disorder. *Journal of Abnormal Psychology, 110,* 553–563.

Norris, F., Smith, T., & Kaniasty, K. (1999). Revisiting the experience–behavior hypothesis: The effects of Hurricane Hugo on hazard preparedness and other self-protective acts. *Basic and Applied Social Psychology, 21,* 37–47.

Norris, F., & Uhl, G. (1993). Chronic stress as a mediator of acute stress: The case of Hurricane Hugo. *Journal of Applied Social Psychology, 23,* 1263–1284.

Park, C. L., Cohen, L., & Murch, R. (1996). Assessment and prediction of stress-related growth. *Journal of Personality, 64,* 71–105.

Perry, R. W., & Lindell, M. K. (1978). The psychological consequences of natural disaster: A review of the research on American communities. *Mass Disasters, 3,* 105–115.

Riad, J., Waugh, W., & Norris, F. (2001). Policy design and the psychology of evacuation. In A. Farazmand (Ed.), *Handbook of crisis and emergency management* (pp. 309–326). New York: Marcel Dekker.

Rauch, S., van der Kolk, B., Fisler, R., Alpert, N., Orr, S., Savage, C., et al. (1996). A symptom provocation study of posttraumatic stress disorder using positron emission tomography and script-driven imagery. *Archives of General Psychiatry, 53,* 380–387.

Sarason, I., Johnson, J., & Siegel, J. (1978). Assessing the impact of life changes: Development of the Life Experiences Survey. *Journal of Consulting and Clinical Psychology, 46,* 932–946.

Schnurr, P., & Green, B. (2004). Understanding relationships among trauma, posttraumatic stress disorder, and health outcomes. In P. Schnurr & B. Green (Eds), *Trauma and health: Physical health consequences of exposure to extreme stress* (pp. 247–275). Washington DC: American Psychological Association.

Selye, H. (1956). *The stress of life.* New York: McGraw-Hill.

Siöberg, L. (2004). Asking questions about risk and worry: Dilemmas of the pollsters. *Journal of Risk Research, 7,* 671–674.

Smith, B. W., & Freedy, J. R. (2000). Psychosocial resource loss as a mediator of the effects of flood exposure on psychological distress and physical symptoms. *Journal of Traumatic Stress, 13,* 349–357.

Smith, S., & Cook, S. (2004). Are reports of posttraumatic growth positively biased? *Journal of Traumatic Stress, 17,* 353–358.

Southwick, S., Morgan, C., Vythilingam, M., Krystal, J., & Charney, D. (2003). Emerging neurobiological factors in stress resilience. *PTSD Research Quarterly, 14*(4), 1–7.

Tobin, G. A., & Montz, B. E. (1997) *Natural hazards: Explanation and integration.* New York: Guilford Press.

Vitaliano, P. P., Maiuro, R. D., Bolton, P. A., & Armsden, G. C. (1987). A psychoepidemiologic approach to the study of disaster. *Journal of Community Psychology, 15,* 99–122.

CHAPTER 5

Ethical Issues
in Disaster Research

ALAN R. FLEISCHMAN, LAUREN COLLOGAN,
and FARRIS TUMA

Disasters, whether unintentional acts of nature or human-made terror, can have profound effects on those who experience them. Research
conducted after various types of disasters (the Oklahoma City bombing,
Hurricane Andrew, the Three Mile Island nuclear accident, the Loma Prieta
earthquake, the terrorist attacks on September 11, 2001) has demonstrated
that adults and children show a wide range of reactions. Some suffer distressing worries, difficulty sleeping and concentrating, and bad memories
that, while disturbing and impairing, most often fade with good emotional
support and the passage of time. Others are more deeply affected and experience long-term problems such as depression, posttraumatic stress disorder
(PTSD), and other anxiety disorders (Norris et al., 2002; Norris, Friedman,
& Watson, 2002). Research focused on the effects of terrorism can provide
important information that may improve long-term survival, help prepare
for subsequent incidents, aid in assessing the physical and emotional needs
of a population, impact on planning and provision of mental health services for victims and other disaster-affected persons, and increase understanding of the human response to trauma more broadly.

Prior studies involving trauma and disaster-affected populations have identified some of the special issues that exist for research in the unique circumstances of terror, but concerns about magnitude of risk to participants of research postdisaster are largely undocumented (Newman & Kaloupek, 2004). Some question whether witnesses to or victims of extreme trauma may be able to anticipate the degree of distress that will accompany research participation (Newman, Walker, & Gefland, 1999; Pope, 1999). The process of institutional review and approval is intended to ensure that adequate procedures are in place to address this and other issues. However, beliefs and knowledge about the potential of these studies to traumatize or upset participants varies greatly among individual investigators and members of review bodies (Newman et al., 1999).

Although the risks and benefits of participation in disaster-focused research are not fully understood, most would agree that there is a significant need for additional research in the aftermath of disaster. This tension points to the importance of balancing the potential benefits to society of activities that seek to enhance knowledge and provide effective services postdisaster and the necessity of protecting the rights of individual human research participants.

FEDERAL REGULATIONS GOVERNING RESEARCH

Federal regulations (The Common Rule—45 CFR 46, subpart A) provide the framework for the protection of the human participants in research. The regulations and additional subparts B through D define the standards for the ethical conduct of research, including the process for proposal review through institutional review boards (IRBs) for research involving human participants. Regulations describe the process of voluntary informed consent and note that additional protections should be afforded vulnerable participants such as children, prisoners, fetuses, the decisionally impaired, and the economically and educationally disadvantaged (Federal Policy for the Protection of Human Subjects, 45 CFR §46.111, 1991). When individuals from these groups are the potential participants of research, there may be limitations on the permissible level of risk to which the participants may be exposed without compensating benefit. In addition, investigators may be required to create special protections to ensure the voluntary nature of the informed consent of the individual or surrogate. IRBs give special scrutiny to such proposals and may create procedural safeguards to protect the interests of the participants.

IRBs are also charged with consideration of the overall burden to specific individuals or populations created by research participation. The burden of research may be additive to other nonresearch burdens being experienced by participants, or it may occur directly as a result of the research, such as when an individual is asked to participate in multiple or redundant studies (Office for Human Research Protections [OHRP], 2001).

Research studies postdisaster take many forms and have a wide range of potential participants, some of whom may require special concern or protections. In each case, investigators and IRB members need to be cognizant of the context of the research, the groups or individuals being studied, and some specific issues related to the protection of human participants who may have experienced traumatic events.

Research involving victims and survivors of acts of violence such as rape and sexual assault, community violence, domestic violence, and child abuse has helped to establish safeguards for the protection of research participants that are useful for IRBs. The terrorist attacks at the Alfred P. Murrah Federal Building in Oklahoma City on April 19, 1995, and in New York City on September 11, 2001, resulted in different approaches to reviewing and regulating the substantial amount of research that ensued. Research in Oklahoma was centrally reviewed and approved through a special process put in place by the University of Oklahoma Health Sciences Center (UOHSC) with the imprimatur of the governor (North, Pfefferbaum, & Tucker, 2002). The result was that the university's IRB became the single body approving research involving the population affected by the bombing, as captured by a registry of victims. The goals of this approach were to protect the survivors of the disaster, maximize the knowledge obtained from the investigations, coordinate the numerous studies, minimize the burden on research participants, and attend to simultaneous needs for acquiring new knowledge and clinical treatment in this population (North, Pfefferbaum, & Tucker, 2002).

In the case of the World Trade Center disaster of September 11, 2001, investigators with interest and expertise from all over the country and internationally wanted to study these events and the aftermath. In the absence of clear recommendations about coordination of research, concern arose about assuring that victims of terror and their families not be subjected to inordinate burdens. Given the massive scope of the disaster and the research that took place afterward, extensive coordination on the scale of Oklahoma City did not take place. This resulted in individual IRBs from across the country reviewing and approving research proposals without the potential to determine the extent of overlap or redundancy of the studies. Balancing out the potential problems related to multiple IRBs, however, was that this process permitted time-sensitive research projects to undergo rapid IRB review and consideration for funding (Fleischman & Wood, 2002).

IRBs facing review of research proposals postdisaster need to utilize the extant regulations and interpret them in a fair and reasonable manner, neither minimizing nor exaggerating the risks of the research to potential participants.

SPECIFIC ISSUES

There are several areas of critical importance to the development, evaluation, and conduct of research protocols postdisaster that require the concern of investigators and review committees in order to assure that participants in research are adequately protected. These include (1) concern about the decisional capacity of potential participants, (2) the vulnerability of research participants postdisaster, (3) evaluating the risks and benefits of research participation, and (4) the ability to obtain voluntary informed consent.

Decision-Making Capacity

There has been a great deal of interest on decision-making capacity in the clinical and research context and the factors that affect an individual's ability to make decisions in the face of acute stress (Rosenstein, 2004). In the clinical setting, adult patients are assumed to have the capacity to make decisions concerning clinical care unless physicians have a reason to question that ability. Even for those with questionable capacity, experience shows that decision-making capacity varies depending on the nature of the question posed and the complexity of the choice. Decision-making capacity can also be improved though intensive educational efforts (Carpenter et al., 2000). Capacity to make decisions is not viewed as a bimodal, yes-or-no, phenomenon and even varies in the same individual over brief periods of time. Appelbaum and Roth (1982) have identified four components of decisional capacity (factual knowledge, ability to communicate a choice, appreciation of information, and ability to manipulate information) that should be considered in evaluating any individual's ability to provide informed consent.

The need to be protective of an individual with questionable capacity to make decisions also varies with what is at stake. The level of risk of the decision and the irreversibility of the choice are important factors in the creation of safeguards to protect the interests of individuals who may have varying or questionable capacity. In the clinical context, physicians are ethically obligated to recommend treatment options deemed to be in the best interests of their patient. The patient evaluates that recommendation and decides whether to proceed, based on his or her own values and assessment of the risks and benefits, while knowing that the physician believes this course of action is consistent with benefiting the patient. This is not always the case in the context of deciding about research participation. There may be no intended direct benefit to the individual participating in research, or potential benefits may be uncertain or unknown. Risk of participation in research may be minimal or vary widely depending on the specific investigation. Thus, the capacity required for participation in research may vary with the level of risk.

There has been a great deal of research in the field of mental health on the assessment of decision-making capacity in both clinical and research settings (Rosenstein, 2004). There are data to support the notion that some potential research participants will have impaired decision-making capacity as a result of their traumatic experience (Marmar, Weiss, & Pynoos, 1995). It would, however, be inaccurate and potentially stigmatizing to assume that all persons who have experienced terror or other disasters are decisionally impaired and unable to make choices for themselves. Although it is reasonable to presumptively accept that potential research participants will have the capacity to make decisions, given the significant impact of experiencing such trauma, the process of informed consent should consider the prospective research participants' ability to provide meaningful and voluntary consent. It is reasonable to consider whether more individuals with impaired decision-making capacity will be encountered in this context than in the general population. However, there is little empirical evidence regarding decision-making capacity in disaster-affected populations. Studies of patients with acute stress disorder and posttraumatic stress disorder offer evidence that decision-making ability in these individuals, as a group, is not significantly compromised. Even individuals who are extremely upset and under significant stress in general are able to make rational decisions about clinical care and research participation (Rosenstein, 2004). Numerous factors influence decision-making capacity under stress, but the extent of the effects of these factors is unclear, and each of these factors is affected by the antecedent mental health of the individual participant, the characteristics of the study, and contextual variables, such as the research site or experience of the investigator.

Vulnerability

The concept of vulnerability has been an important aspect of protection of human participants of research in order to highlight groups of potential participants who may have characteristics that impair their ability to provide voluntary and uncoerced informed consent to participation. The term *vulnerable* is generally applied to groups that are "more likely than others to be misled, mistreated, or otherwise taken advantage of as participants in research studies" (Levine, 2004). In the decades after World War II, in response to the Nazi experiments and various research scandals in the United States, research was viewed as a risky and burdensome enterprise from which individuals needed protection. In 1978, a national commission was convened by Congress to address this problem. It published the Belmont Report, the ethical justification for the regulatory structure for the protection of human participants that exists to this day (National Commission for the Protection of Human Subjects of Biomedical and Behavioral Research, 1978). The report defined vulnerable populations as those groups that might "bear unequal burdens in research" due to their "ready availability in settings where research is conducted," such as prisons, hospitals, and institutions, and it called for extra protections for these groups.

The Code of Federal Regulations, developed as a result of the recommendations of the national commission, does not specifically define vulnerability but creates specific protections for four "particularly vulnerable populations": children, prisoners, pregnant women, and fetuses (§46.201, 1991; §46.301, 1991). In addition, there is reference to other populations whose ability to make voluntary and uncoerced decisions about research participation may be impaired. These include adults who are cognitively impaired or mentally disordered and those who are economically or educationally disadvantaged (§46.111, 1991). When individuals from these groups are potential participants of research, there may be limits on the permissible levels of risk to which the participants may be exposed without compensating benefit, and the IRB may impose procedural safeguards to protect the interests of the participants.

In recent years, the concept of vulnerability has become extraordinarily elastic, capable of being stretched to cover almost any person, group, or situation in which individuals have insufficient power to protect their own interests or are at risk for being "wronged" or treated in ways that assault their dignity (Levine, 2004, p. 396). It gathers people of widely varying characteristics and capacities under one large umbrella without accounting for critical differences among individuals. This has resulted in the belief that labeling a population as vulnerable may be pejorative and potentially stigmatizing. Some have argued that vulnerability ought not be conceived as a characteristic of a group at all, but rather that certain individual characteristics may render persons vulnerable in certain situations (DeBruin, 2001).

Common-sense usage of the term *vulnerability* must be differentiated from its technical meaning in the context of human research protection. Victims of violence and disasters are of course vulnerable in the sense of sometimes requiring additional care and attention, as they have often suffered trauma and loss. Whether it is recognized or not, disaster victims and their families frequently suffer from significant psychological and emotional distress and may show signs of acute anxiety, depression, posttraumatic stress, and severe grief. These emotional factors, combined with the additional stresses of permanent dislocation, social disruption, family and financial strains, environmental worry, and ecological stress, may render some individuals unable to make informed choices. However, available evidence does not indicate that, as a class, disaster victims are unable to participate knowingly and voluntarily in decision making.

Thus, IRBs reviewing research studies involving disaster victims must determine, as they would in all other cases, whether, on balance, the benefits of any particular research endeavor outweigh the cumulative risks to individual participants. Protocols that present novel, high-risk, or uncertain risk–benefit ratios should be examined carefully before being approved. Specific protocols with the possibility of increased risks faced by individual participants should be scrutinized on a case-by-case basis, and additional safeguards or protections may be instituted for some or all participants if warranted. In addition, investigators must be sensitive to the fact that disaster victims have suffered injury and loss and may be more inclined to confuse clinical services and research. This demands a careful explanation of the research to assure that agreement to participate in the study is both informed and voluntary.

Risks and Benefits

The evaluation of the risks and benefits of a research protocol is perhaps the most important aspect of IRB review. There are clearly risks and benefits associated with participation in disaster-focused research, but there has been little empirical research in this area. Newman and Kaloupek (2004) reviewed the evidence of the impact of postdisaster research on participants and the perceptions of participants about their experience.

A number of benefits to participation in postdisaster research have been identified. Such benefits include enhanced awareness of material resources, medical and mental health services, empowerment, learning and insight, altruism, kinship with others, feeling of satisfaction or value after participating, and favorable attention from investigators. However, although there is evidence that benefits exist for at least some research participants, these benefits have not been examined in detail, and it is not known which kinds of participants are most likely to gain from what type of research involvement. In addition, it has been observed that disaster-affected individuals seem to receive greater benefit from interview-based research over questionnaire-based research, or studies that are more biologic in nature (Newman et al., 1999).

There are risks associated with participation in disaster-focused research. Such risks include physical harm, inconvenience, legal action, economic hardship, psychological discomfort, loss of dignity, breach of confidentiality, and unwanted media attention. Unlike findings on the benefits of research participation, researchers have identified several characteristics of participants and protocols that may enhance their potential for risks while taking part in disaster-focused research studies. These characteristics include preexisting distress or mental illness, age (both young and old), history of multiple trauma exposures, social vulnerability, and physical injury. Furthermore, there is evidence to suggest that repetitive research involving the same participants carries a potential for risk. Because disaster-affected persons are limited in number and are of interest to numerous investigators, the potential for overburdening these individuals with multiple or repetitive studies should be considered a risk in this type of research (Newman & Kaloupek, 2004).

Perhaps the most frequently discussed risk is that of emotional distress. Emotional distress is a risk of disaster-focused research participation, but it is not unique to trauma studies, and it varies greatly in degree depending on the individual participant and study. Often, it may be difficult to identify, because the research may not necessarily cause emotional distress but rather may make the participant aware of distress caused by the antecedent trauma (Newman & Kaloupek, 2004). Furthermore, an individual noted to be upset during participation in research might not necessarily regret participation. It is often the act of remembering the past that can induce distress, but at the same time, in the appropriate context, this act can aid individuals in achieving insight into their experiences.

Emotional distress caused by remembering events has sometimes been referred to as "retraumatization." Reactivation or exacerbation of residual stress-related symptoms precipitated by stimuli after the original exposure to a traumatic stressor may be an appropriate component of clinical care in a controlled and safe setting and should not be confused with the actual occurrence of traumatic exposure. Research participation may upset participants, but it does not traumatize them as a disastrous event would (Newman & Kaloupek, 2004). Trauma-inducing events involve unpredictable and uncontrollable experiences, whereas disaster-focused research should be both predictable and highly controlled. The use of the term *retraumatization* is inappropriate in the disaster-research context and may lead to exaggerating the risk involved in participation. Thus, investigators must take special care in assessing the risk–benefit ratio of a research protocol so as not to over- or underestimate risk.

Available evidence demonstrates that negative emotions are experienced by at least some individuals during research posttrauma. Acknowledging that this occurs does not address how such emotional upset compares to the magnitude and frequency of distress that these individuals confront in their daily lives. There are no clear data to define whether research-related upset reflects new symptoms, acute intensification of typical symptoms, or emotional responses that are commonly experienced by the participant. In addition, the majority of participants who experience strong emotional reactions do not regret or negatively appraise research participation, suggesting that distress may be understood as an indicator of emotional involvement in the research project rather than as an indicator of harm (Newman et al., 1999; Ruzek & Zatzick, 2000; Walker, Newman, Koss, & Bernstein, 1997).

Informed Consent

Voluntary informed consent is the cornerstone of research ethics. All research should be viewed as optional and refusal to participate respected. Informed consent was identified as critical to ethical research in the United States after a number of highly publicized research scandals in the 1960s and early 1970s raised public awareness of the risks of research and questioned the motives of investigators. Informed consent is the operationalization of the principle of respect for persons described in the Belmont Report (National Commission, 1978). Although many have focused on the document that is signed by the research participant as the "informed consent," informed consent is a much broader process that includes informing the potential participant of the procedures, potential risks, benefits, and alternatives to the research and then obtaining documentation of permission to proceed.

The history of voluntary and informed participation in research dates back at least to the beginning of the 20th century and the experiments of Walter Reed, who recruited American soldiers to determine the vector of yellow fever (Moreno, 2000). During the 20th century, healthy persons who became experimental medical participants were routinely referred to as volunteers, a term suggesting altruism and praiseworthiness. Patients who became the participants of research were less likely to be viewed as altruistic volunteers and more likely to be seen as deriving benefit from participation. Some maintain that informed consent procedures were less rigorous in these circumstances and sometimes were ignored (Advisory Committee on Human Radiation Experiments [ACHRE], 1996).

There has been a great deal of interest in research involving human participants in the area of public health and prevention of the physical and mental health consequences of war. Members of the armed forces have been exposed to biological, chemical, and nuclear substances to measure effects and determine appropriate responses in the face of attack and have been vaccinated without consent. Other public experiments without consent have subjected whole cities or communities to biological exposures and various measurements and calculations of impact (Moreno, 2000).

Public health research, research in the military, and research post-disaster may all occur in an atmosphere of enhanced patriotism and a sense of civil duty to participate in research in response to public health and national security threats. Given the increased concern for biological warfare and outbreaks of smallpox and anthrax, as well as the greater likelihood for future terrorist attacks, research in these areas may be perceived as a way to lessen the threat to public safety (Lombardo, 2003). This perception is an important factor for investigators and IRBs to consider in order to ensure the voluntary and informed consent of participants in disaster-focused research. Individuals, particularly those directly affected by disaster, may feel pressured to consent to research participation out of a desire not to appear unpatriotic or unhelpful in a time of national need. Such individuals might include firefighters, police officers, and emergency services workers who respond to disaster. These workers, because of historic tradition and media portrayal as strong, brave, and heroic, may feel pressured to contribute to research efforts so as not to appear weak or disappoint their peers or supervisors.

Considering the circumstances of obtaining informed consent in the aftermath of disaster and the substantial need of victims, survivors, and their families for care and comfort, the problem of what has been called the therapeutic misconception is very important in this context. Although research participants may benefit from research participation, it is easy for both the potential participant in the research and the researcher to confuse the purpose of the research, increasing knowledge, with the purpose of clinical care, direct benefit to an individual. Much disaster research is not explicitly therapeutic in intent, and the informed consent process must make the purposes of the research clear and not exaggerate the benefits of interacting with the investigators when treatment is not an intended part of the research and potential benefits may be less predictable (Appelbaum, Roth, Lidz, Benson, & Winslade, 1987).

Compensation of research participants can affect the voluntariness of informed consent and, therefore, requires careful consideration by both investigators and IRBs (Wendler, Rackoff, Emanuel, & Grady, 2002). Some commentators believe that vulnerable participants should never be compensated for research participation, because this may be an undue inducement and affect the voluntariness of participation. However, others argue that it seems unfair to ask participants to bear additional costs that result from participation in research (American Academy of Pediatrics Committee on Drugs, 1995). Reimbursement for expenses such as travel and parking and some modest compensation for time spent in participation has received broad acceptance in the United States. It is generally agreed that individuals who participate in research with no prospect of direct benefit may receive some additional incentive for participation. A small token gift as a thank-you for participation in research is common in postdisaster settings. Because larger gifts may unduly influence participation, it is only acceptable to vary the value of the gift based on the length of time required by the research, not based on the level of risk. In longitudinal studies, a modest incentive for each activity in the study may become an undue inducement if the cumulative amount becomes excessive and able to unduly influence voluntary participation.

CONCLUSIONS

By considering the issues raised in this chapter, investigators, IRBs, and public health and government officials can assure that important research can be reviewed expeditiously and conducted in a manner that protects the interests of participants. Survivors, families of victims, and others who are potential participants in research should play a role in the development and implementation of research projects assuring adequate provisions for confidentiality of the data and sensitivity to the broad range of needs of those affected by the disaster.

Survivors and families are often in need of clinical, legal, and social services. Research should in no way interfere with the delivery of needed services and must respect the needs of individuals who are grieving and suffering. Research participation should be voluntary, and the decision whether or not to participate must not affect access to other needed services or treatments. Researchers must be particularly vigilant to ensure against the so-called therapeutic misconception by helping prospective study participants not confuse research procedures with clinical care and evaluation. In addition, incentives must be carefully considered in order to preserve the voluntary nature of informed consent.

Investigators need to exhibit thoughtful concern for participants who may show emotional or mental health problems that could impair decision making or increase risk. Since research postdisaster is not always intended to benefit present participants, researchers must remember that participants bear the burdens and risks of research in order to benefit future persons who will experience a disaster. Any information-gathering activities in this context must acknowledge and adhere to the imperatives of doing no harm, placing the care and safety of victims and survivors above all else, and coordinating with assistance efforts. Where relevant, this realization should influence research design and IRB review and be reflected in the informed consent process.

Administrators and IRB members who are charged with protecting the interests of human participants in research should accept that there is a low likelihood of significant risk to participants of disaster research when studies are conducted in appropriate settings with sensitivity to the needs of the participants. Realizing that remembering and describing events in the research context, while potentially distressing to some, are quite different from experiencing the original trauma may help reviewers place this type of research in the proper context. Evidence of the important benefits that disaster-focused research participants experience may also be useful to reviewers when weighing the risk–benefit ratio of participation. The degree to which additional protection is afforded should be proportional to the potential risks to which participants are exposed.

Collaboration among investigators and coordination of research in order to decrease redundancy and the burden on individual participants is an important goal in the development of research agendas in the postdisaster time frame. There are several ways in which this cooperation could take place. First, investigators and funders should seek to increase collaboration and decrease redundancy of research as much as possible. Second, local academic or governmental authorities might work with IRBs and researchers on a voluntary basis to assist in coordination and decrease redundancy and participant burden in research. Third, options for a more formalized central structure for protocol review and approval could be considered, as was done in Oklahoma. Whatever approach is taken to address this potential risk, important research should not be delayed by increasing the bureaucracy of the review process.

Finally, careful review of the extant literature in disaster research reveals that there has been insufficient study of specific benefits and risks of research participation, rates and reasons for refusal, various recruitment procedures, methods for involvement of members of affected communities, approaches to integrating provision of clinical and human services with research investigation, and creative and sensitive ways of obtaining informed consent. This is true for virtually all social science, mental health, and health services research and not merely related to research after trauma.

A series of recommendations of points to consider about ethical issues in research with disaster victims and their families was recently published from a group of mental health professionals, trauma researchers, public health officials, ethicists, IRB representatives, and family members from the Oklahoma City and World Trade Center disasters (Collogan, Tuma, Dolan-Sewell, Borja, & Fleischman, 2004):

1. It should be assumed that, as a group, those affected by a disaster have the capacity to provide meaningful and voluntary informed consent to participation in research. When questions arise, individual assessments should be conducted. The decision to participate or not participate in research is entirely within the purview of the competent prospective participant.

2. Capacity assessment tools exist and should be utilized. Capacity might need to be monitored over time; the level of risk of the research should determine the level of concern about capacity. One capacity assessment available to investigators is the the MacArthur Competence Assess-

ment Tool for Clinical Research (McCAT-CR; Appelbaum & Grisso, 2001).

3. Disaster-affected populations should not necessarily be considered "vulnerable" in the regulatory sense. However, research proposals should address the individual psychological state of potential participants and have explicit mechanisms available for timely referral of participants in need of mental health consultation, including training of investigators and research staff to recognize emotional problems in research participants.

4. Specific research proposals should be scrutinized based on the level of risk, the novel nature of the research, and the uncertainty of the risk–benefit ratio; such scrutiny may result in the need for additional procedural safeguards for that specific proposal.

5. There is a critical need for additional research on the risks and benefits of participation in disaster-related research. It is important to study the effect of the research itself on participants and whether their experience of participation was what they had expected based on the enrollment process.

6. Ideally, representatives of the community who will be participants of the research should have some level of involvement in the planning and implementation of the research.

7. Information for potential participants about a research project should make clear whether there is therapeutic intent. Informed consent procedures should reduce the likelihood of participants mistaking research for clinical services (the therapeutic misconception).

8. The setting for the explanation of the research should be a safe, controlled environment conducive to making an informed decision about participation.

9. Provisions for confidentiality of the data and protection of the privacy of the participants should be an explicit part of the research plan.

10. Proposals should have explicit plans for the training and support of research staff who will be exposed to the emotional challenges faced by research participants.

11. Participants in postdisaster research should be informed of the results of studies in which they have participated.

12. Coordination and collaboration among researchers and IRBs may help minimize redundant research and participant burden; various models should be considered to facilitate such coordination without unduly impeding research.

The research community that has focused its attention on assessing and minimizing the impact of terror and disaster on affected individuals and communities has made major contributions to enhancing knowledge, services, and outcomes for countless victims and their families. While continuing with their important work, this research community can best serve victims and survivors of traumatic events by maintaining sensitivity to the needs of this population and striving to understand more about the effects of trauma and trauma-focused research participation.

ACKNOWLEDGMENTS

This chapter is adapted from Collogan et al. (2004). Views expressed are those of the authors and do not necessarily reflect those of the U.S. Department of Health and Human Services, the National Institutes of Health, or the National Institute of Mental Health.

REFERENCES

Advisory Committee on Human Radiation Experiments. (1996). *The human radiation experiments*. New York: Oxford University Press.

American Academy of Pediatrics Committee on Drugs. (1995). Guidelines for the ethical conduct of studies to evaluate drugs in pediatric populations. *Pediatrics, 95*, 286–294.

Appelbaum, P. S., & Grisso, T. (2001). *MacArthur Competence Assessment Tool for Clinical Research (MacCAT-CR)*. Sarasota, FL: Professional Resource Press.

Appelbaum, P., & Roth, L. (1982). Competency to consent to research: A psychiatric overview. *Archives of General Psychiatry, 39*, 951–958.

Appelbaum, P., Roth, L. H., Lidz, C. W., Benson, P., & Winslade, W. (1987). False hopes and best data: Consent to research and the therapeutic misconception. *The Hastings Center Report, 17*, 20–24.

Carpenter, W., Gold, J., Lahti, A., Queern, C., Conley, R., Bartko, J., et al. (2000). Decisional capacity for informed consent in schizophrenia research. *Archives of General Psychiatry, 57*, 533–538.

Collogan, L. K., Tuma, F., Dolan-Sewell, R., Borja, S., & Fleischman, A. R. (2004). Ethical issues pertaining to research in the aftermath of disaster. *Journal of Traumatic Stress, 17*(5), 363–372.

DeBruin, D. (2001). Reflections on "vulnerability." *Bioethics Examiner, 5*, 1–4.

Federal Policy for the Protection of Human Subjects, 45 CFR §46.111(a)(3) (1991).

Federal Policy for the Protection of Human Subjects, 45 CFR §46.201(a) (1991).

Federal Policy for the Protection of Human Subjects, 45 CFR §46.301(a) (1991).

Fleischman, A. R., & Wood, E. B. (2002). Ethical issues in research involving victims of terror. *Journal of Urban Health, 79*(3), 315–321.

Levine, C. (2004). The concept of vulnerability in disaster research. *Journal of Traumatic Stress, 17*(5), 395–402.

Lombardo, P. (2003). "Of utmost national urgency": The Lynchburg hepatitis study, 1942. In J. Moreno (Ed.), *In the wake of terror: Medicine and morality in a time of crisis* (pp. 3–15). Cambridge, MA: The MIT Press.

Marmar, C. R., Weiss, D. S., & Pynoos, R. S. (1995). Dynamic psychotherapy of posttraumatic stress disorder. In M. J. Friedman, D. S. Charney, & A. Y. Deutch

(Eds.), *Neurobiological and clinical consequences of stress: From normal adaptation to posttraumatic stress disorder* (pp. 495–506). Philadelphia: Lippincott-Raven.

Moreno, J. (2000). *Undue risk: Secret state experiments on humans.* New York: Routledge.

National Commission for the Protection of Human Subjects of Biomedical and Behavioral Research. (1978). *The Belmont Report: Ethical principles and guidelines for the protection of human subjects of research* (DHEW Publication No. OS 78–0012). Washington DC: Department of Health, Education, and Welfare. Retrieved January 17, 2003, from Office of Human Subjects Research website: ohsr.od.nih.gov/mpa/belmont.php3

Newman, E., & Kaloupek, D. (2004). The risks and benefits of participating in trauma-focused research studies. *Journal of Traumatic Stress, 17*(5), 383–394.

Newman, E., Walker, E. A., & Gefland, A. (1999). Assessing the ethical costs and benefits of trauma-focused research. *Annals of General Hospital Psychiatry, 21,* 187–196.

Norris, F. H., Friedman, M. J., & Watson, P. J. (2002). 60,000 disaster victims speak: Part II. Summary and implications of the disaster mental health research. *Psychiatry, 65,* 240–260.

Norris, F. H., Friedman, M. J., Watson, P. J., Byrne, C. M., Diaz, E., & Kaniasty, K. (2002). 60,000 disaster victims speak: Part I. An empirical review of the empirical literature, 1981–2001. *Psychiatry, 65,* 207–239.

North, C., Pfefferbaum, B., & Tucker, P. (2002). Ethical and methodological issues in academic mental health research in populations affected by disasters: The Oklahoma City experience relevant to September 11, 2001. *CNS Spectrums, 7,* 580–584.

Office for Human Research Protections. (2001). *Protecting human research subjects: Institutional review board guidebook.* Retrieved July 17, 2003, from the OHRP website: ohrp.osophs.dhhs.gov/irb/irb_chapter3.htm.

Pope, K. S. (1999). The ethics of research involving memories of trauma. *Annals of General Hospital Psychiatry, 21,* 157.

Rosenstein, D. (2004). Decisionmaking capacity and disaster research. *Journal of Traumatic Stress, 17*(5), 373–381.

Ruzek, J. I., & Zatzick, D. F. (2000). Ethical considerations in research participation among acutely injured trauma survivors: An empirical investigation. *Annals of General Hospital Psychiatry, 22,* 27–36.

Walker, E. A., Newman, E., Koss, M., & Bernstein, D. (1997). Does the study of victimization revictimize the victims? *Annals of General Hospital Psychiatry, 19,* 403–410.

Wendler, D., Rackoff, J. E., Emanuel, E. J., & Grady, C., (2002). The ethics of paying for children's participation in research. *Journal of Pediatrics, 141,* 166–171.

PART III

Methods for Sampling and Data Collection

CHAPTER 6

Basic Epidemiological
Approaches to Disaster Research
Value of Face-to-Face Procedures

Evelyn J. Bromet and Johan M. Havenaar

This chapter addresses a number of sampling and fieldwork procedures entailed by mental health studies that use basic epidemiological designs and in-person assessments to determine the impact of disasters and
terrorist attacks. There are many obvious advantages when a disaster study
combines epidemiological strategies with face-to-face interviews. First, epidemiological studies provide generalizable findings because participants are
drawn from clearly defined, representative sampling frames. Second, it is
possible to collect more comprehensive and in-depth information and to
combine quantitative and qualitative data collection strategies. Thus, compared to the constraints of other forms of telephone surveys or mail questionnaires, in-person protocols may involve lengthier assessments, biological measurements (e.g., blood pressure or oral fluid), neuropsychological
testing (which might be relevant for particular toxic exposures), and narrative descriptions that can be rated for content as well as for nonverbal cues
and signs of distress that are manifested as the stories unfold. Third, this
approach presents an opportunity to build personal rapport with members
of the affected community, thus indirectly providing recognition that the
"outside world" cares about their suffering. Of course, such research can

95

be costly and requires considerable planning. On the other hand, the richness, magnitude, scope, and depth of data from epidemiological studies using in-person assessments ensure that the findings will have both theoretical and practical public health value.

In this chapter we first describe the basic epidemiological designs that are used in disaster research, drawing on experiences studying the Chornobyl (also known as Chornobyl) disaster to illustrate key points. These examples are particularly useful for this purpose because the exposure had the potential to have both direct effects on health and indirect effects stemming from the multiple prolonged stresses that ensued. They are also of interest because they show that, even under suboptimal conditions, it is possible to conduct methodologically sound studies. In this context, we also discuss important sources of bias that arise in such disaster research. We then describe the special challenges in designing and executing disaster research, with examples showing how some of these challenges have been met.

DESIGN OPTIONS FOR EPIDEMIOLOGICAL STUDIES

The ultimate goal of epidemiology is to reduce morbidity through appropriate interventions. Epidemiological studies of disasters examine whether the rates of disorder are significantly elevated in the aftermath of a disaster, and, if so, what aspects of the disaster and what other biopsychosocial risk factors are linked to the outcome(s). There are two basic options in designing analytic epidemiological research after a disaster, the retrospective cohort design and the case–control design.

Retrospective Cohort Studies

Most disaster studies seek to determine whether the incidence rate of disorder(s) is significantly higher in exposed as compared to unexposed populations over a specified period of time. The retrospective cohort design is used to address this question. The most informative study is one that is based on representative samples and that differentiates between incident cases (survivors who develop their first episode only after the disaster) and prevalent cases (people with conditions whose onsets predate the disaster) (Maes, Mylle, Delmeire, & Altamura, 2000). Thus, to clarify the temporal order of exposure and disease, this design requires careful retrospective assessments of mental and physical health prior to the disaster. The ideal cohort study, of course, would begin before the disaster occurs so that the risk for mental disorders is obtained prospectively rather than retrospectively. A handful of such "natural experiments" exist (e.g., Bromet, Havenaar, Gluzman, &

Tintle, 2005; Canino, Bravo, Rubio-Stipec, & Woodbury, 1990; Reijneveld, Crone, Verhulst, & Verloove-Vanhorick, 2003; Robins et al., 1986).

Three retrospective cohort studies conducted after the 1986 Chornobyl accident illustrate the retrospective cohort design and its variations. The first, conducted by a Finnish research team (Viinamäki et al., 1995), compared (all) residents of a contaminated village in Russia to a noncontaminated control village 7 years after the accident. Based on the 12-item version of the General Health Questionnaire (GHQ), they found that 48% of exposed women (compared to 34% of unexposed controls) suffered from minor mental disorders, while no differences were detected in the men. Other risk factors for poor mental health included not having a partner, financial inadequacy, and self-rated poor health. The second study was conducted by an international team of Dutch and Russian researchers (Havenaar et al., 1997) and sampled a population ages 18–65 in the Gomel region of Belarus, which was severely polluted by the fallout from Chornobyl, and a socioeconomically comparable uncontaminated region in Russia. Because Belarus had no records from which to draw a representative sample and an extremely low unemployment rate (1%), they creatively adapted the traditional community sampling design by sampling work sites (factories, collective farms, schools, etc.) reflecting the distribution of occupations in the region, supplemented by sites where nonworking people would be found. A total of 3,044 were screened (1,617 exposed) 6.5 years after the Chornobyl accident. The exposed group had significantly greater psychological distress and higher medical service utilization. The highest rates were found among women, particularly mothers with young children. The third study, by American and Ukrainian investigators, focused on children evacuated to Kyiv from the contaminated zone around the power plant (Bromet et al., 2000). For this study, a sampling frame of evacuee children was created from three official lists (including the government registry of Chornobyl "victims"), and a random sample of 300 exposed children who were in utero to age 15 months at the time of the accident was selected. A gender-matched classmate control was chosen for each evacuee child. The measurements included comprehensive symptom and risk factor assessments of the children and their mothers, along with physical examinations and blood tests for the children. The two groups of children did not differ systematically on any of the key measures, but the health concerns of the evacuee mothers were wide ranging.

Under certain circumstances, a retrospective cohort study can serve not just as a stand-alone study but also as the first phase of a two-stage study design aimed at estimating the relative risk of clinical disorder(s) associated with the disaster. There are two conditions that must be met for this type of design to be effective. First, the screening tool administered in the first stage must have demonstrated high sensitivity, specificity, and positive predictive value (the probability that those screening positive will indeed have the clinical disorder of interest) in similar types of populations. Second, respondents should be selected for the second stage using a systematic procedure so that the data on clinical disorder can be weighted and the rates of clinical disorder can be estimated for the entire sample. There are various strategies for selecting respondents for the second stage. Most commonly, respondents who screen positive (i.e., score above a standard cutoff point) on an established screening scale and a random sample who screen negative are selected for the second stage clinical interview. The Gomel study was designed as a two-stage study. In that study, the 12-item General Health Questionnaire, a screening tool with a standard cutoff point determined from studies of untreated populations, was administered in stage 1. Stage 2 involved an examination by psychiatrists using a standardized psychiatric interview and by a specialist in internal medicine using a standardized physical examination. The subsample selected for participation in the second phase included 10% of respondents scoring 0–1, 20% scoring 2–7, and 33% scoring 8–12 (Havenaar et al., 1996). This strategy was chosen in order to oversample potential cases to increase the yield of diagnosed cases. Thus, the two-stage study design is an efficient and cost-effective method for investigating the prevalence of clinical disorders that has been underutilized in disaster research.

The retrospective cohort design also provides an opportunity for subsequent longitudinal research addressing delayed onsets, time to recovery, persistence and fluctuations of disorders, and risk and protective factors. For example, the Kyiv study of evacuees served as the basis for a 7-year longitudinal follow-up study of the 600 exposed and non-exposed mother–child dyads. An advantage of conceptualizing the initial assessment as the first wave of a potential follow-up study, rather than a cross-sectional snapshot, is that tracking information and consent to contact in the future are built into the data collection. That is, as part of the consent procedure, the respondent agrees to future contacts, and information about friends or relatives who could be contacted if the respondent cannot be located is included in the interview. Of course, the procedures must become part of the approval process of the investigator's research compliance board (Institute of Medicine Committee on Assessing Integrity in Research Environments, 2002).

Case–Control Studies

If the aim of a study is to determine whether, after a disaster, the rate of exposure (or exposure severity) is higher in an ill than in a well population, the case–control methodology is used. In contrast to retrospective cohort studies, the starting point of the case–control study is the selection of the cases. Cases can be selected from an existing population cohort (nested case–control study) or from a treatment source (traditional case–control study). Treatment sources can involve settings such as mental health outpatient programs, primary care settings, student health services, employee health services, crisis centers, or disaster-related service programs. Of course, the findings can only be generalized to the source population from which the survivors were drawn. Regardless of the setting, the most informative cases in a case–control study are incident cases, that is, people with no history of disease before the disaster took place. The controls should be chosen to represent, as best as possible, the source population from which the cases derive. This is a powerful and cost-effective method to investigate disaster effects that may be rare (low incidence), yet clinically significant for the population at large.

The case–control method has only rarely been applied in disaster research and was not applied in mental health studies after Chornobyl. However, it was used in studies of physical health consequences. One example is a population-based nested case–control study (Davis et al., 2004) that examined the relationship of radiation exposure to the risk of thyroid cancer in Russian children and adolescents who were 0–19 years old at the time of the accident. The sampling frame was the centralized Chornobyl registry of all exposed persons. The case group was composed of 26 children living in a contaminated region of Russia in 1986 who were diagnosed with thyroid cancer. Two demographically matched controls were selected from the registry for each case. This study found significantly higher radiation dose levels in cases as compared to controls. The second example (Kurjane et al., 2001) is a traditional case–control study of 59 Chornobyl cleanup workers treated at an occupational medicine clinic in Latvia who developed thyroid disease (cases) and 47 age-/sex-matched unexposed healthy controls (described in the study as "healthy blood donors"). The findings on a variety of blood test measures indicated that there were significant long-term impairments indicative of greater exposure to radiation from the accident.

Distinguishing between the Cohort and Case–Control Designs: Sources of Bias

Although the term *case–control study* has been used to describe research comparing exposed to nonexposed groups, we note here that the latter studies are more correctly classified as retrospective cohort studies, whereas studies of "cases," that is, individuals identified by their illness status, fall within the rubric of the case–control design. The distinction is important because in a retrospective cohort study exposure is not subject to misclassification, whereas biased recall of health and mental health problems is of concern. However, in a nonpopulation-based case–control study, exposure is ascertained after the disease has been manifested, and misclassification can occur. A compelling example of misclassification derives from the study by Southwick, Morgan, Nicolaou, and Charney (1997) in which veterans from the first Gulf War were asked about wartime exposures 1 month after returning home and again 2 years later. Eighty-eight percent changed their response to at least one exposure item, in part as a function of their psychological well-being.

Of course, selection bias can arise in both types of studies, albeit for different reasons. In the retrospective cohort study, selection bias may occur if the exposed group has a higher response rate (or lower attrition rate over time) than the controls, which is frequently the case. Selection bias becomes a threat to validity if the reasons for nonparticipation in the exposed group differ from the reasons in the unexposed and these reasons are associated with the outcome. Our study of mental health after the Chornobyl disaster illustrates this point. Suppose that the nonresponse in the evacuee mothers occurred largely because it was too painful for them to discuss their experiences, and the nonresponse among the controls was due to lack of motivation. In this case, differences between the groups in the outcome (mental health) would be reduced by the selection bias in participation. Even though, in most instances, the net result of bias is to decrease the effects of the disaster, effects can also be overestimated (e.g., if participation in a telephone survey is associated with anxiety in the exposed group but not in the controls). Survivor bias can also occur in retrospective cohort studies. Usually we think about the survivors of the disaster as contributing to this source of bias in the same way that we worry about the healthy worker effect in studies of workers and military personnel. However, it can also occur in the controls. For example, we compared workers at the Three Mile Island (TMI) plant with workers at another nuclear power plant. Both groups of workers were members of the International Brotherhood of Electrical Workers, and so we assumed that we had two equivalent groups except for exposure to the disaster. We found that the relative risk of major depression was higher in the TMI workers than the controls. However, when we presented the findings to the union, we learned that our findings were readily explained by selection bias because workers at the control plant, but not at TMI, could transfer to a less stressful work environment (coal-fired plant) with no loss in employment-associated benefits. Thus, because the controls were, in effect, a "super healthy worker" cohort, the differences in mental health that we observed were an artifact of selection bias.

In case–control studies, selection bias will occur if the cases are selected from a treatment program, yet the majority of persons with the disorder are untreated, which would be the case in studies of common mental disorders. One solution is to select three to four times as many controls as cases so that "untreated" cases with the disorder can be distinguished and potentially studied. The case–control study can also be biased by the selection of the control group. This is a special concern for studies of post-traumatic stress disorder (PTSD) because PTSD is comorbid with disorders, such as anxiety disorders, depression, and substance abuse, that can occur independently after disaster exposure. Moreover, patients often seek care because they have more than one disorder. Thus, in a case–control study of PTSD, if the controls are restricted to individuals with no disorder (supernormals), then the control group will have lower rates of comorbid disorders that are also associated with the disaster. Hence, the difference in exposure severity between cases and controls, as reflected in the odds ratio, would be overestimated. Unfortunately, a treatment control group could also be biased and lead to an underestimation of the odds ratio. For example, if the control group were patients treated for new episodes of cardiovascular disease, bias will occur if the disaster increased the likelihood of admission for such treatment.

Thus, each study design brings with it an array of strengths and weaknesses. It is important for disaster researchers to be aware of potential sources of bias as we design and implement our studies and thus to maximize as much as possible the theoretical and public health utility of the research.

SPECIAL CHALLENGES

Having highlighted some major issues in epidemiologically designed disaster research and emphasized the value of in-person assessments, we are acutely aware of the challenges and risks involved in carrying out such research in the aftermath of a disaster. Table 6.1 delineates these challenges. In this section, we describe methods to meet some of these challenges.

Conceptual Challenges

The first challenge that sets the stage for all decisions about the study is formulating the question. This means the question must be clearly articulated and presented in a way that lends itself to being investigated. A good research question should build on the existing knowledge base, fill in gaps or explain inconsistencies in our knowledge, and, most importantly, be worthy of study (see Benight, McFarlane, & Norris, Chapter 4, this volume). Will the answer to the question make a difference, either for stress theory or for postdisaster public health practice?

The formulation of the question will determine whether the study is best done using a case–control design or a cohort design, and will determine what mental health outcomes are included. If the question, for exam-

TABLE 6.1. Challenges in Designing and Executing Epidemiological Disaster Studies with Face-to-Face Assessments

Conceptual challenges
  • Specifying the question → selecting a study design
  • Selecting which outcomes will and will not be measured
  • Building in issues of local concern, including local idioms of distress
  • Developing relevant measures of exposure (disaster severity)
  • Identifying the relevant competing risk factors

Practical challenges
  • Identifying collaborators at all levels, including researchers, survivors, and their trusted representatives, and maintaining objectivity
  • Selling your ideas about study design and interview content
  • Sampling a representative group of victims and relevant unaffected controls
  • Achieving a high response rate in the postdisaster period of turmoil
  • Hiring, training, and monitoring local interviewers who will also be affected by the disaster
  • Transferring money in the face of corruption
  • Exporting Western concepts of informed consent

Disseminating the findings

---

ple, is whether radiation exposure from Chornobyl is a risk factor for schizophrenia, which is a low-prevalence condition, then a case–control study of incident cases of schizophrenia would be appropriate. However, if the question is whether radiation exposure is a risk factor for alcohol abuse, which is highly prevalent in the former Soviet Union, then it is reasonable to conduct a retrospective cohort study.

Even if the outcome is hypothesized to be uniquely caused by the disaster, other competing risk factors will need to be assessed because they could potentially magnify the deleterious effects of the disaster. Indeed, the advantage of focusing on a specific outcome is being able to assess the full array of competing risk factors. However, disaster studies are often seen as an opportunity to explore various outcomes, and in reality a broad-brush approach to mental health is typically used. A related decision, how best to assess the disorder(s), is often made on practical grounds. Assuming that the study uses face-to-face interviews, two linked questions are frequently asked:

1. What tools have been used successfully in prior disaster studies?
2. Who is available to collect the data? Are local psychologists and social workers available who can be trained to administer a semi-structured clinical interview or a neuropsychological test battery? Are there teachers, nurses, college students, or other sufficiently educated individuals who can be trained to administer a structured

interview and some simple cognitive tasks? Are experts available to train others and to monitor these complex interview schedules? Or is it most parsimonious to administer self-report symptom questionnaires primarily?

For our Chornobyl study in 1997, we had an educated interviewing staff, but there was no tradition of conducting mental health interviews, or even lengthy interviews. Thus we relied primarily on self-administered symptom scales and only a single interviewer-administered mental health module on depression.

It is also important to reflect on whether the choice of mental health outcomes is unduly influenced by the popular tools available for studying them, and hence whether sufficient consideration has been given to all potentially relevant outcomes that could arise from the event. It is very easy to blur these issues. For example, two common responses after disasters are headache and anger. Yet, compared to PTSD and depression, for which many well-known scales are available, headache and anger are rarely studied in their own right. Indeed, when a mental health evaluation package was quickly assembled and administered to more than 10,000 workers exposed to the World Trade Center disaster, it included several widely used self-report measures of depression, anxiety, and general well-being but no scales for headaches or anger.

Disasters occur all over the world. The idioms of expressing distress differ widely, and the cross-cultural applicability of our mental health concepts and assessment tools is not always known. Moreover, in many cultures, physical symptoms are the normative means for expressing distress. From the respondent's point of view, they would be interpreted as physical health consequences of the disaster. These issues have direct implications not just for conceptualizing and selecting the mental health end points but also for selecting and comprehensively evaluating physical health end points. Thus, if the local population is concerned that a disaster, like Chornobyl, causes headaches, dizziness, and cardiovascular problems, these need to be evaluated not just in the context of anxiety disorder but also as potential medical conditions in their own right. For this reason, our Chornobyl studies included physical examinations and blood tests.

As discussed by McFarlane and Norris (Chapter 1, this volume), operationalizing the concept of "disaster severity" is also challenging. For events like the Amsterdam El Al air crash occurring in multiethnic communities with substantial immigrant populations, disaster severity is best treated as a multidimensional concept. Local members of the research team are obviously an important resource for developing these measures. Focus groups with representative samples of the affected community are another. The reliability and validity of the disaster severity measures need to be established. This issue is often overlooked in the rush to field a disaster study. However, since these are the most crucial risk factors, their development needs to be a prominent part of the pretesting phase of the disaster study.

For each of the key outcomes to be studied, the relevant competing risk factors and potential confounding variables, as noted above, must be carefully measured as well, and they too should reflect local knowledge about unique risk factors. For the respondents, however, being asked about an array of risk factors may be perceived as "missing the point"—since their concern is with the exposure. For example, in a study of psychological and neuropsychological effects of solvent exposure in an American plant (Parkinson et al., 1990), the majority of the respondents were smokers. They were irritated by the questions about smoking since their participation was based on their concerns about the adverse effects of solvent exposure.

Practical Challenges

The first practical challenge is to identify collaborators and organize a research team. By research team, we do not mean just the investigators but also the individuals on-site who can play a role in shaping the content of the study, ensuring that it will be successfully executed, and assisting with creating suitable feedback for the community when the study is completed. We use the word *team* here to underscore the cooperative spirit, mutual trust, and mutual respect that must be maintained within the research group. In disaster studies, the team is likely to be assembled quickly and at the same time to find itself having to operate under extremely difficult circumstances and with major time constraints. Also, it is not unusual for some members of the research team or their relatives to be directly affected by the event. The challenge then is to maintain scientific objectivity in a situation where both the research team and the affected population share the shock and devastation of the event.

When we developed our research program on the mental health of residents after the 1979 nuclear power plant accident at Three Mile Island, there were no psychiatric epidemiological forerunners that could provide guidance. Most previous disaster mental health studies were anecdotal or focused on samples of convenience, such as litigants and hospitalized patients. Moreover, one of the high-risk groups that we chose to study, mothers of young children, had the same demographic profile as the principal investigator, field director, and many of the interviewers. All of us were deeply affected and confused by the contradictory and worrisome news reports about the severity of the accident and the possible adverse health consequences for the children. We therefore worked especially hard at self-awareness of our own level of bias and how it could encroach on the research effort. In the end, in order to have an objective portrait of the mental health consequences of Three Mile Island, we decided, perhaps wrongly, to ask the respondents about their attitudes only at the very end of the interview and to limit the number of questions, especially in the first waves of data collection in 1979 and 1980 (Bromet, 1991).

Even though selecting a representative sample may be obviously advantageous from a scientific point of view, as discussed above, this idea and its rationale are not readily appreciated by disaster communities, especially after extreme physical and mental injuries have occurred. In the case of disasters involving toxic exposures and harm to children, it is almost impossible to convey why the assessments would be limited only to those who are "selected" for the study. While the research team may view the endeavour as a "study," the community will often view it as an opportunity to obtain high-level health evaluations that are not otherwise available. One reasonable way to respond is to reserve room within the project to evaluate these "nonstudy"individuals. This builds goodwill and shows that the researchers understand and respect the community's needs. Thus, as part of the Kyiv children's study of Chornobyl, physical examinations and blood tests were provided not just to the 600 children who were preselected for the study but to any family member or neighbor who requested it. Similarly, in the Gomel study, respondents not selected for the second phase of the study, which involved a physical examination by a Dutch physician, were given the opportunity to participate. Dozens of people made use of this possibility, sometimes bringing relatives or friends. Needless to say, the results of these examinations were excluded from the data analysis.

Defining, selecting, and recruiting the affected population and the controls are among the most challenging and important tasks in disaster studies. The chaotic situation that occurs immediately after a disaster, as exemplified by Hurricane Katrina, can make it impossible to determine who exactly was affected and where they went. Immediately after the crash of the El Al Boeing 747 into a housing block in Amsterdam in 1992, the authorities estimated that between 1,000 and 1,500 persons directly experienced the crash. This included rescue workers who arrived during the early hours after the event. Six years later, even though the endless rumors that toxic agents were present in the cargo had been proven false, more than 6,000 people came for a medical checkup because they feared that their health might have been compromised by the event (Yzermans & Gersons, 2002). Because of the chaos and the need to maximize the number of people available at the disaster site, even tightly run organizations, such as police and fire departments, may be unable to produce accurate lists of officers who participated in relief work.

Some disaster studies have had very low response rates (Weisaeth, 1989). Obviously, it is difficult to achieve a high response rate when the postdisaster period is one of great turmoil, food and housing shortages, economic hardships, and battles for benefits. However, there are methods for optimizing response rates. One incentive, as noted above, is to provide physical examinations as part of the package. Another is to provide financial remuneration or a meaningful gift. Yet a third is to offer medical referral for individuals found to be at risk. A fourth incentive, and perhaps the key to optimizing the response rate, is training the interview staff on why a high response rate is important and on techniques to motivate participation, handle resistance, and to convert reluctant individuals. This should be an ongoing process as the fieldwork takes place.

Once the target sample is defined, it can be difficult to identify an unaffected comparison group that is similar in all respects except for exposure to the disaster, as illustrated above by the TMI worker study. This is particularly true for disasters that are threatening to the population at large (not just the direct victims), that are repeatedly replayed on television, or that draw rescue workers from distant communities. In disasters involving toxic exposures, the comparison sites should be screened for other contaminants that could lead to the same end points. For example, one of the first Western epidemiological studies of Chornobyl (International Atomic Energy Association, 1991) evaluated the health status of five age groups living in rural contaminated communities with that of controls from "nonexposed" villages and found no significant differences in physical health (hematological, thyroid, and general health measures). After the study was completed, the Ukrainian government revealed that the control villages were polluted by dangerous levels of pesticides.

The execution of disaster studies can be equally challenging. Many disasters occur in remote areas, but even regions that are easily accessible under normal conditions might be difficult to reach because of disrupted transportation systems or restrictions imposed by the authorities regarding entry to the area. Telephones may not work reliably, and communication among the research team and between the team and potential respondents becomes difficult to maintain. In 1986, when the Chornobyl accident occurred, many people in the former Soviet Union had shared phone lines, and thus there was no guarantee that confidentiality could be maintained if study recruitment was handled over the telephone. Of course, it is even more difficult to assemble the exposure group when affected populations are evacuated, and the evacuees are not systematically documented or registered.

Many disasters happen in settings where the government is corrupt and where Western concepts of informed consent are not just alien but give rise to suspicions about the research. This may mean that a quick disaster study immediately following an event is impossible and that long-term planning is a necessity. Thus, it was impossible to execute an unbiased study of the mental health consequences of Chornobyl during the Soviet era. It was only after the Soviet Union collapsed in 1991 that major epidemiological investigations could be undertaken and be monitored by Western investigators. For these studies, Western concepts of informed consent were implemented in spite of initial resistance. Methods for transferring funds and supervising expenditures may also require creativity, watchful vigilance, and trust.

Disseminating the Findings

Once the study is completed, the interviewers and respondents should be the first to hear about and react to the findings. In the past, many investigators failed to budget for this aspect of a study, but it is an obligation that is now widely assumed. How best to accomplish the dual goals of full (and appropriate) disclosure and response to the community is often the final challenge. There are many options, including presentations at community meetings (especially meetings that include question-and-answer periods), letters, sharing findings with the media (after informing the participants), and/or giving presentations at local churches and other types of meeting places. The most important issue here is to share the findings honestly and respectfully together with local collaborators. This is not always as easy as it would appear. When the Chornobyl study was completed, the U.S. and Kyiv investigators presented the findings at a "town hall" style of meeting in downtown Kyiv. We discussed the fact that no differences were found between evacuee children and controls in their blood tests and physical examinations, and we left considerable time for questions and answers. The meeting ended with strong overt displays of emotion between participants and the research team. However, during the week preceding the presentation, our Kyiv colleagues were refusing to participate because they were convinced that the negative findings would outrage the public and cause a riot in the lecture hall. The resolution we reached was that we presented what we found, emphasized the limits of our measurements, and offered to pursue additional blood tests and physical examinations to anyone who requested it. Such "out-of-pocket" expenses are not unusual in disaster studies.

REWARDS OF DISASTER STUDIES INVOLVING IN-PERSON INTERVIEWS

Face-to-face interviews provide a rich resource for public health planning. Beyond the obvious uses of epidemiologically collected health data, in-depth disaster studies offer the victims and the researchers some unique rewards (see Table 6.2). These include knowing that the community has a forum

TABLE 6.2. Why the Challenges Are Worth Meeting

- Victims want and need to talk
- Possibility of developing new insights that have public health implications
- Theoretical value of understanding disasters as "natural" experiments
- Confirming for the victims that they have a voice and are not forgotten

for expressing distress, anger, somatic symptoms, and worries that will be conveyed to public health authorities, and having the privilege of learning firsthand about the raw experiences that disaster victims face. As scientists, the reward also comes from knowing that the data will provide objective stepping stones for future research on traumatic stress.

We commented earlier that descriptive studies employing the usual set of measures may not add incrementally to our arsenal of knowledge, while studies that integrate physical and mental health and use neuropsychological and other biological measures will indeed be valuable for understanding the mechanisms involved in the evolution of health problems after traumatic events. We would also emphasize, in closing, the importance of active listening. An in-person interview gives an implicit message that the disaster community's stories are important. When participants are encouraged to use their own words, we can better understand what the disaster experience has meant for their health and well-being (Speckard, 2002). Clinicians who interview disaster victims do this routinely. Past research has been remiss when there is a bias in presuming to know both the questions and the answers that should be addressed.

ACKNOWLEDGMENTS

Preparation of this chapter was supported in part by Grant No. R01 MH051947 to Evelyn J. Bromet.

REFERENCES

Bromet, E. (1991). The psychologic effects of the radiation accident at TMI. In R. C. Ricks & M. D. Berger (Eds.), *The medical basis for radiation accident preparedness: III. Psychological Perspective* (pp. 61–70). New York: Elsevier.
Bromet, E. J., Goldgaber, D., Carlson, G., Panina, N., Golovakha, E., Gluzman, S. F., et al. (2000). Children's well-being 11 years after the Chornobyl catastrophe. *Archives of General Psychiatry, 57,* 563–571.
Bromet, E. J., Havenaar, J. M., Gluzman, S. F., & Tintle, N. L. (2005). Psychological after-

math of the Lviv air show disaster: A prospective controlled study. *Acta Psychiatrica Scandinavica, 112*, 194–200.

Canino, G., Bravo, M., Rubio-Stipec, M., & Woodbury, M. (1990). The impact of disaster on mental health: Prospective and retrospective analyses. *International Journal of Mental Health, 19*, 51–69.

Davis, S., Stepanenko, V., Rivkind, N., Kopecky, K. J., Voilleque, P., Shakhtarin, V., et al. (2004). Risk of thyroid cancer in the Bryansk Oblast of the Russian Federation after the Chornobyl Power Station accident. *Radiation Research, 162*, 241–248.

Havenaar, J. M., Poelijoe, N. W., Kasyanenko, A. P., van den Bout, J., Koeter, M. W. J., & Filipenko, V. V. (1996). Screening for psychiatric disorders in an area affected by the Chornobyl disaster: The reliability and validity of three psychiatric screening questionnaires in Belarus. *Psychological Medicine, 26*, 837–844.

Havenaar, J. M., Rumyantseva, G. M., van den Brink, W., Poelijoe, N. W., van den Bout, J., van Engeland, H., et al. (1997). Long-term mental health effects of the Chornobyl disaster: An epidemiological survey in two former Soviet Regions. *American Journal of Psychiatry, 154*, 1605–1607.

International Atomic Energy Association. (1991). *The International Chornobyl Project: An assessment of radiological consequences and evaluation of protective measures.* Unpublished report, Vienna, Austria: IAEA.

Institute of Medicine Committee on Assessing Integrity in Research Environments. (2002). Washington, DC: National Academy of Sciences.

Kurjane, N., Bruvere, R., Shitova, O., Romanova, T., Jaunalksne, I., Kirschfink, M., et al. (2001). Analysis of the immune status in Latvian Chornobyl clean-up workers with nononcological thyroid diseases. *Scandinavian Journal of Immunology, 54*, 528–533.

Maes, M., Mylle, J., Delmeire, L., & Altamura, C. (2000). Psychiatric morbidity and comorbidity following accidental man-made traumatic events: Incidence and risk factors. *European Archives of Psychiatry and Clinical Neuroscience, 250*, 156–162.

Parkinson, D., Bromet, E., Cohen, S., Dunn, L., Dew, M. A., Ryan, C., et al. (1990). Health effects of long-term solvent exposure in blue collar women. *American Journal of Industrial Medicine, 17*, 661–675.

Reijneveld, S. A., Crone, M. R., Verhulst, F. C., & Verloove-Vanhorick, S. P. (2003). The effect of a severe disaster on the mental health of adolescents: a controlled study. *Lancet, 362*, 691–696.

Robins, L. N., Fischbach, R. L., Smith, E. M., Cottler, L. B., Solomon, S. D., & Goldring, E. (1986). Impact of disaster on previously assessed mental health. In J. H. Shore (Ed.), *Disaster stress studies: New methods and findings* (pp. 21–48). Washington, DC: American Psychiatric Press.

Southwick, S. M., Morgan, C. A., III, Nicolaou, A. L., & Charney, D. S. (1997). Consistency of memory for combat-related traumatic events in veterans of Operation Desert Storm. *American Journal of Psychiatry, 154*, 173–177.

Speckhard, A. (2002). Voices from the inside—psychological responses to toxic disasters. In J. M. Havenaar, J. G. Cwikel, & E. J. Bromet (Eds.), *Toxic turmoil: Psychological and societal consequences of ecological disasters* (pp. 217–236). New York: Kluwer/Plenum Press.

Viinamäki, H., Kumpusalo, E., Myllykangas, M., Salomaa, S., Kumpusalo, L., Kolmakov, S., et al. (1995). The Chornobyl accident and mental wellbeing—a population study. *Acta Psychiatrica Scandinavica, 91*, 396–401.

Weisaeth, L. (1989). Importance of high response rates in traumatic stress research. *Acta Psychiatrica Scandinavica Supplement, 80* (Suppl. 355), 131–137.

Yzermans, J., & Gersons, B.P.R. (2002). The chaotic aftermath of an airplane crash in Amsterdam: A second disaster. In J. M. Havenaar, J. G. Cwikel, & E. J. Bromet (Eds.), *Toxic turmoil: Psychological and societal consequences of ecological disasters* (pp. 85–99). New York: Plenum Press.

CHAPTER 7

Telephone-Based Research Methods in Disaster Research

SANDRO GALEA, MICHAEL BUCUVALAS,
HEIDI RESNICK, JOHN BOYLE,
DAVID VLAHOV, and DEAN KILPATRICK

Telephone-based research methods have gained prominence as a potential tool in the armamentarium of the disaster researcher. Telephone-based methods allow for the rapid sampling and assessment of large populations and offer particular advantages for researchers interested in the consequences of disasters. This chapter provides a practical introduction to these methods. We focus here on how such research can be conducted and identify key issues that researchers should consider before and during the course of such research. We discuss the potential advantages and disadvantages of telephone-based research with reference to the situations when such methods may be more or less appropriate. We refer to "telephone-based research methods" as study methods that involve recruitment and interviewing of study participants through telephones. It is possible to recruit participants by telephone and interview them in person or using other methods, or vice versa, to recruit participants using other methods (e.g., off lists containing particular subgroups such as college students) and then interview these persons by telephone. We use the terms *telephone sampling* or *telephone interviewing*, respectively, to refer to these special instances.

DESIGN ISSUES IN TELEPHONE SURVEYS

Sampling

Choosing a Sampling Frame

The first practical question when considering the application of a telephone-based research method in the postdisaster context is the particular sampling frame that is the target of the survey. It is the goal of all research to obtain information on persons who are of interest to answer a particular scientific question. The characteristics of these persons (i.e., the "sampling frame") dictate both the methods that are applied to assess this population and how these methods are implemented. For example, if a particular research question pertains to the psychopathology among a small group of rescue personnel who assisted disaster victims, a list of these rescue personnel may exist, and it may be feasible to contact all these persons and interview them in person (by having interviewers visit them) or having them all come to be interviewed at a central location.

Telephone-based research methods, on the other hand, are particularly well suited to the sampling of large populations that are difficult to contact, or to interview, using other modalities. For example, a study that intends to sample all residents of a large city will have to devise a method to access persons who validly represent this sampling frame. In this context, problems about accessing buildings in dense urban areas and the size of the population to be sampled frequently make telephone-based recruitment and interviewing the only feasible option. Overall, investigator judgment that combines an awareness of the sample of interest, the key research questions and the assessment modalities that are needed to address them, and the practical and logistical (e.g., financial, time) parameters that bound the research will best guide choice of research method. In the rest of this chapter we will discuss considerations about the use of telephone-based research methods that may help inform such decisions.

Generating a Sample: List-Based Sampling, Random Sampling, and Oversampling

There are three principal methods of sample recruitment that are in use in telephone-based research, each with particular advantages and disadvantages. List-based samples involve the use of preexisting lists of all persons in a particular sampling frame. Such lists are useful when they represent the entire universe of persons in the sampling frame. For example, in research about mental health among families of the victims of the Pan Am 103 explosion over Lockerbie, researchers used a list of all family members, provided by official government sources, to contact all family members of victims (Smith, Kilpatrick, Falsetti, & Best, 2002). Telephone interviewing then provides an opportunity to contact persons on these lists cost-effectively, particularly if these persons are geographically dispersed.

List-based sampling rapidly loses utility if the lists available are not comprehensive but rather include only a subgroup of all the persons in a particular sampling frame. For example, telephone directories provide a list of all persons within a particular city or region with listed telephone numbers. However, only about two-thirds of all U.S. households have listed telephone numbers (Survey Sampling Inc., 1990). In addition, the proportion of telephone numbers that are listed or unlisted in given areas throughout the United States varies, with a higher proportion of unlisted numbers in central cities than in suburban/rural areas. Therefore, if a telephone directory list is used as the primary means of characterizing a sampling frame, the sample will then best be construed as representative of *listed* telephone numbers. Epidemiologically, such samples are subject to *selection bias*. Given that we cannot adequately characterize the nature of this bias (e.g., are persons with listed telephone numbers younger or older than those with unlisted numbers?), the consequences of this bias are difficult if not impossible to assess, making it difficult to draw conclusions from the study. Therefore, list-based samples are useful only in a narrow subset of studies where a comprehensive list of persons in the sampling frame of interest is indeed available.

Random digit dialing (RDD), first proposed in the early 1960s, is a group of probability sampling techniques that provide an opportunity of reaching any household with a telephone within a sampling frame (Cooper, 1964). The primary advantage of RDD is that it removes the problem of selection bias arising from unlisted telephone numbers in specific areas. The science of generating random digit number lists is sophisticated, and a full discussion of the pros and cons of various techniques of generating random digit numbers is beyond the scope of this chapter (see Lavrakas, 1993). In brief, RDD surveying generally makes use of a sample frame that involves phone numbers that have been generated at random. These numbers include a combination of 3-digit area code and 3-digit prefix (sometimes called the telephone "exchange") that includes the area of interest for the survey (e.g., city or country), and a randomly generated series of 4-number suffixes. In the early inception of the U.S. phone systems 3-digit prefixes were tightly correlated with precise geographic areas. Therefore, given a particular geographic sampling frame selecting numbers within a given prefix made it possible to generate a random list of all numbers within a particular area. However, with the increasing mobility of telephone numbers, 3-digit prefixes are becoming less reliable in terms of identifying specific geographic areas. Increasingly, particular geographic areas are covered by multiple telephone prefixes, requiring that all prefixes be included in the

RDD sampling frame in order to ensure that all households in the frame have a nonzero probability of selection.

Generation of RDD lists for surveying includes simple random sampling (i.e., the generation of numbers within a given area code and prefix), modifications of a technique often referred to as the Mitofsky–Waksberg method, or list assisted sampling. The Mitofsky–Waksberg method uses two-stage sampling (Waksberg, 1978). In the first stage a telephone number is selected from a simple random list and dialed. If the number proves to be a residential number, the set of 100 numbers that include the same eight digits as the number dialed (called the primary sampling unit, or PSU) is retained for the second stage. Surveying then can be carried out within the second-stage PSUs, increasing the likelihood of working numbers and minimizing phone calls to nonworking numbers (Potthoff, 1994). List-assisted sampling further refines this method to cost-effectively sample number banks that contain the majority of working telephone numbers (Tucker, Lepkowski, & Pierkarski, 2002).

Although generally the goal is to sample subgroups of the population in proportion to their size, sometimes a small group, such as an ethnic group, is of particular interest for the research. In this case, the research design can involve *oversampling* of persons within that racial/ethnic group. This will then result in a greater number of persons within this group, allowing for more power for within- and between-group analyses. Such oversampling results in a sample with differential probability of selection, and such differential probability of selection must be accounted for by appropriate weighting.

Special Issues: Sampling Telephones versus Sampling People

Telephone-based sampling relies on sampling *telephones* rather than sampling people or households. There are three important considerations that arise from this. First, telephone-based research methods rely on persons having a telephone in their house. Therefore, by definition, persons who are homeless or who are living in institutions (e.g., prisons, long-term care facilities) are not part of the sampling frame. Another concern in this regard is the growing use of cellular telephones and, particularly, the proportion of persons who use only cellular telephones and do not have a home telephone. It is not current practice to include telephone numbers for cellular telephones in telephone sampling frames. The Telephone Consumer Protection Act of 1991 (TCPA) prohibits placing calls from automated dialing systems to numbers with services for which the called party is charged for the incoming call. Practically, since many cellular telephone calling plans still bill the plan holder for calls received (at least insofar as deducting airtime minutes), it is a potential violation of the law to include cell phone numbers as part of a telephone-based sampling frame. In 2003, approxi-mately 3% of persons in the U.S. used a cellular telephone as their only telephone, with up to 6% among certain groups, particularly persons under the age of 25 (Blumberg, Luke, & Cynamon, 2004). As the use of cellular telephones grows, newer techniques in telephone sampling may need to be developed.

Second, a household with more than one telephone has a higher likeli-hood of being sampled than a household with only one telephone. Statisti-cal adjustment in the form of sample weights have to be applied to deal with this differential probability of selection.

Third, persons also have a probability of selection inverse to the num-ber of people in the household. This is not an issue in telephone-based stud-ies of entire households, but if the focus of the investigation is persons, this introduces an important differential probability of selection of persons liv-ing in different-sized households. For example, persons living in households with two persons have twice the likelihood of being sampled as persons liv-ing in households with four persons. There are two considerations that are relevant in this regard. First, once again, statistical adjustment for this dif-ferential probability of selection is needed. Second, it is not sufficient to sample whomever may answer the phone since this introduces selection bias (e.g., women may be more likely to answer the phone than are men). Rather, a system needs to be put in place to randomly select persons from a household for participation in the telephone-based assessment. The most commonly used methods in this regard are the Kish procedure, which asks interviewers to enumerate all eligible persons in a household and then uses an algorithm to randomly select a person in the household (Kish, 1949, 1965), and the birthday selection method, which asks for the person with the birthday closest to the interview date; both methods produce quasi-random assessments of respondents within a household (Groves & Lyberg, 1988).

CONDUCT OF TELEPHONE-BASED RESEARCH

General Principles regarding Telephone-Based Survey Development and Interviewing

The art of constructing good survey instruments has been the subject of several excellent reference texts (Dillman, 1978; Fowler, 1993). In planning surveys intended for telephone use, the principles that apply to the design of all good surveys apply here also. However, perhaps more than in-person interviews, telephone-based surveys need to be as simple as possible, at a sixth-grade reading level at the most, relying on straightforward communi-cation of question concepts that can be effective on the telephone. Given the absence of face-to-face contact, the interviewer cannot rely on visual aids, gestures, or demonstrations to explain a particular question, hence making clarity of questions paramount. In our experience, interviews that are designed with closed-ended questions are more effective for telephone-based assessments than are open-ended questions. It is simpler and ideal if respondents can respond to questions with a simple "yes" or "no," a number (as in age), or one-word answers or phrases that are selected from rating scales or fixed-answer alternatives. In addition to minimizing mistakes in responses and inter-interview variability, such question wording increases the likelihood that participant responses are confidential since, even if someone were listening to the respondents' answers, they would be unable to determine the meaning of the responses.

Keeping telephone-based surveys as brief as possible is critical to maximize participant survey completion. One of the principal contrasts between telephone-based surveying and in-person interviews is that the rapport between participant and interview is more limited in telephone-based surveying. In addition, the burden is on the interviewer to keep the participant on the telephone. If the survey becomes too burdensome, it is easy for the participant to disconnect the phone and end the survey. Therefore, surveys must encourage participant engagement and minimize participant fatigue. In our experience, more than 95% of participants who start participation in postdisaster research will complete surveys that are approximately 30 minutes in length (Galea et al., 2004).

Conduct of Surveys

Interviews must be designed in such a manner as to make participants comfortable with the interview process, to ensure that participants understand questions that they are being asked, and to allow them the option of stopping the interview at any time and requesting help if they need it, particularly in the immediate postdisaster context.

Upon contact with a potential respondent, telephone surveys typically include an opening script that is designed to (1) introduce the purpose of the call, (2) explain who is calling, (3) disclose how long the interview will take, (4) explain any relevant survey procedures, (5) notify participants of institutional review board oversight of the research and their rights as participants in research studies, and (6) offer a telephone number (ideally toll-free) that a participant can call to verify survey authenticity. Such opening scripts, carefully and concisely worded, are the first contact between an interviewer and a participant and are critical in establishing a rapport between the two that will serve the research well throughout the course of the interview. Verbal informed consent is typically obtained as part of the opening script. In some telephone-based studies, particularly ones that consist of telephone-based interviewing of participants recruited off existing contact lists, written information about the study is sent to participants ahead of the actual telephone contact, facilitating both the opening script and the consent process. After the opening script is read, permission to proceed with the interview is obtained from all participants. It is helpful for interviewers to have available to them scripts for how to deal with frequently asked questions (e.g., "How did you get my number?"). All numbers in a telephone-based sampling frame are dialed 10–15 times at several different times of day in academic surveys (although frequently fewer numbers of times in market research) before being declared nonanswers.

Interviews are conducted as efficiently as possible, with the interviewers reading preset scripts and deviating as little as possible from the scripts and questions as written. Procedures should be in place for participant callback if participants need to stop during the call at any time. In the context of postdisaster research where there is a concern about participant distress, it is important to have mental health support systems in place that can provide assistance if participants are distressed and/or request such help. Generally, participation in trauma research is well tolerated, and participants report positive effects of participation that compensate for any modest levels of upset or distress experienced during research assessments (Newman & Kaloupek, 2004, p. 383; see also Fleischman, Collogan, & Tuma, Chapter 5, this volume). Given the greater anonymity afforded by telephone-based assessments, it is plausible that distress is further minimized using these techniques, although we are not aware of assessments that have compared distress after telephone and other forms of assessment after disasters. However, the presence of even a small number of respondents who may want mental health assistance suggests the need for a mental health backup system for research conducted soon after a mass trauma (Galea et al., 2002; Galea et al., in press).

One of the key questions that often confront researchers conducing postdisaster assessments is whether there is a need to provide a financial incentive to participants. Nominal financial incentives ($10–$25) probably do not substantially improve outcome rates for short cross-sectional surveys or limited assessments but may be helpful as part of a tiered approach to recruiting, and retaining, persons in a telephone-based cohort study (Bucuvalas, Morgan, & Galea, 2002). If a decision is made to provide an incentive, the respondent's address needs to be obtained, usually at the end of the survey, for mailing of the incentive. Safeguards must be put in place to ensure that addresses and other unique identifiers are kept in a separate database from the actual survey responses, thus maintaining participant anonymity. This, properly explained, helps to increase respondent confidence in the confidentiality of their responses.

Professional Survey Management

The conduct of a telephone-based research study, like all studies, requires daily management and careful supervision. In that regard one of the more common questions faced by academic researchers in considering this work is whether such work can or should be carried out by trained professional surveyors or by volunteer surveyors (frequently students or trainees). Although, in theory, a rigorously trained staff of surveyors could carry out a telephone-based research project optimally regardless of whether they are paid or unpaid, paid staff are clearly incentivized to do well and can be better monitored and corrected when deviating from standard procedure. In addition, the intricacies of day-to-day management of telephone-based research methods are copious and may be challenging for nonprofessionals or researchers who are not immersed in a high volume of telephone-based surveys on a day-to-day basis.

As such, many telephone-based research projects are conducted by professional market research firms with research experience who work in collaboration with researchers on devising a research plan, developing a survey, and training surveyors. The professional firms then typically supervise day-to-day conduct of the survey and provide data to the researchers for analysis. These collaborations can be productive and highly efficient in the postdisaster context, maximizing the skills of both researchers and survey professionals, both bringing invaluable insights that can improve the conduct of telephone-based research (Galea et al., 2002).

Regardless of the management brought to bear on any particular research project, all interviewers must be trained and adept at administering the interview and dealing with potential participant questions. If a particular survey is being conducted in more than one language, interviewers who are fluent in the languages of the survey need to be available and a system in place to make sure interviewers who can speak a particular language are available to handle respondents who may request an interview in that language. Data monitoring for inter-interviewer variability and for internal survey consistency is essential on a day-to-day basis. Typically a certain proportion of interviews are audiotaped or listened to by supervisors to ensure fidelity to study protocols and the written interview. Recruitment and refusal rates should be monitored by supervisors and the project director daily.

Most telephone surveys are currently conducted using computer-assisted telephone interviewing (CATI). CATI systems control the handling of the sample telephone numbers and program the survey questions to be presented to the interviewer on a computer screen with controls for skip patterns, item rotation, and acceptable response ranges. In this way CATI-coded questionnaires can restrict possible responses to questions (hence minimizing both erroneous answers and interviewer coding errors) and, in more so-phisticated uses of CATI systems, include algorithms that carry out checks for internal consistency on an ongoing basis through the survey. CATI-coded surveys can also be particularly useful in special contexts, such as longitudinal cohort studies where the CATI program can embed informa-tion about the respondent obtained in previous survey waves that can in-form question administration in an ongoing wave (Lavrakas, Settersten, & Maier, 1991). With the sophistication of computer-controlled scripts, CATI telephone interviews can also use complex skip logic and qualifications to route respondents through question series that would be very distracting for an interviewer to administer without the assistance of a computer. Can-tor and Lynch (2000) identify several other advantages of using CATI for telephone interviews. The first is that it permits greater quality control over interviewer behavior because of the standardization of how questions are presented in sequence to the interviewer. A second advantage is that CATI interviews usually occur in a centralized facility, which permits direct real-time monitoring of interviewers. One study randomly assigned interviewers to either a CATI condition or a standard interview condition in which in-terviewers used a regular interview to collect information via telephone from the interviewer's home (Hubble & Wilder, 1988). Respondents in the CATI interview condition had substantially higher disclosure rates for vio-lent and nonviolent crimes.

Calculation of Telephone Survey Outcome Rates

There are two primary considerations with regard to the calculation of out-come rates in telephone-based research methods. The first of these is the calculation of outcome rates, and the second pertains to the significance of these rates. Pinpointing an exact outcome rate in telephone surveys is often difficult due to the challenge in classifying indeterminate cases. An exhaus-tive list of potential methods for calculating response rates is provided by the American Association for Public Opinion Research (AAPOR, 2003).

Briefly, the all-encompassing term that should be used (but is seldom encountered in academic research) is *outcome rates*; this term includes sev-eral other rates, including response rates, cooperation rates, and refusal rates. *Response rates* are the number of completed interviews divided by the number of all possible interviews. *Cooperation rates* are the proportion of all cases interviewed divided by all eligible cases. *Refusal rates* are the proportion of all cases in which a respondent refuses to be interviewed or cuts off contact before some predetermined point in the survey that repre-sents completion. There are several ways to calculate each of these outcome rates. There are six different types of response rates, depending primarily on how partial interviews are considered. Since all possible interviews are included in the denominator in these calculations (including cases of unknown eligibility), response rates are the most conservative outcome rate that can be provided. Cooperation rates are outcome rates among those eligible and therefore are higher than response rates; there are two cooperation rates that generally can be calculated, depending primarily on assessment of eligibility. There are three types of refusal rates that differ primarily on how the disposition of cases of unknown eligibility is treated. It is advisable to report several outcome rates, together with careful explanation of how they were calculated, in academic research publications.

The second key question in this regard pertains to the significance of outcome rates and whether there is a relationship between outcome rates and telephone-based methods' ability to provide valid estimates of population-based prevalences or associations of interest. Some of the best evidence that can be applied to answer this question arises from large surveys that have been ongoing for several decades and across regions, hence allowing comparisons of survey validity with changing response rates. The Behavioral Risk Factor Surveillance Survey (BRFSS) conducted by the Centers for Disease Control and Prevention (CDC) is an annual telephone survey aimed at assessing a range of behavioral risk factors nationwide (CDC, 2005). The BRFSS response rates vary from year to year and from state to state, but the overall decrease in BRFSS response rates is well documented, with median response rates across states falling from a high of 71.4% in 1993 to a low of 48.9% in 2000. Surveys conducted by official organizations, such as health departments and the government, typically have higher response rates than research surveys conducted by academic or nonprofit institutions (Mariolis, 2001).

Importantly, recent analyses of BRFSS data have shown that for a range of response rates for telephone surveys between 30 and 70%, the response rates were at most weakly associated with bias (Mariolis, 2002). In one analysis, it was shown that although a larger difference in response rate was associated with a larger difference in estimates of cigarette smoking prevalence between the BRFSS and the in-person Current Population Survey (CPS), the effects were small (Mariolis, 2002). Further evidence in this regard comes from an analysis that was designed to test potential differences associated with different response rates obtained from identical surveys. Keeter, Miller, Kohut, Groves, and Presser (2000) compared data from two surveys with response rates of 61% and 36% and found very few significant differences across 91 comparisons. In the field of mental health, analysis of data from the National Comorbidity Survey showed that the impact on population prevalence estimates of response rates differing between 74 and 82% were small (Kessler, Little, & Groves, 1995).

There are two last considerations with respect to outcome rates. First, extreme effort to recruit more reluctant nonparticipants may itself introduce bias, since the reluctantly recruited participants potentially have reasons for providing false or misleading responses. This concern has long been raised by experts on psychological measurement and response-bias scales have been developed to allow for adjustment for or exclusion of inaccurate responses from survey assessments (Drasgow, Levine, & McLaughlin, 1987; Reise & Due, 1991). Large national surveys that invest substantial effort in maximizing response rates also include measures such as extensive interviewer training to increase rapport with participants in order to attempt to minimize this concern (Kessler, Mroczek, & Belli, 1999). Second, overzealous efforts to increase response rates may well be unethical if they violate respondents' stated desire not to participate in a particular survey assessment.

Telephone Surveys and Sampling Weights

Survey weights ensure that each person in the sampling frame has an equal probability of selection. These weights are inverse to the number of telephones in a household (to account for the fact that households with more telephones are more likely to be selected) and proportional to the number of persons within a household (to account for the fact that a single person represents other noninterviewed persons in the same household).

Other forms of sample weights also can be developed. In telephone-based samples that are recruiting persons in the general population from a particular geographic area, poststratification weights are frequently developed to account for discrepancies between the sample as recruited and anticipated distributions of persons within specific strata as expected based on U.S. Census data. For example, if young whites are undersampled, a sample weight is developed that is inverse of the proportional undersampling of this subgroup. Caution must be exercised in developing such weights for several reasons. In small samples, subgroup estimates may rely on very small sample sizes, and any deviation from the anticipated census distribution may be a function of random variability more than of any systematic undersampling. Sample weights reduce computational efficiency in standard statistical programs and, as such, should be used judiciously and only when clearly indicated. A final practical note in this regard is that certain statistical programs are not capable of accurately dealing with complex survey weights in many of their advanced procedures. For example, standard statistical procedures in SAS 8.0 with weights applied result in overestimation of sample size and in artificially low estimates of standard errors. SUDAAN (Shah, Barnwell, & Bieler, 1997) and STATA 8.2 (2004) are both statistical software packages that adequately take into account weighted survey designs.

ADVANTAGES AND DISADVANTAGES OF
TELEPHONE-BASED RESEARCH METHODS

Advantages of Telephone-Based Research Methods

The principal advantage afforded by telephone-based research methods is the opportunity for a cost-effective and valid means of assessing persons in a large sampling frame. Starting with cost issues, the principal factor driving costs in data collection is typically personnel costs, primarily in the form of pay for interviews and data collectors. In-person interviewing, widely considered the gold standard in psychiatric epidemiology because it allows the administration of clinician-administered structured clinical interviews, is also the most personnel-intensive, and therefore most expensive, form of data collection. Although costs for all surveys vary tremendously, given a multitude of factors, in our experience in-person interviews can be as much as five times as expensive as telephone surveys.

The costs involved in any research method are largely a function of the length of time it takes to collect data on any given participant. The time per participant also then affects how long it will take to complete data collection on a given desired sample size. In-person recruitment or interviewing requires interviewers to go to a participant's address (be it home or otherwise) and incur substantial travel time between interviews. Alternatively, in-person interviews that rely on participants coming to a central research site require substantial coordination on the part of the research team to ensure that participant transportation is facilitated to, and that participants arrive at, a designated research site. In telephone surveying, interviewers can move from one interview to the next without leaving a central telephone surveying facility. It is also worth noting that in many densely populated urban areas access to residential buildings is difficult and, absent official permission or fiat, makes the reliable sampling of these residences infeasible.

Therefore, when compared to in-person recruitment, telephone-based methods allow researchers to contact more persons in a particular time for less money. These particular advantages make phone research methods particularly suitable for the postdisaster context. In many instances after disasters, an early postdisaster assessment that can establish baseline mental health estimates is a critical part of the research. In addition, delays in obtaining funding and the relatively limited availability of short-term funds make cost considerations paramount. Therefore, a survey technique that can be implemented relatively quickly and cost-effectively can enable research to be conducted in the postdisaster context that may otherwise not be feasible to implement. Telephone interviews using CATI in a centralized facility also offer quality control over data collection that is not possible in in-person interviews.

It is worth noting that there are other methods of recruiting participants that provide alternatives to either in-person or telephone-based recruitment. The reader is referred to other chapters in this volume for coverage of some of these methods, including Web-based research (Schlenger & Silver, Chapter 8, this volume). The ultimate decision about which study design optimally may be employed to address a particular research question rests not only on evidence of a method's feasibility and costs but also on evidence that a particular method can assess mental health reliably and validly. In that regard, a substantial body of evidence suggests that telephone research methods are a reliable form of epidemiological assessment.

Validity of Telephone-Based Assessments as Compared to In-Person Assessments

One assessment conducted both in-person and telephone interview surveys simultaneously in the same area using the same interview schedule (Weeks, Kulka, Lessler, & Whitmore, 1983). Response rates for the telephone survey were lower than for the in-person surveys, and telephone respondents tended to be younger, better educated, and more likely to be white than in-person respondents. However, and most importantly, the same assessment showed that there were no substantial differences in the accuracy of self-reported conditions or in health utilization questions. In fact, the assessment showed that internal consistency between responses was higher in the telephone surveys than in the in-person surveys. This study also showed that telephone surveys were appreciably cheaper to conduct than in-person surveys. A similar study (Aneshensel, Frerichs, Clark, & Yokopenic, 1982) found no statistically significant differences between the two interview methods for overall assessment of health status, illnesses reported for the preceding 4 months, or reports of hospitalization. In a recent analysis comparing national estimates of data from the BRFSS and the National Health Interview Survey (NHIS; which obtains information on medical conditions and health risk factors via within-household in-person interviews), it was shown that BRFSS estimates were similar to NHIS estimates for 13 of 14 measures examined, suggesting that any effect of telephone versus in-person interview on the quality of the information obtained was negligible (Nelson, Powell-Griner, Town, & Kovar, 2003). Specific to mental health, several studies have shown that telephone assessment of Axis I disorders (including depression and anxiety disorders) produced nearly identical results to in-person assessments using a variety of instruments (Simon, Revicki, & vonKorff, 1993; Paulsen, Crowe, Noyes, & Pfohl, 1988).

Another recent study compared in-person and telephone interviews with respect to their ability to detect exposure to violent victimization and several DSM-IV disorders among a sample of older adults (ages 55–85) who were randomly assigned to be interviewed using a highly structured interview either via telephone or in person (Acierno, Resnick, Kilpatrick, & Stark-Riemer, 2003). There were no significant differences associated with interview mode for prevalence of victimization experiences or prevalence of DSM-IV disorders.

Limitations of Telephone-Based Research Methods

The absence of in-person contact limits the potential for biometric assessment that may increasingly be the key to answering important questions regarding the biological underpinnings of the psychological consequences of disasters. However, it is possible to locate and interview respondents via telephone and then collect biological samples by other means.

The dynamics of telephone-based interviewing are also different than those inherent in in-person interviewing. As noted previously, the absence of visual cues, the ease with which participants may terminate a telephone-based survey, and the need to keep the survey brief are all potential limitations to use of the method. In addition, telephone survey outcome rates have been falling over the past several decades, and the introduction of new technologies, including caller identification, and cellular phones are new challenges that may reduce outcome rates even further in coming years. Although the best evidence suggests that there is little evidence of systematic bias inherent in lower response rates that are obtained through best survey practice, greater effort may need to be expended in telephone-based sampling to obtain satisfactory outcome rates in order to provide confidence that a given study sample adequately reflects the underlying sampling frame.

Problems can also arise in telephone sampling when the sampling frame of interest is restricted to particularly small geographic areas, as in sometimes the case in studies of localized disasters. Frequently it is difficult for persons to accurately identify whether they live within or outside a survey's geographic boundaries, and it is challenging for an interviewer on the telephone to narrow down such boundaries absent visual aids (e.g., maps) that are relatively easy to use in in-person interviews. Algorithms can be developed and implemented through CATI coding that offer respondents dichotomous choices about where they live anchored to familiar features of the local landscape (e.g., are you closer or further from the park than this street?) that can narrow down respondent location to ensure it is within a desired sampling frame. Such algorithms however are time-intensive to implement.

Ultimately, the reliance on functioning telephones for this mode of data collection may limit the use of telephone-based methods in particular postdisaster contexts. In disasters that result in widespread system disruption or massive relocation, telephone surveys soon after an event may not be an appropriate method of participant recruitment. Of course, the same factors are present and present serious challenges to door-to-door or mail samples in similar contexts. In our experience, in the United States, telephone service is generally rapidly restored, and even persons who are displaced have telephone numbers forwarded, enabling contact relatively soon after a disaster. However, in the global context, particularly outside the Western world, the utility of telephone-based methods remains limited to countries with reliable telephones that can access a suitably high proportion of the population.

FUTURE OF TELEPHONE-BASED RESEARCH METHODS

We conclude with a note about the future of telephone surveys. As discussed in this chapter, telephone-based survey methods offer particular advantages for researchers interested in the consequences of disasters, particularly in large general population sampling frames. However, these advantages are offset by disadvantages that to some extent limit the appli cability of these methods. We suggest that most of the promise of telephone-based methods lies in the innovative use of telephone-based methods and the combination of research methods to maximize the advantages of different techniques.

In terms of innovative use of telephone-based methods, the application of telephone-based methods to study designs such as longitudinal cohort studies or case–control studies can make substantial contributions to the postdisaster research literature. For example, there is a paucity of research that has used telephone-based recruitment of general population representative samples for the purposes of longitudinal cohort studies in the aftermath of disasters. As a result we have little empiric evidence to inform our understanding of the general population consequences of disasters. Similarly, telephone-based methods can be used to recruit population-based controls for case–control studies where cases are persons with psychopathology after disasters, be it posttraumatic stress disorder in the long term or distinct patterns of psychopathology. Such study designs, facilitated by telephone-based methods, can push the envelope in postdisaster research and address questions that currently remain unanswered.

Combinations of research methods may hold particular promise. For example, persons in the general population can be recruited using telephone-based methods and invited to participate in subsequent research stages that involve biometric or in-person assessments. This combination of population-representative sampling and the opportunity for in-depth or biological assessments may allow the extension of biological research in the postdisaster context to population-based samples, an extension that currently remains highly unusual.

Finally, the proliferation of Web-based and electronic forms of participant communication also presents an opportunity for telephone-based methods. In this case electronic communication with participants may be used both to assist in recruitment and to obtain ancillary participant data. In addition, it may be feasible to assess participants by using telephone-based methods after provision of information through the Internet, allowing the researcher to provide large amounts of information but to preserve person-to-person questionnaire administration.

ACKNOWLEDGMENTS

Preparation of this chapter was supported in part by Grant Nos. R25 MH070552, R01 DA 017642, R01 MH 66081, and R01 MH 066391 from the National Institutes of Health.

REFERENCES

Acierno, R., Resnick, H., Kilpatrick, D., & Stark-Riemer, W. (2003). Assessing elder victimization. *Journal of Social Psychiatry and Psychiatric Epidemiology, 38,* 644–653.

American Association for Public Opinion Research Standard Definitions. (2003). *Final dispositions of case codes and outcome rates for surveys.* Retrieved February 11, 2005, from www.aapor.org/pdfs/newstandarddefinitions.pdf

Aneshensel, C. S., Frerichs, R. R., Clark, V., & Yokopenic, P. A. (1982). Telephone versus in-person surveys of community health status. *American Journal of Public Health, 72*(9), 1017–1021.

Blumberg, S. J., Luke, J. V., & Cynamon, M. L. (2004, May). *The impact of wireless substitution on random-digit-dialed health surveys.* Paper presented at American Association for Public Opinion Research Annual Conference, Phoenix.

Bucuvalas, M., Morgan, M., & Galea, S. (2002, May). *Tracking continuing psychological outcomes from the World Trade Center Disaster among New Yorkers.* Paper presented at the American Association of Public Opinion Research Annual Conference, Nashville, TN.

Cantor, D., & Lynch, J. P. (2000). Self-report surveys as measures of crime and criminal victimization. *Criminal Justice 4,* 85–138.

Centers for Disease Control and Prevention. (2005). *Behavioral Risk Factor Surveillance System.* Retrieved February 2, 2005, from www.cdc.gov/brfss/

Cooper, S. L. (1964). Random sampling by telephone: An improved method. *Journal of Marketing Research, 1*(4), 45–48.

Dillman, D. A. (1978). *Mail and telephone surveys: The total design method.* New York: Wiley.

Drasgow, F., Levine, M. V., & McLaughlin, M. E. (1987). Detecting inappropriate test scores with optimal and practical appropriateness indices. *Applied Psychological Measurement, 11,* 59–79.

Fowler, F. J., Jr. (1993). *Survey research methods* (2nd ed.). Newbury Park, CA: Sage.

Galea, S., Nandi, A., Stuber, J., Gold, J., Bucuvalas, M., Rudenstine, S., et al. (2005) Public reactions to survey research after terrorist attacks. *Journal of Traumatic Stress, 18*(5), 461–465.

Galea, S., Vlahov, D., Resnick, H., Kilpatrick, D., Bucuvalas, M., & Morgan, M. (2002). An investigation of the psychological effects of the September 11th attacks on NYC: Developing and implementing research in the acute postdisaster period. *CNS Spectrums, 7*(8), 593–596.

Galea, S., Vlahov, D., Tracy, M., Hoover, D., Resnick, H., & Kilpatrick, D. G. (2004). Hispanic ethnicity and post-traumatic stress disorder after a disaster: Evidence from a general population's survey after September 11. *Annals of Epidemiology, 14*(8), 520–531.

Groves, R. M., & Lyberg, L. E. (1988). An overview of nonresponse issues in telephone surveys. In R. M. Groves, P. P. Biemer, L. E. Lyberg, J. T. Massey, W. L. Nicholls, & J. Waksberg (Eds.). *Telephone survey methodology* (pp. 191–212). New York: Wiley.

Hubble, D., & Wilder, B. E. (1988). Preliminary results from the National Crime Survey CATI Experience. New Orleans, LA: Proceedings of the American Statistical Association, Survey Methods Section.

Keeter, S., Miller, C., Kohut, A., Groves, R. M., & Presser, S. (2000). Consequences of reducing nonresponse in a national telephone survey. *Public Opinion Quarterly, 64*(2), 125–148.

Kessler, R. C., Little, R. J. A., & Groves, R. M. (1995). Advances in strategies for minimizing and adjusting for survey nonresponse. *Epidemiologic Reviews, 17*(1), 192–204.

Kessler, R. C., Mroczek, D. K., & Belli, R. F. (1999). Retrospective adult assessment of childhood psychopathology. In D. Shaffer, C. P. Lucas, & J. E. Richters (Eds.), *Diagnostic assessment in child and adolescent psychopathology* (pp. 256–285). New York: Guilford Press.

Kish, L. (1949). A procedure for objective respondent selection within the household. *Journal American Statistical Association, 44,* 380–387.

Kish, L. (1965). *Survey sampling.* New York: Wiley.

Lavrakas, P. J. (1993). *Telephone research methods* (2nd ed.). Applied Social Research Methods Series, Vol. 7. Newbury Park, CA: Sage.

Lavrakas, P. J., Settersten, R. A., Jr., & Maier, R. A., Jr. (1991). RDD panel attrition in two local area surveys. *Survey Methodology, 17,* 143–152.

Mariolis, P. (2001, October). Data accuracy: How good are our usual indicators? In *Achieving data quality in a statistical agency: A methodological perspective.* Symposium conducted at the meeting of Statistics Canada, Ottawa, Canada.

Mariolis, P. (2002, May). *Response rates and data accuracy.* Paper presented at the American Association of Public Opinion Research, Nashville, TN.

Nelson, D. E., Powell-Griner, E., Town, M., & Kovar, M. G. (2003). A comparison of national estimates from the National Health Interview Survey and the Behavioral Risk Factor Surveillance System. *American Journal of Public Health, 93*(8), 1335–1341.

Newman, E., & Kaloupek, D. G. (2004). The risks and benefits of participating in trauma-focused research studies. *Journal of Traumatic Stress, 17,* 383–394.

Paulsen, A. S., Crowe, R. R., Noyes, R., & Pfohl, B. (1988). Reliability of the telephone interview in diagnosing anxiety disorders. *Archives of General Psychiatry, 45,* 62–63.

Potthoff, R. F. (1994). Telephone sampling in epidemiologic research: To reap the benefits, avoid the pitfalls. *American Journal of Epidemiology, 139*(10), 967–978.

Reise, S. P., & Due, A. M. (1991). The influence of test characteristics on the detection of aberrant response patterns. *Applied Psychology Measurement, 15*, 217–226.

Shah, B., Barnwell, B., & Bieler, G. (1997). *SUDAAN User's Manual, Release 7.5.* Research Triangle Park, NC: Research Triangle Institute.

Simon, G. E., Revicki, D., & vonKorff, M. (1993). Telephone assessment of depression severity. *Journal of Psychiatric Research, 27*(3), 247–252.

Smith, D. W., Kilpatrick, D. G., Falsetti, S. A., & Best, C. L. (2002). Postterrorism services for victims and surviving family members: Lessons from Pan Am 103. *Cognitive and Behavioral Practice, 9*, 280–286.

Stata/SE 8.2 for Windows. (2004). College Station, TX: StataCorp LP.

Survey Sampling Inc. (1990). *A survey researcher's view of the U.S.* Fairfield, CT: Survey Sampling.

Tucker, C., Lepkowski, J. M., & Pierkarski, L. (2002). The current efficiency of list-assisted telephone sampling designs. *Public Opinion Quarterly, 66*, 321–338.

Waksberg, J. (1978). Sampling methods for random digit dialing. *Journal of the American Statistical Association, 73*, 40–46.

Weeks, M. F., Kulka, R. A., Lessler, L. T., & Whitmore, R. W. (1983). Personal versus telephone surveys for collecting household health data at the local level. *American Journal Public Health, 93*(12), 1389–1394.

CHAPTER 8

Web-Based Methods in Disaster Research

WILLIAM E. SCHLENGER and
ROXANE COHEN SILVER

Conducting methodologically rigorous studies of responses to disasters is extraordinarily challenging in several important ways. As Silver (2004) has discussed, research in the natural laboratory is typically expensive, labor-intensive, and time-consuming. Obtaining external funding—particularly quick-response funding following a national or community disaster—is often difficult. Obtaining samples of traumatized populations can be challenging, and research on entire groups of traumatized individuals is sometimes restricted. Institutional review boards are often appropriately (but sometimes inappropriately) uncomfortable with trauma-related research. As a result, studies are often conducted with small nonrepresentative samples of individuals who are willing to answer sensitive questions posed by a stranger. Many studies are conducted within clinical settings with individuals who seek professional help for their mental health symptoms. The conclusions drawn from these studies do not readily generalize to the broader population.

The design and implementation of research following major disasters and terrorist attacks thus present formidable scientific and logistical challenges, many of which result from the fundamental unpredictability of these events. This chapter addresses the use of Internet-based approaches to community epidemiological studies following such events. Although clearly not a cure-all, use of Internet-based methods provides at least partial solutions to some of the important challenges. In what follows we identify some critical challenges for epidemiological studies of major disasters or terrorist attacks, discuss how Internet-based studies can reduce them, summarize briefly some of the advantages and drawbacks of Web-based sampling and data collection, and provide some details of how Internet-based studies can be implemented.

CHALLENGES OF STUDYING THE AFTERMATH OF MAJOR DISASTERS AND TERRORIST ATTACKS

Community epidemiological studies in the aftermath of disasters and other large-scale traumatic events today typically involve surveys conducted with probability samples of a specific population (e.g., people living in the neighborhood or city in which the event took place, the U.S. population). These surveys are aimed at estimating the prevalence and/or incidence of one or more specific conditions and of important comorbidities, identifying specific "risk factors" that convey vulnerability to the condition(s), etc. The prevalence of posttraumatic stress disorder (PTSD) and associated risk factors has been relatively well documented in community studies that cover a broad range of potentially traumatic events (e.g., Kessler, Sonnega, Bromet, Hughes, & Nelson, 1995) or that focus on a specific event (e.g., Resnick, Kilpatrick, Dansky, Saunders, & Best, 1993), but the incidence of PTSD and its course have been less well studied. Additionally, the relationship of PTSD to other psychiatric and substance use disorders has also been relatively well documented, but less attention has been paid to other potentially important comorbidities (e.g., chronic health conditions).

The primary scientific and logistical challenges of conducting such studies, however, result from the unpredictability of many of the exposures of interest, that is, the fact that disasters and other large-scale traumatic events typically occur with little or no warning. North and Pfefferbaum (2002) have identified a number of issues involved in conducting such studies and offer helpful guidelines and recommendations. Some of the more challenging design problems arise from two specific characteristics of studies of sudden and unanticipated large-scale traumatic events: the necessarily observational nature of the studies, and the need for them to be designed and implemented quickly (Schlenger, Jordan, Caddell, Ebert, & Fairbank, 2004). The studies are observational because researchers cannot (and, we hope, *would* not) randomly assign people to exposed versus nonexposed conditions. This necessary lack of random assignment limits the ability to draw *causal* inferences about the link between exposure and observed outcomes.

Further, the unpredictability of these events often results in the studies being *post-only* designs—that is, designs in which all assessments are conducted *after* exposure to the event (see Silver, Holman, McIntosh, Poulin, & Gil-Rivas, 2002, for an exception). Post-only designs provide limited ability to rule out preexisting symptomatology as an explanation of the study findings and open the door to confounding of symptom reports with exposure levels, which also weakens the ability to draw causal inferences about the exposure (see Silver et al., 2006). When designs are both observational and post-only, inferential power is further eroded.

The need for rapid response, which arises from the unpredictability of the exposure and the desire to document both degree of exposure and postexposure adjustment as fully and accurately as possible, creates both scientific and pragmatic challenges to the research team. For example, assessments of specific features of an individual's exposure are best when made with little time lapse between the exposure and assessment. Doing so, however, requires mounting a major field data collection effort, including developing assessment interviews and sampling plans and hiring and training interviewers, in days or weeks rather than months or years.

The need for rapid response following disasters has pushed the field in recent years away from traditional in-person survey interview methods and toward data collection methods that can be implemented quickly, such as telephone surveys and Internet-based surveys. For example, papers describing findings related to the bombing of the Alfred P. Murrah Federal Building in Oklahoma City in April 1995 began to appear in the literature in 1999 (North et al., 1999). Conversely, four papers (Galea et al., 2002; Schlenger et al., 2002; Schuster et al., 2001; and Silver et al., 2002) describing reactions to the September 11, 2001, terrorist attacks appeared in top-tier health journals in the first 12 months following the attacks. All four of these studies used either telephone- or Internet-based survey methods.

Moreover, the threat of future terrorist attacks and the likelihood of future community disasters demands that a higher level of urgency and research sophistication be directed at understanding the psychological effects of such events over time. As noted by others (Norris, Friedman, & Watson, 2002), empirical evidence concerning the adjustment process following disaster exposure can aid clinicians by identifying potential risks and may facilitate the design of interventions for individuals coping with negative outcomes.

HOW INTERNET USE CAN ENHANCE DISASTER STUDY DESIGN

Despite the scientific and pragmatic challenges, it is important that disaster and terrorism studies be conducted in the strongest feasible designs. In the following sections we describe how using the Internet can enhance the design of these studies, focusing on three specific design features: probability sampling, psychometrically sound assessment of primary outcomes, and use of longitudinal designs.

Probability Samples

All community epidemiological studies of disasters should include adequately sized population-based probability samples of persons representing the full range of exposure levels (e.g., from *very high* to *none*). Probability sampling is critical to these studies because it is the foundation of the study's external validity. That is, the fundamental scientific basis for external validity (i.e., generalizability of results) flows from the principle that estimates from samples are unbiased estimates (i.e., representative) of population parameters to the extent that every member of that population has a known and nonzero probability of being in the sample. The external validity of estimates based on study samples that are not probability samples of the population to which inference is intended is completely unknown, and the estimates from such studies generalize only to the people who participated in the study. Stated in a different way, samples are not representative of a given population because of who *is* in them, but rather because of who *could have been* in them.

Unfortunately, much of the Internet-based research conducted to date has used volunteer rather than probability samples. As the Internet has become more popular, many have sought to use it to obtain information from large samples. Thus, Internet "instant polls" have become ubiquitous. Harris Interactive maintains a panel with "multimillion participants" recruited primarily via their website (www.harrisinteractive.com) who have "expressed interest in participating in clinical trials and/or market research studies." As a result, they can provide large numbers of people with specific characteristics for market research or other studies. Although the panel is huge and samples drawn from it can be large, estimates from random samples drawn from it generalize only to the full panel of volunteers, not to the U.S. general (or any other) population.

In addition, a large number of commercial software systems that manage online data collection have become available in recent years. These systems are designed to facilitate rapid and relatively inexpensive hosting of a survey. As a result, announcements about Web-based surveys are now commonly broadcast on listservs or through emails or other recruitment materials that provide links to an online questionnaire. Although the numbers of respondents to such efforts can be very large, these samples of convenience are also not probability-based, and therefore the generalizability of findings from such studies is very limited, and the selection biases unknown.

These facts point to an important truth about using the Internet for epidemiological studies today: the Internet can offer tremendous advantages as a *data collection medium*, but is rarely useful in drawing samples for such studies. Census figures indicate that, although Internet use has been growing over the years, only 60% of the U.S. population over age 18 had use of a computer at home, school, or work as of 2001 (U.S. Census Bureau, 2001). Thus, those individuals with easy access to the Internet cannot be considered representative of the national population.

The primary exception to concerns about using the Internet to draw a study sample involves circumstances in which a list of a population of interest is available and includes a current e-mail address for each person on the list. Examples where this is the case are typically limited to establishment surveys, such as a large corporation that wants to assess job satisfaction among its employees without the burden and expense of surveying *every* employee, or a university seeking information about student attitudes related to an important policy topic.

Psychometrically Sound Assessment of Primary Outcomes

Although the specific outcomes included depend on the study's specific aims, disaster and terrorism studies will typically include comprehensive assessment of PTSD, depression, and selected other health and psychosocial outcomes. For pragmatic reasons, most or all of these assessments will necessarily be made via survey-based (i.e., screening) measures. These measures must, however, have been well validated against comprehensive clinical assessment in community (i.e., not treatment-seeking) samples.

A growing literature has documented that sensitive topics, such as psychiatric symptoms, substance use and reports of details of trauma exposure, are more likely to be acknowledged in self-report assessments than in interview-based assessments. Findings from randomized experiments document that any method that reduces the relevance of an interviewer appears to increase the willingness of respondents to reveal sensitive and/or personal information (Lau, Thomas, & Liu, 2000). In fact, research comparing interview modalities demonstrates that Web-based data collection improves the accuracy of reports respondents provide over less anonymous interview modalities, particularly telephone interviews (Chang & Krosnick, 2001; Krantz & Dalal, 2000; Reips, 2000). This is especially true when the reports in question are sensitive, whereas Web-based data collection appears to reduce social desirability bias. To the extent that the admission of trauma-related symptoms, as well as distress, is uncomfortable in the presence of an interviewer, a Web-based methodology provides an excellent alternative. In fact, Web-based survey methodology offers enormous potential for improving the state of the art in survey research (Batinic, Reips, & Bosnjak, 2002; Couper, 2000).

Given that this new method provides important and perhaps previously untapped information, it is possible that data collection via the Internet allows a more "honest" reporting of symptomatology after terrorism or a community disaster than has previously been available. This advantage for Internet-based assessment over telephone and in-person interview methods, however, raises potential participant safety concerns (e.g., that focusing on the details of these topics with an already distressed participant may increase distress to dangerous levels) that must be addressed in the study protocol.

Longitudinal Design

When possible, disaster and terrorism studies should use longitudinal designs that include at least one preexposure assessment of key constructs (e.g., specific exposures, outcomes, potential moderators) and multiple postexposure assessments. Longitudinal designs provide for both within- and between-subjects comparisons, which helps counter some of the inference problems associated with observational and post-only designs. Additionally, new methods for analyzing longitudinal data developed over the past few decades, including applications of the random ("mixed") effects approach (Laird & Ware, 1982) and the generalized estimating equations (GEE) approach (Zeger & Liang, 1986), model more comprehensively the multiple sources of variance in repeated measures designs and are more tolerant of missing data than traditional methods (e.g., repeated measures analysis of variance). As a result, these approaches are more powerful and less subject to bias than the traditional approaches.

Using the Internet can facilitate the implementation of longitudinal studies. Internet-based data collection is cost-effective for longitudinal research because the marginal cost of additional rounds of assessment is small relative to telephone or face-to-face interview methods. Additionally, maintaining contact with a panel over the course of a long-term longitudinal study via e-mail offers many advantages over the traditional reminder postcards, newsletters, phone calls, etc. Finally, longitudinal data collection is possible with the use of identifiers that link survey responses over time.

How Can Web-Based Studies Meet All These Criteria?

Although there are some clear advantages associated with Internet surveys for disaster studies—including rapid response and relative ease of conducting longitudinal follow-up—selecting samples via the Internet remains problematic. The authors of this chapter both have experience with a probability-based research panel created by Knowledge Networks, Inc. (KN), that is "Web-enabled" (Schlenger et al., 2002; Silver et al., 2002). KN is a survey research firm specializing in Web-based surveys that uses multistage probability sampling methods to create survey samples, using random-digit-dialing (RDD) telephone sampling methods to recruit a large "standing" panel of potential research subjects. These methods provide a known nonzero probability of selection for every person in the United States living in a household that has a telephone (census data indicate that 94% of U.S. households have telephones). For specific studies, KN typically selects a (simple or stratified random) sample from the panel, so that representation of the U.S. population is maintained. Estimates from KN samples for other studies have closely tracked census-based distributions of sociodemographic characteristics such as age, gender, race, Hispanic ethnicity, employment status, income, education, and regional distribution.

The KN panel is currently the only ongoing Internet-based cohort that was started as a nationally representative probability sample (Couper, 2000; Dennis & Krotki, 2001). As part of their agreement with KN to participate in a panel, respondents are offered free Internet service and a WebTV appliance by KN as an incentive to participate, or other financial incentives if the household is already Web-enabled. In return, panel members participate in 10- to 15-minute Internet surveys three to four times a month. The panel does not respond significantly differently over time to surveys than more "naive" survey respondents (Dennis, 2001, 2003). Survey responses are confidential, with identifying information never revealed without respondent approval. When surveys are assigned to panel members, they receive notice in their KN-provided password protected e-mail account that the survey is available for completion. Surveys are self-administered and accessible any time of day for a designated period (typically 3 weeks), and participants can complete a survey only once. Each survey includes written informed consent, including a reminder that "you are always free to refuse to answer a particular question or survey." Moreover, participants may leave the panel at any time, and receipt of the WebTV and Internet service is not contingent on completion of any particular survey.

When such a panel is created in advance of the disaster or terrorist event (essentially mimicking the formation of a postevent RDD sample), several challenges are addressed. First, these preexisting samples provide known sampling characteristics and can enable population estimates. Second, a great deal of information can be collected from the sample before a disaster or terrorist attack occurs. On occasions where the sampling frame matches that of interest in the aftermath of a disaster, these premeasures can be linked to postevent response. For example, Silver et al. (2002, 2006) were able to utilize mental and physical health information (ailments and health care utilization) and behaviors (degree of television exposure, religious attendance, voting patterns) that were collected prior to the terrorist attacks of September 11, 2001, as predictors of postattack outcomes in the nation, avoiding retrospective (and often biased) reporting of this information. Third, longitudinal data collection is possible because a preevent relationship has been established with participants, and the ongoing panel is monitored through a preestablished e-mail account. Thus, attrition that occurs as a result of participants moving and/or changing telephone numbers is minimized. For example, Silver et al. (2006) were able to follow their national sample from 2 weeks through 3 years postattacks, collecting data approximately every 6 months and securing participation rates averaging around 80% per wave across seven waves of data collection.

MECHANICS OF WEB-BASED DATA COLLECTION

Space does not permit a full explication of the nuts and bolts of survey design on the Web, and excellent resources are available elsewhere to address many specific aspects of Internet-based data collection (see, e.g., Dillman, 2000; Dillman & Bowker, 2001; Norman, 2005). Some features of Web-based data collection are worth noting, however. Because there is no interviewer and thus no opportunity for clarification during data collection, questions must be clear, written at a basic reading level, and the use of jargon should be avoided. Instructions must be detailed, explaining the specific kinds of questions to follow and providing clarification as to how individual items should be completed. The full range of response options (including "not applicable"), as well as skip patterns out of irrelevant questions, must be clearly specified in advance and programmed accordingly. The visual aspect of the survey becomes extremely important with Web-based methods, and the browser employed, hardware utilized, and screen size all impact the way the survey appears to the respondent. Thus, formatting must be flexible and adaptable to these various possibilities. Unlike telephone or face-to-face interviews, the researcher must be particularly attentive to visual features, such as font size and color, background color, screen layout (e.g., the number of questions provided per screen page vs. using one long screen), whether the respondent needs to scroll across the screen to see the entire question or response option at one time, and so on. Decisions must be made regarding a number of other formatting issues, such as whether to use pull-down menus, whether the response options are provided horizontally or vertically, as well as the number of items that are visible on a screen at any one time. Investigators must also decide whether respondents will be allowed to skip a particular question, whether its completion will be requested more than once if it is not answered, or whether a response will be required before the next screen appears. Finally, because of the flexibility of the Web-based design, open-ended responses can supplement closed-ended questions as long as respondents are able to type their answers in adequate and flexible response fields that are provided.

A LOOK TOWARD THE FUTURE

Internet-based research offers a strong advantage over other data collection methods in the flexibility and anonymity it allows respondents. Surveys can be completed in the privacy of a respondent's home, at a time that is convenient. Question delivery can be standardized, avoiding the challenges of interviewer training and the biases inherent in interviewer questioning. The time-consuming and error-prone steps of data coding and data entry are avoided, as respondents complete answers on their own, and data files are clean and complete at the conclusion of the data collection effort.

Nonetheless, several potential pitfalls of Internet-based data collection must be considered. They include respondents' concerns about being identified (which requires assurances that "cookies" will not be used to link individuals to their answers), the need to ensure a strategy by which respondents cannot complete a survey more than once, and the need to develop a strategy that maximizes the chance that the person who completed the survey was the targeted respondent. Finally, sometimes the very population that one might want to target may suffer infrastructure disruptions that make Web-based data collection impossible (e.g., the Internet service goes down, electricity is shut off).

Notwithstanding their many strengths, potential limitations of Web-based methods must be acknowledged. First, because panel respondents are requested to complete repeated surveys as part of their "contract," it is important to consider the possibility that respondent overload influences response in a fashion that may be difficult to assess. At this early stage in the use of this data collection modality, we also have too little information about the impact of the "professional respondent" on population estimates in general, and we have limited information as to how frequent survey completion may bias respondents for subsequent survey data collection. In addition, it is important to recognize that the use of existing Web-enabled panels can be expensive (although not necessarily more expensive than face-to-face or telephone-based data collection methods), and in order to collect immediate response data, funding must be made available to potential researchers very quickly.

Despite these and other limitations, the critical nature of the topic and the need for research evidence to guide the design of interventions for terrorism and other community disasters has led to the recognition of the value of innovative methods. The continuing increase in the availability of Internet access makes it clear that Internet data collection will be an important part of research on these topics for the foreseeable future. Until the Internet penetration rate exceeds 90% of the population, however, it is likely that we will see a growth in the use of mixed modes of data capture, in which survey participants have the opportunity to choose from a variety of response modes (e.g., Internet, telephone, pencil-and-paper) the one that best suits their circumstances. Nonetheless, with thoughtful applications of theory, careful design and implementation, and appropriate caveats, it is likely that Web-based survey research methods can be a useful tool, and perhaps the eventual method of choice, in the repertoire of trauma researchers for many years to come.

REFERENCES

Batinic, B., Reips, U.-D., & Bosnjak, M. (Eds.). (2002). *Online social sciences*. Seattle: Hogrefe & Huber.

Chang, L., & Krosnick, J. A. (2001, May). *The accuracy of self-reports: Comparisons of an RDD telephone survey with internet surveys by Harris Interactive and Knowledge Networks*. Paper presented at the American Association for Public Opinion Research Annual Meeting, Montreal, Canada.

Couper, M. P. (2000). Web surveys: A review of issues and approaches. *Public Opinion Quarterly, 64,* 464–494.

Dennis, J. M. (2001). Are Internet panels creating professional respondents?: The benefits of online panels far outweigh the potential for panel effects. *Marketing Research,* Summer, 34–38.

Dennis, J. M. (2003). *Panel attrition impact: A comparison of responses to attitudinal and knowledge questions about HIV between follow-up and cross-sectional samples*. Menlo Park, CA: Knowledge Networks.

Dennis, J. M., & Krotki, K. (2001, August). *Probability-based survey research on the Internet*. Paper presented at the Conference of the International Statistical Institute, Seoul, South Korea.

Dillman, D. A. (2000). *Mail and Internet surveys: The tailored design method* (2nd ed.). New York: Wiley.

Dillman, D. A., & Bowker, D. K. (2001). The Web questionnaire challenge to survey methodologists. In U. D. Reips & M. Bosnjak (Eds.), *Dimensions of Internet science* (pp. 159–178). Lengerich, Germany: Pabst Science Publishers.

Galea, S., Ahern, J., Resnick, H., Kilpatrick, D., Bucuvalas, M., Gold, J., et al. (2002). Psychological sequelae of the September 11 terrorist attacks in New York City. *The New England Journal of Medicine, 346,* 982–987.

Kessler, R. C., Sonnega, A., Bromet, E., Hughes, M., & Nelson, C. B. (1995). Posttraumatic stress disorder in the National Comorbidity Study. *Archives of General Psychiatry,* *52,* 1048–1060.

Krantz, J. H., & Dalal, R. (2000). Validity of Web-based psychological research. In M. H. Birnbaum (Ed.), *Psychological experiments on the Internet* (pp. 35–60). San Diego, CA: Academic Press.

Laird, N. M., & Ware, J. H. (1982). Random-effects models for longitudinal data. *Biometrics, 38,* 963–974.

Lau, J. T. F., Thomas, J., & Liu, J. L. Y. (2000). Mobile phone and interactive computer interviewing to measure HIV-related risk behaviours: The impacts of data collection methods on research results. *AIDS, 14,* 1277–1278.

Norman, K. L. (2005). *Online survey design guide.* Retrieved May 10, 2005, from lap.umd.edu/survey_design/index.html

Norris, F. H., Friedman, M. J., & Watson, P. J. (2002). 60,000 disaster victims speak: Part II. Summary and implications of the disaster mental health research. *Psychiatry, 65,* 240–260.

North, C. S., Nixon, S. J., Shariat, S., Mallonee, S., McMillen, J. C., Spitznagel, E. L., et al. (1999). Psychiatric disorders among survivors of the Oklahoma City Bombing. *Journal of the American Medical Association, 282,* 755–762.

North, C. S., & Pfefferbaum, B. (2002). Research on the mental health effects of terrorism. *Journal of the American Medical Association, 288,* 633–636.

Reips, U.-D. (2000). The Web experiment method: Advantages, disadvantages, and solutions. In M.H. Birnbaum (Ed.), *Psychological experiments on the Internet* (pp. 89–117). San Diego, CA: Academic Press.

Resnick, H. S., Kilpatrick, D. C., Dansky, B. S., Saunders, B. E., & Best, C. L. (1993). Prevalence of civilian trauma and posttraumatic stress disorder in a representative national sample of women. *Journal of Consulting and Clinical Psychology, 61,* 984–991.

Schlenger, W. E., Caddell, J. M., Ebert, L., Jordan, B. K., Rourke, K. M., Wilson, D., et al. (2002). Psychological reactions to terrorist attacks: Findings from the National Study of Americans' Reactions to September 11. *Journal of the American Medical Association, 288,* 581–588.

Schlenger, W. E., Jordan, B. K., Caddell, J. M., Ebert, L., & Fairbank, J. A. (2004). Epidemiologic methods for assessing trauma and PTSD. In J. P. Wilson & T. M. Keane (Eds.), *Assessing psychological trauma and PTSD* (2nd ed., pp. 226–261). New York: Guilford Press.

Schuster, M. A., Stein, B. D., Jaycox, L. H., Collins, R. L., Marshall, G. N., Elliott, M. N., et al. (2001). A national survey of stress reactions after the September 11, 2001 terrorist attacks. *New England Journal of Medicine, 345,* 1507–1512.

Silver, R. C. (2004). Conducting research after the 9/11 terrorist attacks: Challenges and results. *Families, Systems and Health, 22*(1), 47–51.

Silver, R. C., Holman, E. A., McIntosh, D. N., Poulin, M., & Gil-Rivas, V. (2002). Nationwide longitudinal study of psychological responses to September 11. *Journal of the American Medical Association, 288,* 1235–1244.

Silver, R. C., Holman, E. A., McIntosh, D. N., Poulin, M., Gil-Rivas, V., & Pizarro, J. (2006). Coping with a national trauma: A nationwide longitudinal study of responses to the terrorist attacks of September 11th. In Y. Neria, R. Gross, R. Marshall, & E. Susser (Eds.), *September 11, 2001: Treatment, research and public*

   mental health in the wake of a terrorist attack. New York: Cambridge University
      Press.
U.S. Census Bureau (2001). *Computer and Internet use in the United States, September,*
      2001. Accessed May 2005 from www.census.gov/population/www/socdemo/com-
      puter/ppl-175.html.
Zeger, S. L., & Liang, K.-Y. (1986). Longitudinal data analysis for discrete and continuous
      outcomes. *Biometrics, 42*, 121–130.

CHAPTER 9

School-Based Studies of Children Following Disasters

ANNETTE M. LA GRECA

Children represent an understudied yet vulnerable population in the aftermath of disasters and terrorism. For example, the effects of natural disasters have often been documented in terms of the costs for rebuilding homes and replacing possessions, but natural disasters also may take a toll on children's academic, social, and emotional development (see Silverman & La Greca, 2002). The loss and disruption of life that ensues after a disaster may lead to school closings, school absences, and reductions in academic functioning; to reduced opportunities for social interactions with friends; and to increased exposure to major life stressors such as family illness, divorce, family violence, and substance use. Furthermore, although many children are affected, adults may not realize the extent to which this occurs or may underestimate the problem. Especially when parents and other significant adults in children's lives are affected by disaster and have problems coping, children and adolescents may lack available personal resources to deal with disasters and their aftermath. Thus, children may be substantially affected by disaster, and affected in ways that raise substantial concern for their welfare.

Elsewhere, my colleagues and I have discussed the main types of reactions displayed by children as a consequence of their exposure to disasters and terrorism, as well as a general framework for considering the risk and

141

protective factors that influence the development and maintenance of children's postdisaster reactions (see La Greca, Silverman, Vernberg, & Roberts, 2002; Silverman & La Greca, 2002). We have also discussed approaches to interventions with children following disaster events (La Greca, 2001; La Greca & Silverman, 2006). In this chapter, the focus is on the considerations surrounding efforts to conduct research on the effects of disasters and terrorism within school settings. Schools are a logical setting in which to evaluate children's disaster reactions, because most children are enrolled in school, and thus schools provide an opportunity to obtain community estimates of the effects of disasters and terrorism on children. Many studies of the effects of natural disasters on children have, in fact, been school-based studies of children and adolescents (see La Greca & Prinstein, 2002; Silverman & La Greca, 2002). Similarly, studies of children's and adolescents' reactions following the 1995 bombing of the Federal Building in Oklahoma City (Gurwitch, Sitterle, Young, & Pfefferbaum, 2002) and some of the key studies emerging from the 2001 terrorist attack on the World Trade Center (Applied Research & Consulting LLC and the Columbia University Mailman School of Public Health, 2002) have evaluated children and adolescents in school settings. This approach to child disaster research is extremely common and valuable.

Although there is a vast range of topics that can be covered in a chapter such as this one, the present chapter is designed to highlight several key issues that are pertinent to study design and implementation. It is organized as follows. The first section discusses the types of disaster-related research questions that are well suited to a school-based approach, and also describes some of the potentials and challenges associated with conducting disaster research in school settings. The second section focuses on issues related to study design, including sampling strategies for selecting schools and assessment strategies for evaluating children and adolescents. The third section deals with selected issues in study implementation, and especially the recruitment and retention of participants and considerations for training research assistants. The final section provides a brief summary and conclusion. For simplicity, the text refers to "children," but this is meant to include "children and adolescents."

USING A SCHOOL-BASED APPROACH
TO STUDYING CHILDREN AND DISASTERS

One of the key advantages of a school-based approach to studying children following disasters and terrorist events is the potential access to a large representative sample of participants who were affected by the disaster. Because children are required to attend school, school-based studies can examine a population of children that have a broad range of demographic characteristics. Unlike studies conducted in mental health settings, or that recruit community samples via advertising, school-based studies are less likely to recruit samples that are biased in terms of family socioeconomic status, the willingness or financial ability of families to seek help for mental heath concerns, or other similar considerations.

In general, school-based studies are particularly well suited to disaster or terrorist events that affect an entire community or geographic area, as is often the case with natural disasters (e.g., hurricanes, earthquakes, tornadoes, floods, fires, tsunamis), school shootings, or certain terrorist attacks. Because school-based studies capture children in their natural environment, with the full range of possible reactions, they are particularly useful for epidemiological studies of children's reactions to disaster and terrorist events (e.g., Pfefferbaum et al., 2003; Shannon, Lonigan, Finch, & Taylor, 1994) as well as for prospective studies of risk and resilience following such events (e.g., La Greca, Silverman, Vernberg, & Prinstein, 1996; La Greca, Silverman, & Wasserstein, 1998). School-based studies may also be appropriate for disseminating and evaluating the effectiveness of prevention programs (i.e., to prepare children for disasters or to build resilience) and for evaluating universal or selected interventions in the aftermath of disasters (Vernberg, 2002).

In contrast, mass transportation disasters (e.g., ferry sinking, plane crash) that affect individuals from a very broad geographic area are not likely to be conducive to a school-based research approach (see Yule, Udwin, & Bolton, 2002). Similarly, events that affect a small number of children and families (e.g., motor vehicle crashes, house fires, abuse victims) may be better understood by focusing on the victims and their families rather than on children residing in community settings (see Scotti, Ruggiero, & Rabalais, 2002). In addition, school-based studies may not be desirable for evaluating interventions that focus on children and families that have severe postdisaster trauma reactions or psychopathology, as such individuals typically represent a small proportion of the school population, and studying them in the school-environment could potentially be stigmatizing. Moreover, children and families experiencing severe and persistent posttraumatic stress may need intensive psychological interventions that are more typically delivered in mental health settings (Vernberg, 2002).

School-based research approaches also have a number of challenges that should be considered before designing a study. First, schools and school systems are often in chaos after a disaster and initially may need to focus on rebuilding efforts and/or ensuring that children are safe and secure. This is especially true for communitywide or school-specific disasters (e.g., massive natural disasters, school shootings), where rebuilding efforts or safety are likely to take precedence over research. (For example, Hurricane Andrew struck south Florida in August 1992 at the beginning of the school year. Because of the widespread destruction, many schools were uninhabitable, and a priority for the local school system was to repair and rebuild the damaged schools so that they could reopen. Similarly, in September 2004, two hurricanes struck the east coast of Florida; as a result, schools in some Florida counties were closed for more than a month for major repairs.) Moreover, school teachers and administrators may be directly affected by the disaster and have to deal with the psychological, financial, and personal effects of the disaster on themselves and their families. In many cases, there is considerable disruption in schools immediately following disasters that may present a challenge for investigators who are trying to initiate a research protocol. In particular, it may be difficult to recruit schools (or school systems) in the first place, and even when administrators are very interested in research participation, it may be difficult to obtain letters of support or parental permissions in a timely manner.

Second, research is secondary to a school's priorities, which are primarily academic in focus. As a result, school-based research needs to fit within the school context or system. When schools lose instructional time due to a disaster or terrorist event, the pressure is likely to be even greater than usual to focus on academic activities and "make up for lost time" during the school day. Many school systems, such as those in Florida and Texas, also participate in high-stakes achievement testing on an annual basis, which determines the type and amount of funding available for individual schools. As a result, many teachers, administrators, and students experience considerable stress and pressure to perform well on the tests and are reluctant to take time away from preparation activities. Moreover, the pressures are likely to be greatest in the month or two immediately preceding the annual achievement testing, thus making it very difficult to implement research protocols during certain periods of the academic year.

Third, in school-based studies, it may be difficult to ask children sensitive or distressing questions (especially on issues that don't pertain to communitywide events). If testing is conducted in groups, it may be difficult to identify children who are having problems or exhibiting distress; this may limit the kinds of questions that are asked. Alternatively, individual interviews with children may provide a better forum for assessing sensitive material, but require considerable personnel to implement. In either case, it is essential to establish a protocol for handling distressed children and for making appropriate referrals (e.g., to school counselors) and notification (i.e., letting parents know if their child is distressed).

Fourth, a common challenge to school-based research is devising a protocol that minimizes the demands on teachers' time and resources. (Teachers are likely to be distressed and overloaded already, for the reasons delineated above.) At the same time, teachers are often critical to a study's success, as many school-based studies rely on teachers to distribute and collect parental consent forms, and possibly to complete measures on how the children are functioning.

Fifth, it may be difficult or impossible (and undesirable) to control the kinds of support and assistance that children receive following disasters. However, this situation presents a challenge for school-based research that is aimed at evaluating an intervention or prevention program, or even for understanding the natural course of children's reactions following disasters. As a result, it is often necessary to monitor and keep records of the kinds of school-based support activities and assistance that are provided, and to "control for" such events in subsequent analyses.

Finally, a big challenge for school-based research is the complexity of conducting research studies in diverse, multilingual, multicultural school systems. Although research that focuses on diverse children and adolescents is highly desirable and enhances the external validity of a study, it may require a number of complex research strategies, such as sending parental permission forms home in multiple languages; adjusting recruitment strategies to deal with parents who are unfamiliar with (and possibly wary of) research; and translating measures into multiple languages.

Notwithstanding these challenges, school-based research is an incredibly important approach for understanding children's postdisaster reactions. The sections below address some of the specific details that are involved in developing a school-based protocol.

SELECTED ISSUES PERTINENT TO STUDY DESIGN

Sampling Strategies

Once an investigator has developed a research question that is conducive to a school-based study, a critical issue becomes how to select schools for participation. To some extent, this depends on the type of disaster that has occurred and the kind of research question that is being asked. In general, for research questions that focus on the percentage of children who are affected, the types of reactions they have, and the factors that are predictive of outcomes (either immediately or over time), investigators will want to recruit schools that enroll children who were directly affected by the disaster. Specifically, for natural disasters that cause physical destruction and affect a large community, typically investigators will want to select schools that are in close proximity to the disaster—such as those that are in the direct path of a hurricane, or schools that enroll children from a neighborhood that was directly affected by a fire, flood, or tornado. In making school selections, it is desirable to enumerate all the schools that were affected by the disaster and then use a standard sampling procedure for selecting the specific target schools for participation (e.g., choose the target schools at random from those most affected, or sample all the schools if resources allow). In selecting schools, efforts should be made to ensure that the included schools would provide a representative sampling of the diverse demographics (e.g., socioeconomic status, ethnicity) of the disaster-affected area. Moreover, if the research design calls for control or comparison children who were *unaffected* by the disaster, it would be desirable to recruit additional schools that were not directly affected by the disaster (i.e., more physically removed from the actual event) but that share similar demographics (e.g., enroll children from similar ethnic backgrounds; are equivalent in socioeconomic status (SES); are similar in size and academic level). To select comparison schools, it is desirable to first enumerate all the unaffected schools and then identify the unaffected schools that match each target school (in terms of demographics or other relevant factors). Then the comparison school(s) could be selected at random from those that are a suitable match for the target school(s). Within the target and comparison schools, it is desirable to assess the entire population of children that fall within the eligible age range. If that is not possible, an alternative strategy is to sample classrooms at random from each appropriate grade level. (For further discussion of sampling issues, see Cicchetti & Rogosch, 1999, and Tolan, 1999.)

For controlled intervention studies, investigators will want to select schools in affected areas that are matched on demographic characteristics (ethnicity, SES) and degree of exposure to the event (e.g., experienced a similar amount of physical destruction). All possible pairs of such schools could be enumerated and then the pairs randomly selected for participation in the study. Within each pair selected for participation, schools then can be randomly assigned to intervention or control conditions.

One important consideration for school-based studies is that the data analytic plan will need to address the nesting of children within classroom groups and within schools in evaluating the data (see Kendall, Butcher, & Holmbeck, 1999). Potential "school effects" should be routinely evaluated and controlled in studies that include children from multiple schools.

In the case of a terrorist attack or bombing, it could be useful to select schools that are most likely to enroll students who are "psychologically affected" (i.e., had many children who lost family members in the attack or bombing) as well as those who were in direct "proximity" of the event. For example, Pfefferbaum and colleagues (2002) studied a large sample of middle school children following the 1995 bombing of the Federal Building in Oklahoma City, finding that children who were in close proximity to the blast, as well as those who knew direct victims of the bombing (i.e., family members, friends), displayed high levels of posttraumatic stress (see Gurwitch et al., 2002, for a detailed review).

As noted, in selecting schools for research participation, it is important that efforts be made to include schools with diverse populations to enhance the generalizability of the study's findings. However, diversity within the sample poses additional challenges for recruitment and/or retention (e.g., translating measures and permission forms into multiple languages). Diversity within the sample also is an issue that will need to be considered and/or controlled in data analytic plans.

Assessment Strategies for Evaluating Children and Adolescents in School Settings

Developing appropriate assessment strategies is an important consideration in designing a study. When assessing children's postdisaster reactions in school settings, three key interrelated issues are likely to arise. These are *when* to conduct the assessment (i.e., timing), *what* to assess (i.e., constructs or variables of interest), and *whom* to assess (i.e., child, parent, teacher).

When to Assess

The timing of the assessment will be influenced both by practical constraints (e.g., how soon you can obtain school permission or cooperation postdisaster; when the testing can occur within the constraints of the school calendar) as well as by conceptual issues, such as the type of research question that is being evaluated. For questions that pertain to the immediate impact of a disaster, often referred to as peritraumatic reactions, assessments need to be conducted within the first few weeks after the event. For example, in the study of middle school children's reactions to the bombing of the Federal Building in Oklahoma City, Pfefferbaum and colleagues (2002) evaluated youngsters' reactions 7 weeks after the bombing. In general, relatively few studies of children have focused on this initial postimpact period (see Norris & Elrod, Chapter 2, this volume; Vernberg, 2002; Vogel & Vernberg, 1993).

By and large, because of the formidable challenges and logistics of conducting research in the immediate aftermath of a disaster, the vast majority of studies of children's postdisaster reactions have conducted assessments 3 months or more postdisaster, during the "recovery and reconstruction" phase (see La Greca & Prinstein, 2002; Silverman & La Greca, 2002). In fact, some investigators have conducted their initial assessment a year or more postdisaster (e.g., Garrison, Weinrich, Hardin, Weinrich, & Wang, 1993). Studies conducted 3 months or more after the event are likely to be evaluating persistent disaster reactions.

What to Assess

In terms of the types of postdisaster reactions that have been evaluated, the most frequently studied have been those associated with posttraumatic stress disorder (PTSD) or related posttraumatic stress (PTS) symptoms (see Silverman & La Greca, 2002). The diagnostic criteria for PTSD require that the symptoms be present at least 1 month after the disaster-event for a diagnosis of acute PTSD, and three months or longer for a diagnosis of chronic PTSD (American Psychiatric Association, 1994). Thus, studies conducted earlier than 3 months postdisaster cannot really evaluate the prevalence of chronic PTSD.

In addition to PTS symptoms or diagnoses, there has been considerable interest in related, or "comorbid," symptoms and disorders. Specifically, symptoms of depression and anxiety (especially separation anxiety, agoraphobia, and panic) may be of interest to evaluate (e.g., Asarnow et al., 1999), as well as externalizing behavior problems (Silverman & La Greca, 2002; Vogel & Vernberg, 1993). In describing children's disaster reactions, some consideration should be given to how reactions may vary with the child's age and development, and how issues of gender and ethnicity may be linked with children's reactions (American Academy of Child and Adolescent Psychiatry, 1998).

In addition to negative psychological reactions, it is important to evaluate whether children's disaster reactions are associated with functional impairment (e.g., deteriorating grades, problems with peer relationships). Moreover, positive outcomes and personal growth may also result from trauma (e.g., Sears, Stanton, & Danoff-Burg, 2003), although this has not been considered in the context of child disaster research. In particular, "positive psychology" is devoted to creating a science of human strengths that act as buffers against mental illness (Seligman, 2002), and it seems logical to extend this concept to include buffers against exposure to natural disasters and other trauma. Potential outcome variables of interest include instilling hope, the active pursuit of goals, optimistic cognitive processing, self-efficacy, and skillful coping. Although measures exist to assess some positive psychological concepts, further instrument development is needed for positive psychology to be applied to child disaster research.

Finally, if resources permit, investigators could broaden the assessment protocol to incorporate variables that might *contribute to* children's disaster reactions. These variables include, but are not limited to, the availability of social support, parental reactions to the disaster, and the occurrence of other life stressors (see Silverman & La Greca, 2002).

Whom to Assess

To a large extent, the assessment methods used in child disaster research will be dictated by the research question and the types of constructs/variables that are of interest (see above). Although it is beyond the scope of this chapter to provide a detailed review of the various assessment measures that are used in child disaster research, the reader is referred to several sources (American Academy of Child and Adolescent Psychiatry, 1998; Saylor & De Roma, 2002).

It is considered critical to obtain children's and adolescents' reports of their own disaster reactions, as parents and other adults may be biased or unaware of the extent to which children are affected (Saylor & De Roma, 2002). Such assessments typically have included self-report questionnaires, such as the PTSD Reaction Index (Pynoos, Rodriguez, Steinberg, Stuber, & Frederick, 1999; see Saylor & De Roma, 2002, for other examples), although structured psychiatric interviews are critical for obtaining formal diagnoses of PTSD.

In terms of other informants, school-based studies may be conducive to obtaining teacher reports of children's functioning, especially for elementary school students who spend most of the day with one teacher. However, for middle school and high school students (ages 13 years and older), teacher reports may be more difficult to obtain, as the students change classes frequently and teachers may not know the students well (see La Greca & Lemanek, 1996). Thus, teachers become much less useful as informants for adolescent youths because they have limited daily contact with their students. Adolescents and their parents are much more valuable as informants at this point in development (La Greca & Lemanek, 1996). Moreover, even with preadolescents, teachers may have difficulty reporting on children's subjective, internal feelings, such as feelings of anxiety, depression, or traumatic stress (e.g., Kazdin, 1990; Loeber, Green, & Lahey, 1990).

Finally, depending on the specific research question, it may be important to obtain parent ratings of children's or adolescents' functioning and disaster-related experiences and reactions, and possibly even the parents' disaster reactions. However, unless there are considerable resources to carry out the research protocol, it can be a challenge to obtain parent reports. Sending questionnaires home to parents typically results in a much smaller sample of parents who participate than is desirable. In addition, it is difficult to control the "testing situation" when parents complete questionnaires at home. Funding resources might allow other strategies, such as conducting phone interviews or group-testing sessions after school, although these may require considerable resources for personnel and incentives for parental participation.

SELECTED ISSUES IN STUDY IMPLEMENTATION

Recruitment and Retention of Participants

After a study design has been developed, there are particular issues that come into play in implementing a school-based study. Paramount among these issues are the recruitment strategies that will be used to obtain the largest and most representative sample of children possible, and procedures for obtaining parental consent for child participation. In addition, for studies that assess children at multiple time points (i.e., longitudinal studies, intervention studies), participant retention is also critical. Several resources that discuss recruitment and retention issues may be useful (Dilworth-Anderson & Williams, 2004; Hinshaw et al., 2004; Rice & Broome, 2004).

The recruitment process can be challenging, as there are many levels of communication and interaction that must be considered, including the overall school system; administrators and teachers at the specific schools that are involved in a research project; parents (or legal guardians) of the participants; and the child or adolescent participants themselves. Because many school systems have their own review process, or may have a centralized office for considering research requests, an important first step is to contact the main administrative offices for the school system in question and inquire about their procedures for research approval. Large school systems may have a standard application form, but even if not, it is likely that the school administration will request a copy of the research proposal (explaining study goals and specific aims), a description of the study measures and procedures, and a copy of the informed consent for parents before they allow a project to proceed. Often, this part of the approval process may be conducted concurrently with seeking approval from the appropriate Institutional Review Board (IRB).

The next challenge for recruitment is securing the support and enthusiasm of key school personnel (e.g., the principal or assistant principal; the school counselor) and the classroom teachers in the particular schools in which the research will be conducted. In this regard, it is especially important that the study procedures not be burdensome to schools or to children and families (Riesch, Tosi, & Thurston, 1999).

For many school-based studies, children are provided with information about the study and a parental consent form to bring home to parents; signed consent forms (indicating permission for participation or not) are often returned to the school setting. Because of this procedure, school administrators can be extremely helpful to investigators by conveying their support for the school-based study in the materials that are sent home to parents, and by encouraging the teachers to assist in the research process. The enthusiasm of the teachers is important for gaining their cooperation in implementing the study, and especially for encouraging children to discuss the study with their parents and to return the parental consent forms. Teachers often help to distribute consent forms, answer questions children may have about the study, and keep track of which children do and do not return the consent forms. In some cases, schools may allow the investigators to explain the study to students and teachers, although even in such cases the teachers are often the "front line" for collecting consent forms.

Especially after traumatic events like disasters, school personnel (e.g., teachers, counselors) may have reservations about research participation because they may fear that the assessment process will lead to or exacerbate children's distress. Because of this common concern, it is critical for the investigator to thoroughly explain to school personnel that there is no evidence for iatrogenic effects resulting from assessing children's reactions following traumatic events.

Several additional strategies may be useful in securing the school's support for the study. If possible, it may be useful to offer incentives or valued services to the school in return for their participation. Examples of incentives that could be offered to school personnel include gift certificates (i.e., for books or leisure activities), money, food, plants, school materials, or items that are donated by local businesses. Examples of school services that might be of interest are talks or workshops for school personnel on relevant topics (i.e., classroom behavior management; stress management; relaxation) and providing teachers and principals with "feedback" on how their students are doing overall (i.e., overall school statistics) immediately after the data are collected and analyzed. In order to provide timely feedback to schools, and also to identify children who are distressed, investigators often will need to score, enter, and analyze data (at least in a preliminary manner) very soon after data collection. This may represent an additional but necessary challenge to the research effort.

When parental permission forms are distributed through the classroom teachers, it may be helpful to have small incentives for the children to return the forms (regardless of whether they receive permission to participate or not). For examples, fun stickers, small erasers, cute pencils, or other age-appropriate items might encourage children to remember to return the consent forms. It is important to emphasize to teachers that they should encourage children *to return* the parental consent forms *regardless* of whether or not the children are given consent to participate.

In terms of obtaining parental consent and child assent for participation, this process is facilitated when schools and teachers support the research project (as outlined above). In addition, investigators should explicitly communicate with families about research procedures, risks, and benefits in the consent form (see Hinshaw et al., 2004) and let parents know what procedures are in place if their child should display distress. Because of the potentially sensitive nature of postdisaster research with children, "passive consent" procedures (i.e., parents are informed about the study and contact the investigators only if they do not want their child to participate) typically are not considered appropriate for this type of research.

In order to encourage active parental consent for child participation, or for parents' own participation in research, additional recruitment strategies may be needed. For example, it may be helpful to "spread the word" about the study to parents via PTA meetings or other school-based functions that parents attend; in this way the researchers can answer questions that parents may have about the research protocol. In general, it is useful to involve "stakeholders" in developing ideas for recruitment and retention of study participants. For example, Riesch and colleagues (1999) advocated for consulting adolescents regarding appropriate recruitment and retention strategies to use with other adolescents. For schools that enroll students from multicultural backgrounds, it may also be helpful to recruit parents from diverse backgrounds who support the study and who could demonstrate their enthusiasm to other parents who might otherwise be wary of research participation. Letters or flyers about the study that are sent home to parents may also help to disseminate information, but they should be translated into multiple languages (for diverse school settings) so that they can be understood by parents from different language backgrounds.

When funding allows, incentives for child and parent participation are also helpful in recruiting and retaining participants. Investigators should consider the use of incentives early in the research design, paying attention to developmental and ethical considerations (see Rice & Broome, 2004). If funds are limited, participants could be entered in a lottery for several prizes that might be attractive to children or parents (e.g., coupons for movie rentals, gift certificates for a bookstore). Because parents may be concerned about how their child is functioning, and because ethical considerations dictate that parents be notified when children display significant signs of psychological distress, it may be reassuring to parents to let them know that they will be contacted if the study procedures identify significant distress in their child.

For studies that evaluate children at multiple time points, such as longitudinal follow-up studies, or studies of the effectiveness of postdisaster interventions, it will be especially important to create incentives so that the participants do not drop out over time. Financial incentives are often potent. However, with limited resources, the "lottery system" mentioned above might be useful. Other strategies to encourage children and families to become invested in a project might be to have a special project logo or theme ("Coping Kids Project") that is printed on tee shirts, certificates, or other items to show appreciation to the participants.

Given the importance of participant retention for longitudinal, intervention, and prevention studies, it is also important to have some mechanism in place for tracking and recontacting participants over time, especially if they move or change schools. For example, once parental permission and consent to participate have been obtained, it may be useful to ask parents to provide the names and contact information for family members or friends who will know how to contact them in the future if they move.

Considerations for Training Research Assistants

This section briefly reviews a few issues that pertain to training research assistants (RAs) for school-based protocols, to ensure continued cooperation by school personnel and that all study procedures run smoothly. First, RAs typically need an orientation to the complexities of school systems and school "etiquette" before beginning a research protocol, especially with the security issues that are paramount in most U.S. schools today. For example, RAs should be introduced to the principal and key teachers, and should check in (with appropriate identification) at the main school office each time they enter the school for data collection purposes. If a team of assistants is working with a key RA, the RA in charge should make a point of letting the school personnel know who the assistants are and why they are there. The RAs should also understand that it could be upsetting or disruptive to teachers to interrupt academic lessons or "pull out" students from class for testing. RAs should be taught to be flexible and polite to teachers at all times, recognizing that they are on "school turf" and that the research study may be secondary to other more pressing academic needs. Study procedures should not disrupt or burden the schools.

Second, RAs will need to have a solid grounding in ethics and research issues such as confidentiality (of students' responses, of protocol forms, etc.) and methods for protecting confidentiality; in treating participants with respect; and in avoiding coercion, especially if a child decides not to participate. Most institutional review boards (IRBs) require that all research personnel who interact with human subjects participate in formal training (often via an online course) on the ethics and procedures of human subjects research. Even if such instruction is not required, it is extremely valuable to include as part of an RA's training. Assistants who do not come into contact with participants, but who may be involved with data entry and management, also need to be aware of procedures to protect participants' confidentiality and other rights.

Third, presumably RAs will be chosen because they have an interest in and experience with children and adolescents. Nevertheless, it is important to provide training on how to recognize signs of discomfort and distress in children and adolescents, especially because the study procedures are likely to ask about upsetting events and reactions that occurred following a traumatic event. There should also be a specific procedure in place for RAs to follow when a participant does become distressed (e.g., let them know that you understand they are distressed; ask if they would like to take a break or stop; ask if they would like to talk with a teacher or counselor). A record should be kept of all distressing or unusual events; in fact, IRBs now require that such events be reported.

Finally, depending on the specific study protocol and measures, it is possible that some participants might report incidents of child abuse. Because of this, training for RAs should include education on the legal and ethical requirements associated with abuse reporting. There should be a procedure in place for how such reports are to be handled, even if they are unlikely to occur. Investigators are encouraged to seek advice from local child maltreatment specialists who are aware of local legal issues and relevant resources.

SUMMARY AND CONCLUSION

As noted at the outset of the chapter, children and adolescents represent an understudied but vulnerable population in the aftermath of disasters and terrorism. School-based studies that address the kinds of reactions that children display following disasters, the mediators and moderators of these stress reactions, and the variables that put children at risk for adverse reactions in the long term are especially important research interests (La Greca et al., 2002). In particular, efforts to develop conceptual models to predict children's disaster reactions are needed, especially ones that elucidate the causal risk factors that lead to children's disaster reactions and that begin to delineate the likely processes underlying their reactions.

School-based studies are also needed that consider the effectiveness of postdisaster interventions and the prevention of long-term distress. Although a number of promising treatment and prevention manuals now exist (see La Greca & Silverman, 2006), they await further testing and evaluation. There is a critical need for evidence-based and transportable interventions that are appropriate for different phases of disaster recovery (e.g., acute versus long-term) and that can be implemented in various settings, including schools (La Greca et al., 2002).

At the same time, as outlined in this chapter, there are a number of practical challenges to implementing child disaster research in school settings. Several recommendations are offered, based on the material contained in this chapter. *First,* investigators are encouraged to be patient but persistent in their efforts to engage schools in the research endeavor, recognizing the enormous difficulties that disasters and other traumatic events pose to schools, teachers, students, and families. Understand that it will be important to be flexible and accommodating in planning the study procedures. *Second,* efforts to design protocols that are not burdensome to schools and participants and that are sensitive to developmental and cultural issues are especially needed. *Third,* school-based child disaster research requires viewing school personnel as collaborators in the research process. The input supplied by school personnel and participants may prove extremely useful in developing appropriate protocols as well as in identifying appropriate strategies for participation and retention. *Fourth*, given the sensitive nature of assessing children's postdisaster reactions, it is essential to establish a protocol for handling distressed children and for making appropriate referrals in case a child becomes distressed. *Fifth*, because it will not be possible to control the kinds of support that children receive following disasters, it is important to monitor the assistance that children receive and consider such events in statistical analyses. *Finally*, when working in a multicultural school system, one must plan to make adjustments in recruitment, retention, and study procedures, as discussed in the chapter, to ensure that the protocol will be inclusive and sensitive to cultural issues.

REFERENCES

American Academy of Child and Adolescent Psychiatry (1998). AACAP Official Action: Practice parameters for the assessment and treatment of children and adolescents with posttraumatic stress disorder. *Journal of the American Academy of Child and Adolescent Psychiatry, 37*(Suppl.), 4S–26S.

American Psychiatric Association (1994). *Diagnostic and statistical manual of mental disorders* (4th ed.) (DSM-IV). Washington, DC: Author.

Applied Research & Consulting LLC and the Columbia University Mailman School of Public Health. (2002). *Effects of the World Trade Center attack on NYC public school students: Initial report to the New York City Board of Education.* Retrieved January 25, 2005, from www.nycenet.edu/offices/spss/wtc_needs/firstrep.pdf

Asarnow, J., Glynn, S., Pynoos, R. S., Nahum, J., Guthrie, D., Cantwell, D. P., et al. (1999). When the earth stops shaking: Earthquake sequelae among children diagnosed for pre-earthquake psychopathology. *Journal of the American Academy of Child Adolescent Psychiatry. 38*, 1016–1023.

Cicchetti, D., & Rogosch, F. A. (1999). Conceptual and methodological issues in developmental psychopathology research. In P. C. Kendall, J. N. Butcher, & G. N. Holmbeck (Eds.), *Handbook of research methods in clinical psychology* (2nd ed., pp. 433–465). New York: Wiley.

Dilworth-Anderson, P., & Williams, S. W. (2004). Recruitment and retention strategies for longitudinal African American caregiving research: The Family Caregiving Project. *Journal of Aging and Health, 16*(5 Suppl.), 137S–156S.

Garrison, C. Z., Weinrich, M. W., Hardin, S. B., Weinrich, S., & Wang, L. (1993). Posttraumatic stress disorder in adolescents after a hurricane. *American Journal of Epidemiology, 138*, 522–530.

Gurwitch, R., Sitterle, K. A., Young, B. H., & Pfefferbaum, B. (2002). The aftermath of terrorism. In A. M. La Greca, W. K. Silverman, E. M. Vernberg, & M. C. Roberts (Eds.), *Helping children cope with disasters and terrorism* (pp. 327–358). Washington, DC: American Psychological Association.

Hinshaw, S. P., Hoagwood, K., Jensen, P. S., Kratochvil, C., Bickman, L., & Clarke, G. (2004). AACAP 2001 research forum: Challenges and recommendations regarding recruitment and retention of participants in research investigations. *Journal of the American Academy of Child and Adolescent Psychiatry 43*, 1037–1045.

Kazdin, A. E. (1990). Assessment of childhood depression. In A. M. La Greca (Ed.),

Through the eyes of the child: Obtaining self-reports from children and adolescents (pp. 189–223). Boston: Prentice Hall.

Kendall, P. C., Butcher, J. N., & Holmbeck, G. N. (Eds.), (1999). *Handbook of research methods in clinical psychology* (2nd ed.). New York: Wiley.

La Greca, A. M. (2001). Children experiencing disasters: Prevention and intervention. In J. N. Hughes, A. M. La Greca, & J. C. Conoley (Eds.) *Handbook of psychological services for children and adolescents* (pp. 381–402). New York: Oxford University Press.

La Greca, A. M., & Lemanek, K. L. (1996). Assessment as a process in pediatric psychology. *Journal of Pediatric Psychology, 21,* 137–151.

La Greca, A. M., & Prinstein, M. J. (2002). Hurricanes and tornadoes. In A. M. La Greca, W. K. Silverman, E. M. Vernberg, & M. C. Roberts (Eds.), *Helping children cope with disasters and terrorism.* (pp. 107–138). Washington, DC: American Psychological Association.

La Greca, A. M., & Silverman, W. K. (2006). Treating children and adolescents affected by disasters and terrorism. In P. C. Kendall (Ed.), *Child and adolescent therapy: Cognitive-behavioral procedures* (3rd ed., pp. 356–382). New York: Guilford Press.

La Greca, A. M., Silverman, W. K., Vernberg, E. M., & Prinstein, M. (1996). Symptoms of posttraumatic stress after Hurricane Andrew: A prospective study. *Journal of Consulting and Clinical Psychology, 64,* 712–723.

La Greca, A. M., Silverman, W. K., Vernberg, E. M., & Roberts, M. C. (2002). Children and disasters: Future directions for research and public policy. In A. M. La Greca, W. K. Silverman, E. M. Vernberg, & M. C. Roberts (Eds.) *Helping children cope with disasters and terrorism.* (pp. 405–424). Washington, DC: American Psychological Association.

La Greca, A. M., Silverman, W. K., & Wasserstein, S. B. (1998). Children's predisaster functioning as a predictor of posttraumatic stress following Hurricane Andrew. *Journal of Consulting and Clinical Psychology, 66,* 883–892.

Loeber, R., Green, S. M., & Lahey, B. B. (1990). Mental health professionals' perception of the utility of children, mothers, and teachers as informants on child psychopathology. *Journal of Clinical Child Psychology, 19,* 136–143.

Pfefferbaum, B., Doughty, D. E., Reddy, C., Patel, N., Gurwitch, R. H., Nixon, S. J., et al. (2002). Exposure and peritraumatic response as predictors of posttraumatic stress in children following the 1995 Oklahoma City bombing. *Journal of Urban Health, 79,* 354–363.

Pfefferbaum, B., North, C. S., Doughty, D. E., Gurwitch, R. H., Fullerton, C. S., & Kyula, J. (2003). Posttraumatic stress and functional impairment in Kenyan children following the 1998 American Embassy bombing. *American Journal of Orthopsychiatry, 73,* 133–140.

Pynoos, R. S., Rodriguez, N., Steinberg, A. M., Stuber, M., & Frederick, C. (1999). *PTSD Reaction Index—Revised.* Unpublished psychological test, University of California, Los Angeles.

Riesch, S. K., Tosi, C. B., & Thurston, C. A. (1999). Accessing young adolescents and their families for research. *Image Journal of Nursing Scholarship, 31,* 323–326.

Rice, M., & Broome, M. E. (2004). Incentives for children in research. *Journal of Nursing Scholarship, 36,* 167–172.

Saylor, C., & De Roma, V. (2002). Assessment of children and adolescents exposed to disaster. In A. M. La Greca, W. K. Silverman, E. M. Vernberg, & M. C. Roberts (Eds.). (2002). *Helping children cope with disasters and terrorism* (pp. 35–54). Washington, DC: American Psychological Association.

Scotti, J. R., Ruggiero, K. J., & Rabalais, A. E. (2002). The traumatic impact of motor vehicle accidents. In A. M. La Greca, W. K. Silverman, E. M. Vernberg, & M. C. Roberts (Eds.), *Helping children cope with disasters and terrorism* (pp. 259–291). Washington, DC: American Psychological Association.

Sears, S. R., Stanton, A. L., & Danoff-Burg, S. (2003). The yellow brick road and the emerald city: Benefit finding, positive reappraisal coping and posttraumatic growth in women with early-stage breast cancer. *Health Psychology, 22,* 487–497.

Seligman, M. E. (2002). How to see the glass half full. *Newsweek, 140*(12), 48–49.

Shannon, M. P., Lonigan, C. J., Finch, A. J., Jr., & Taylor, C. M. (1994). Children exposed to disaster: I. Epidemiology of post-traumatic symptoms and symptom profiles. *Journal of the American Academy of Child and Adolescent Psychiatry, 33,* 80–93.

Silverman, W. K., & La Greca, A. M. (2002). Children experiencing disasters: Definitions, reactions, and predictors of outcomes. In A. M. La Greca, W. K. Silverman, E. M. Vernberg, & M. C. Roberts (Eds.), *Helping children cope with disasters and terrorism* (pp. 11–34). Washington, DC: American Psychological Association.

Tolan, P. H. (1999). Research methods in community-based treatment and prevention. In P. C. Kendall, J. N. Butcher, & G. N. Holmbeck (Eds.), *Handbook of research methods in clinical psychology* (2nd ed., pp. 403–418). New York: Wiley.

Vernberg, E. M. (2002). Intervention approaches following disasters. In A. M. La Greca, W.K. Silverman, E. M. Vernberg, & M. C. Roberts (Eds.), *Helping children cope with disasters and terrorism* (pp. 55–72). Washington, DC: American Psychological Association.

Vogel, J., & Vernberg, E. M. (1993). Children's psychological responses to disaster. *Journal of Clinical Child Psychology, 22,* 464–484.

Yule, W., Udwin, O., & Bolton, D. (2002). Mass transportation disasters. In A. M. La Greca, W. K. Silverman, E. M. Vernberg, & M. C. Roberts (Eds.), *Helping children cope with disasters and terrorism* (pp. 223–240). Washington, DC: American Psychological Association.

CHAPTER 10

Qualitative Approaches to Studying the Effects of Disasters

LAWRENCE A. PALINKAS

Disaster research is often viewed as a largely quantitative enterprise in which the effects on individuals, communities, and societies are enumerated in terms such as rates of morbidity and mortality or financial losses and costs of reconstruction. However, there is another research tradition, rooted primarily within the disciplines of sociology and anthropology, that has employed qualitative methods to examine the effects of disasters on the behavior of individuals, groups, and organizations (Oliver-Smith, 1996). Moreover, when used in an integrated fashion through mixed method designs (Teddlie & Tashakkori, 2003), the quantitative and qualitative research traditions each possess enormous potential to complement each other, providing a more comprehensive level of insight and understanding through combinations of breadth and depth, exploration, and confirmation. This chapter describes the use of qualitative methods in research on the mental health effects of disasters and terrorism, examines the rationale for using such methods, outlines the types of methods that have been used in the past and might have potential for use in the future, and offers recommendations for their use in disaster research.

RATIONALE FOR QUALITATIVE METHODS

As conceptualized by Miller and Crabtree (1992), scientific inquiry in general has at least five aims: identification, description, explanation generation, explanation testing, and control. The first three of these comprise what is often termed *exploratory* research, while the latter two are more appropriately referred a *confirmatory* research. Qualitative methods usually are used for identification, description, and explanation generation, whereas quantitative methods are used most commonly for explanation testing and control.

Within the context of investigating the mental health effects of disasters and terrorism, qualitative methods have been used to accomplish several distinct aims or objectives. First, they are ideal for obtaining a "thick description" (Geertz, 1973) of phenomena. Thick descriptions are rich, detailed, and concrete accounts of communities, societies, and events that illustrate the complex interactions among key variables within a specific social and cultural context. For instance, in the early 1970s, Tony Oliver-Smith and Barbara Bode independently conducted ethnographic fieldwork in Yungay, Peru, in the aftermath of an earthquake that destroyed the city and left 70,000 dead and 140,000 injured. Each provided a thick description of the event through their detailed accounts of the community before, during, and after the earthquake. In turn, each used this thick description as the foundation for understanding specific elements of the psychosocial impacts of the disaster on the survivors. Oliver-Smith (1992), for instance, argued that the aid provided to survivors of the earthquake may have compounded their psychological trauma by undermining their sense of autonomy. Bode (1989) demonstrated the importance to mental health of cultural explanatory models underlying the efforts of victims to understand the event and cope with the aftermath. These methods provide a depth of understanding of an issue or topic that complements the breadth of understanding afforded by quantitative methods. Such a thick description aids in the interpretation of results obtained from the use of quantitative methods and best illustrates the complexity of social interactions both before and after a traumatic event (Oliver-Smith, 1996).

Related to the character and value of the thick description, a second reason for the use of qualitative methods in understanding the mental health effects of disasters is to place such effects within their social and cultural context. Kleinman (1995) and Young (1995) have argued that an understanding of the local context is essential to the interpretation of the idioms of distress that are transformed by the clinical construct into a diagnosis of posttraumatic stress disorder (PTSD). As is the case with all expressions of emotion, the symptoms that characterize the PTSD diagnosis are subject to local variations in their expression (presence or absence of specific symptoms), interpretation as to their meaning (bereavement or pathology), and social significance (acceptance or isolation) (Eisenbruch, 1991; Kleinman, 1995). These local variations are often reflected in differences in patterns of response to standardized diagnostic instruments (Bolton, 2001; Marsella & Christopher, 2004), making the interpretation of these responses as evidence of a valid clinical construct somewhat problematic.

An illustration of the use of qualitative methods to study the sociocultural context of mental health effects of disasters is the East County Ethnographic Study (Palinkas, Prussing, Landsverk, & Reznik, 2003; Palinkas, Prussing, Reznik, & Landsverk, 2004). In March 2001, two shootings at high schools located in East San Diego County, California, left 2 dead and 23 injured. Analyses of data collected through participant ob servation, extended interviews, and focus groups revealed three community-wide patterns of response to the two events: (1) intrusive reminders of the trauma associated with intense media coverage and subsequent rumors, hoaxes, and threats of additional acts of school violence; (2) efforts to avoid thoughts, feelings, conversations, or places (i.e., schools) associated with the events; negative assessment of media coverage; and belief that such events in general cannot be prevented; and (3) anger, hypervigilance, and other forms of increased arousal (Palinkas, Prussing, et al., 2004). In addition, embedded within the community explanatory models of the cause (etiology), course (symptoms and consequences), and cure (prevention) of youth violence were four distinct explanations for the shootings: (1) unique or idiosyncratic characteristics of the two shooters (both of whom were outsiders, one because he was a newcomer to community and a victim of bullying, and the other, who was a victim of child abuse with a history of mental illness); (2) universal factors (living in a culture of violence, widespread exposure to violence in the media); (3) family-centered characteristics of the two shooters, the target communities, and society at large (single-parent households exhibiting dysfunctional relationships); and (4) community-specific characteristics (the prevalence of a "frontier mentality," reputation for social intolerance, widespread access to guns). Both the idioms of distress and the explanations for youth violence embedded within these cultural explanatory models could be attributed to the rapid pace of urbanization experienced over the past decade in East San Diego County; the concomitant decline of a rural lifestyle; an increase in the number of "outsiders," single-parent households, and social problems; and changing values associated with these social and demographic changes (Palinkas et al., 2003; Palinkas, Prussing, et al., 2004).

Third, qualitative research is used to clarify the values, language, and meanings attributed to people who play different roles in disasters (Oliver-Smith, 1996). As described by Sofaer (1999, p. 1105), "They allow people to speak in their own voice, rather than conforming to categories and terms imposed on them by others." By working to elicit the perspective of the victims and aid workers alike, for instance, qualitative methods help to "ground" (Glaser & Strauss, 1967) the research and thereby enhance the validity of the data being collected. For example, Norris and colleagues (2001) elicited symptom descriptions corresponding to the criterion symptoms of PTSD through unstructured interviews with Mexican survivors of disasters in Mexico and the United States and identified clusters of symptoms corresponding to *ataque de nervios* as well as depression, lasting trauma, and somatic complaints.

The employment of such methods also requires that the researcher and the objects of that research (i.e., study participants or subjects) collaborate to generate understanding of the phenomena of interest through the iterative process of data collection and analysis. Hence, they are ideal for participatory research. The East County Ethnographic Study, described above, relied upon community partners to assist in the recruitment of participants, the collection and analysis of data, and the interpretation of the results and their policy implications (Palinkas et al., 1993). Furthermore, qualitative research has traditionally been used to give voice, in particular, to those who are otherwise rarely heard (Sofaer, 1999). As such, they are ideal for investigating the causes and consequences of the health disparities that afflict these groups, including disparities in disaster impacts. For instance, quantitative data collected in a household survey conducted 1 year after the *Exxon Valdez* oil spill revealed several ethnic differences in the association between exposure to the oil spill and subsequent cleanup efforts and the prevalence of PTSD, as well as a host of other adverse physical and mental health outcomes (Palinkas, Downs, Petterson, & Russell, 1993; Palinkas, Petterson, Downs, & Russell, 2004). Qualitative data collected during the ethnographic fieldwork phase of the project revealed that the oil spill and cleanup represented the death of a traditional way of life for Alaska Natives who depended upon traditional subsistence activities to maintain their individual and social identity and who spent prolonged periods away from the community, and hence from critical sources of social and emotional support, when employed in cleanup activities (Palinkas et al., 1993).

Fourth, because of its value in conducting exploratory research, qualitative methods have often been used during the initial stages of a project to enable the investigator to acquire background and understanding of the issues; to obtain "pilot data" in the form of case studies, case series, or focus groups; and to provide guidance in the development of theories and the formulation of hypotheses when little or no previous research has been conducted on the phenomena of interest. These methods have often proven to be invaluable in the development of valid and reliable quantitative methods for investigating these phenomena. For instance, Bolton (2001) used formal ethnographic methods (free-listing and pile sorts) and key informant interviews to investigate how Rwandans perceived the mental health effects of the 1994 genocide and the local validity of Western mental illness concepts in an effort to adapt existing assessment instruments for local use. These methods are used to ensure that the items and response options on a survey or psychometric instrument are interpreted consistently and as intended by the developers of such measures across potential respondents.

Finally, although the collection and analysis of both quantitative and qualitative data is a labor-intensive process that requires a considerable investment in time and resources, ethnographic fieldwork offers certain advantages in disaster research in that it can be launched soon after the event occurs with minimal disruption to an already traumatized community. The East County Ethnographic Study, for instance, was initiated within days after the second shooting (Palinkas et al., 2003).

QUALITATIVE METHODS

Sample Selection

One of the key differences between quantitative and qualitative research methods lies in the criteria used to determine who and how many people to include as study participants. The assumptions, derived from statistical probability theory, which underlie the random selection of a specified number of participants necessary to ensure representativeness and eliminate the possibility of a Type I and Type II error differ from the assumptions that underlie the purposeful selection of "information-rich" participants for study in depth. Patton (2002) listed 16 different purposeful nonrandom sampling strategies used in qualitative research. These include extreme or deviant case sampling, used to learn from unusual manifestations of the phenomenon of interest (such as those who survived an event of natural disaster or act of terrorism with no obvious emotional effects versus those who were completely disabled by the event); maximum variation sampling, used to select participants from a wide variety of groups or segments of a population to get variation on dimensions of interest; critical case sampling, used to permit logical generalization and maximum allocation of information to other cases because if it's true in one case, it's likely to be true in other cases; and snowball sampling, used to identify cases of interest from sampling individuals who know other individuals with detailed knowledge of cases that are information-rich—that is, that serve as good examples for study and are likely to be good interview participants (Patton, 2002, pp. 243–244). The selection of any of these sampling strategies depends, in part, on logistical constraints (such as the number of available participants and the time available for identification of sampling domains and recruitment) and, in part, on the correspondence between study objectives and the logic of data collection (i.e., can the study objectives be accomplished with the information obtained from participants recruited through a specific sampling strategy?).

With respect to the number of participants to be sampled, Patton (2002) observed that there are no rules for sample size in qualitative inquiry. Rather, "sample size depends on what you want to know, the purpose of the inquiry, what's at stake, what will be useful, what will have credibility, and what can be done with available time and resources" (p. 244). Based on these criteria, Deren, Shedlin, Hamilton, and Hagen (2002) conducted three focus groups with 26 active drug users in New York City to assess the impact of the September 11, 2001, terrorist attacks on the perception of changes in drug use, drug availability, police activities, and access to services. Analyses conducted as part of the East County Ethnographic Study were based on data collected from 85 community residents who participated in semistructured interviews and focus groups (Palinkas et al., 2003; Palinkas, Prussing, et al., 2004). Lincoln and Guba (1985) provided some elaboration to these criteria in the form of a principle of "saturation," or redundancy, when the purpose is to maximize information. Under these conditions, "the sampling is terminated when no new information is forthcoming from newly sampled units" (p. 202). However, because qualitative research is an iterative process where data collection and analysis often occur concurrently, researchers are required to initiate qualitative inquiry with a considerable amount of uncertainty as to how many participants to recruit. Even with the experience of having conducted similar research in the past as a guide, such uncertainly is only likely to be reduced once data collection gets under way.

Data Collection

Two of the best-known methodological techniques for the collection of qualitative data are ethnographic fieldwork and focus groups. Ethnography is an approach to learning about the social and cultural life of communities, institutions, and other settings that is scientific, investigative, uses the re searcher as the primary tool of data collection, uses rigorous research methods and data collection techniques to avoid bias and ensure the accuracy of data, emphasizes and builds on the perspectives of those being studied, and is inductive, building local theories for testing and adapting them for use both locally and elsewhere (LeCompte & Schensul, 1999; Spradley, 1979; Bernard, 2002). Ethnography traces its roots to cultural anthropology, where it was developed for the purposes of describing and understanding another culture or way of life from the native point of view (Spradley, 1979). However, it has also been used to investigate the values, attitudes, and behaviors of people living in our own culture, including those components of our culture involved in the causes and consequences of disasters and terrorism (Oliver-Smith, 1996; Bolton & Tang, 2004).

Ethnography is not a method per se but rather a strategy that facilitates the collection and analysis of data acquired through fieldwork (Bernard, 2002). This strategy incorporates several different methods that may be used independently or in combination as a way of triangulating or verifying the accuracy of data obtained from any one particular method. Among the most commonly used methods in ethnographic fieldwork are participant observation, extended interviews and elicitation methods, and case studies.

Participant observation has been used in disaster research to understand the social and cultural context of postdisaster recovery (e.g., Bode, 1989; Oliver-Smith, 1992). This method offers several advantages in studies of the mental health effects of disasters and terrorism. As people get used to having you around, you have a greater chance of observing behavior or events as it actually occurs, thereby increasing the validity of the data collected. The differences between what people say and what they actually do become apparent. Sensible questions can be formed in the language of the people being studied. The sequence and connectedness of events that contribute to the meaning of a phenomenon can be identified. Observation enables the researcher to acquire an intuitive understanding of what's going on and allows one to speak with confidence about the meaning of data. Finally, many research problems cannot be adequately investigated by any other means. Participant observation is generally useful and appropriate for addressing any research question that requires an understanding of processes, events, relationships, and context (Bernard, 2002).

Disaster research has also made extensive use of semistructured interviews to collect data on mental health effects. For instance, Palinkas and colleagues (2003) conducted semistructured interviews with 85 individuals representing each of the major target groups in the community: students, parents, teachers and school administrators, physical and mental health service providers, and community leaders and public safety officials. Interviews were conducted with the use of a guide developed in conjunction with the study team's community representatives and specifically intended to elucidate people's perceptions of what caused these shootings, what might have prevented them, what was being or should be done in response to the events, and the impact of these events on individuals, families, and communities. These techniques were designed to elicit the community's perception on these issues, thereby enhancing the external validity of the information obtained. The average interview was approximately 1 hour in length.

Nevertheless, semistructured interviews reflect a "middle ground" of a continuum of techniques for conducting extended interviews. At one end of this continuum is the unstructured interview, to be applied when few if any issues related to the phenomenon of interest have been identified and when the primary intent is to obtain the informant's perception of what issues are important or relevant (LeCompte & Schensul, 1999). This information can be used to develop questions for semistructured or structured interviews. For instance, Tobin and Whiteford (2002) conducted informal interviews with government officials and survivors of a volcanic eruption in Ecuador to inform the development of a survey to a larger, more representative sample of survivors, and to facilitate the interpretation of the results from this survey. More importantly, they are an essential first step in building the rapport with the informant necessary to obtaining valid and reliable data in the future (Bernard, 2002).

At the other end of the continuum is the structured interview. Structured interviews rely upon techniques such as formal ethnographic methods and cognitive domain elicitation (Johnson & Weller, 2002; Weller & Romney, 1988). In general, these techniques are utilized when the universe of issues related to a phenomenon of interest are identified a priori and when the intention is to validate or confirm the hypothesis or perspective of the investigator (Bernard, 2002). These techniques are designed to identify items within a cultural domain (i.e., language, beliefs, values, knowledge, and behaviors) and to identify interrelationships within and among domains. Data for these domains are collected by exposing several informants to the same set of stimuli, which can be the same set of questions or completion of an identical task. These tasks include free-listing, pile sorts, triad tests, paired comparisons, frame substitution tasks, and ranking and rating tasks. As noted earlier, Bolton (2001) invited survivors of the 1994 genocide in Rwanda to list and describe the main problems caused by this event. For problems that seemed mental or emotional, participant respondents were asked who people consulted about these problems. Informants were also asked to sort cards containing the names of symptoms into piles based on which symptoms "go together." Together, these methods helped to elucidate local idioms of distress related to the event and their correspondence to the idioms contained in standardized diagnostic assessment instruments.

Case studies provide an in-depth understanding of the mental health impacts of a disaster or act of terrorism through an intensive examination of a single person, experience, or organization. For instance, Oliver-Smith (1992) helped to illustrate the mental health effects of the Yungay earthquake by describing its impact on Roberto Falcón, one of the survivors. Through Roberto's life story, the reader is able to witness the emotional strain and struggle to cope with loss in the aftermath of the event and to gain perspective in contrasting his life before and after the disaster. Although such studies are rarely generalizable, they are often used to obtain greater depth of understanding of a particular phenomenon through description. Case studies are also used to illustrate general principles obtained through other methods. Case studies are usually based on data collected from extended interviews, but may also incorporate data obtained through direct and indirect observation.

The focus group approach is designed to use group interactions to generate data and insights on a more restricted (focused) range of issues or topics that are less accessible in individual interviews. It is a technique for developing rich exploration of content with a group of 6–10 "homogeneous strangers" (i.e., people who share similar social or demographic characteristics or experiences but who do not know one another), allowing for observation of interaction on the subject, providing evidence of how people discuss a topic, and making certain that key issued are not overlooked (Morgan, 1988). Focus groups have been used to explore issues related to novel areas of inquiry, evaluate new products or ideas for research, confirm results obtained from other methods, and develop and pilot-test items to be used in questionnaires (Morgan, 1988). Tobin and Whiteford (2002) conducted four focus groups with 7–10 participants per group to assess the impact of a volcanic eruption on survivors in Ecuador. The participants were all adult women recruited through contacts made at local organizations, communities, and shelters. The sessions lasted about 2 hours and were used to establish baseline data regarding issues associated with the evacuation and health effects. Although this technique is often perceived as a cost-effective strategy for collecting data from a large number of respondents at the same time, it is not intended to replace a series of individual interviews with the same number of people. Rather, it is intended to generate insight on the part of both investigator and group members gained through the exchange of information that does not typically occur in the context of individual interviews.

Data Analysis

Miller and Crabtree (1992) described qualitative data analytic strategies as falling along a continuum with quasi-statistical techniques that are more objective (separating the researcher from the object of research), scientific (valid, reliable, reproducible, accurate, and systematic), general (exhibiting lawlike regularities), technical (procedural, mechanical) and standardized (measurable, verifiable) at one extreme; and immersion/crystallization techniques that are subjective (emerging from the researcher), intuitive (involving experiential insight), particular (personal, context-dependent), existential (concerned with everyday existence), and interpretative (related to meaning) at the other extreme. In between these two extremes are strategies that involve editing and use of templates to identify core meanings and consistencies within the content of the qualitative data. Editing and template analyses are generally rooted within one or more intellectual traditions such as phenomenology (seeking to understand the meaning, structure, and essence of the lived experience of a phenomenon for a person or group of people; Husserl, 1931), hermeneutics (seeking to understand the political, historical, and sociocultural context of that lived experience; Ricoeur, 1981), symbolic interactionism (seeking to understand how people use symbols to give meaning to their social interactions; Blumer, 1969), and grounded theory (seeking to understand social psychological and/or social structural process derived from data collected within a given social scene and then illustrated by characteristic examples of data; Glaser & Strauss, 1967).

Perhaps the most commonly used of all qualitative analytic approaches, template strategies are distinguished by a process in which data are coded, and themes are elicited from the meanings and consistencies embedded in these codes. This process is initiated when the empirical material contained in the interviews and field notes are independently coded by the project investigators at a very general level in order to condense the data into analyzable units. Segments of interviews, ranging from a phrase to several paragraphs, are assigned codes based on a priori (i.e., based on questions in the interview guide) or emergent (i.e., based on the data themselves) themes. In many instances, the same text segment is assigned more than one code. Ideally, each interview is independently coded by at least two investigators. Disagreements in the assignment or description of codes are resolved through discussion between investigators and enhanced definition of codes. In a study of the mental health effects of disasters or terrorism, the final list of codes, constructed through a consensus of team members, might consist of a numbered list of themes, issues, accounts of behaviors, and opinions that relate to the event itself, its causes and consequences, and the likelihood of preventing similar events from occurring in the future. Based on these codes, computerized text analysis software such as Atlas.ti (2004) or QSR NVivo (Fraser, 2000) may be used to generate a series of categories arranged in a treelike structure connecting transcript segments grouped into separate categories, or "nodes." These nodes and trees can be used to examine the association between different a priori and emergent categories and to identify the existence of new, previously unrecognized, categories. The number of times these categories occur together, either as duplicate codes assigned to the same text or as codes assigned to adjacent texts in the same conversation, are recorded, and specific examples of co-occurrence are illustrated with transcript texts. Finally, and perhaps most importantly, through the process of constantly comparing these categories with one another, the different categories are further condensed into broad themes distinguished on the basis of those qualities or meanings they share in common and those that distinguish them from categories belonging to other themes.

RAPID ASSESSMENT PROCEDURES

Despite their potential for addressing many important issues relating to the effects of disasters, qualitative methods are often criticized for being too labor-intensive and taking too long to complete, a constraint that is of particular concern to the time-limited nature of mental health effects subsequent to a traumatic event (Bolton & Tang, 2004). Rapid Assessment Procedures (RAP) offers a potential solution to these concerns. This approach has been used successfully by anthropologists and sociologists in conducting both process and outcome evaluations of community development and health services delivery programs at home and abroad, and is designed to provide depth to the understanding of organizations or programs and their community context that is critical to the development and implementation of more quantitative (cross-sectional or longitudinal) approaches involving the use of survey questionnaires (Scrimshaw & Hurtado, 1987; Harris, Jerome, & Fawcett, 1997). Distinguishing features of RAP include: (1) formation of a multidisciplinary research team including a member or members of the target organizations and their clients; (2) development of materials to train community members in data collection; (3) use of several data collection methods (e.g., focus groups, informal interviews, newspaper accounts, agency reports, statistics) to verify information through triangulation; (4) iterative data collection and analysis to facilitate continuous adjustment of the research question and methods to answer that question; and (5) completion of the project quickly, usually in 4–6 weeks (Harris et al., 1997). The methodology relies heavily on techniques of participant observation and semistructured interviewing.

RAP has been used in the past to study the effects of both technological disasters and incidents of mass violence. The East County Ethnographic Study (Palinkas et al., 2003; Palinkas, Prussing, et al., 2004) used RAP to assess the impact of the school shootings on students, families, and communities as well as to elicit community explanatory models of youth violence and violence prevention. Bolton (2001) conducted a rapid ethnographic study in two rural communes in Rwanda to assess the mental health effects of the 1994 genocide. In each instance, RAP enabled a timely collection of data through community participation that allowed for an enhanced role of the perspective of the victim in the interpretation of study results.

To apply RAP or some other form of compressed qualitative research design efficiently, however, certain assumptions must be adequately addressed (LeCompte & Schensul, 1999). First, the researchers must already be familiar with the field setting and/or cultural context and, ideally, speak the language. Second, the research should have limited focus and not strive to comprehensively cover a wide spectrum of beliefs and behaviors in different cultural domains. Third, the researchers must collaborate with local or indigenous "experts" who can assist in establishing the context for data collection, designing the research, and interpreting the results, thereby helping to avoid mistakes resulting from a lack of familiarity with the setting. Finally, data collection techniques must be suitable for convenient use in a brief period of time. For instance, participant observation in the aftermath of a disaster may be a less efficient means of collecting information on the mental health effects (because of the demands placed on investigators to spend an extended period of time before coming to an understanding of the significance of what is observed) than more quasi-statistical approaches using structured interviewing techniques such as free-listing and pile sorts.

MIXED-METHOD DESIGNS

Stallings (1997) observed that disaster research requires a special hybrid research methodology, because the circumstances of studying disasters are unique and methods must vary according to the stage of the unfolding disaster process. Such a hybrid methodology is potentially available in the form of mixed-method designs that enable the researcher to simultaneously answer confirmatory and exploratory questions, and therefore verify and generate theory in the same study (Teddlie & Tashakkori, 2003). They are particularly suited for the examination of complex social phenomena that cannot be understood using either purely quantitative or qualitative techniques. Examples of mixed-method designs in studying the mental health effects of disasters include the use of focus groups with drug users and surveys of service providers to assess the impact of the September 11, 2001, attacks on drug users in New York City (Deren et al., 2002); the use of interviews with government officials, focus groups with survivors, and a survey of evacuees to assess the mental health impacts of a volcano eruption in Ecuador (Tobin & Whiteford, 2002); and the use of formal ethnographic methods, key informant interviews, and standardized questionnaires to assess the mental health effects of the Rwandan genocide (Bolton, 2001).

Typically, mixed-method designs are those that combine qualitative and quantitative methods in a single study or multiphased study. Most typologies of mixed-method designs distinguish between (1) the timing or sequencing of data collection, for example, quantitative preceding qualitative, qualitative preceding quantitative, both operating simultaneously; (2) the priority given to quantitative or qualitative methods, for example, qualitative preceding quantitative if the intent is to first explore the problem under study prior to confirming working hypotheses; qualitative succeeding quantitative if the intent is to explore possible explanations for unanticipated findings; quantitative occurring simultaneously with qualitative if the intent is to triangulate findings; (3) the stage in the research process at which integration of quantitative and qualitative research occurs, for example, specification of research questions, data collection, data analysis, interpretation of results; and (4) the potential use of a transformational value- or action-oriented perspective in the study, for example, to effect social change by placing central importance on the experiences of individuals who suffer from discrimination or oppression, describing reality in its multiple (cultural, political, economic, historical) contexts, and developing understanding and trust between researcher and participant (Cresswell, Clark, Gutmann, & Hanson, 2003).

Mixed methods may serve multiple functions. Among those, the first is triangulation—the corroboration of findings generated through the quantitative analyses with qualitative data collected through semistructured interviews and focus groups. Triangulation is especially important when a small sample size limits the power of hypothesis testing even though the study can provide effect size estimates that are quite valuable for calibrating sample and cluster sizes for subsequent studies.

Related to triangulation, the second function often served by mixed-method designs is complementarity, in which the findings from qualitative studies are employed to assess external as well as internal validity in the absence of sufficient statistical power for an independent assessment of validity. For instance, the administration of survey measures may provide a starting point for semistructured interviews and, conversely, to enhance the validity of the instrument by expanding on domain content to incorporate issues not addressed in the survey measure and place the domains within the specific context of mental health and well-being.

The third function of mixed methods is expansion, in which the results derived from such qualitative methods as semistructured interviews and focus groups are presented side by side with quantitative results to determine whether similar or different conclusions are drawn, based on the data collection strategy employed.

CONCLUSIONS

Qualitative methods are not intended to supplant or replace quantitative methods. For instance, one would never assess the prevalence of PTSD using data collected from open-ended responses to semistructured interviews or from comments made during focus group sessions (Palinkas, Prussing, et al., 2004). To do so would violate fundamental assumptions implicit in the application of quantitative methods (e.g., generalizability, exposure to same stimuli) and would minimize the advantages implicit in the application of qualitative methods (e.g., uncovering the unexpected through exploration, understanding meaning and context, observing interactions). Nevertheless, whether used independently or in combination with quantitative methods, qualitative methods offer enormous potential in understanding the causes and consequences of mental health effects of disasters and terrorism. The application of such methods, however, requires greater communication and collaboration between qualitative and quantitative methodologists as members of multidisciplinary teams of investigators dedicated to examining the social and cultural context of traumatic events as a critical element to understanding their mental health consequences. Such communication and collaboration do not necessarily require the mastery of both sets of methods so much as they require the development of a common understanding as to what each set of methods brings to the research enterprise.

REFERENCES

Atlas.ti. (2004). Berlin: ATLAS.ti Scientific Software Development GmbH. Available online at www.atlasti.com

Bernard, H. R. (2002). *Research methods in anthropology: Qualitative and quantitative approaches* (3 ed.). Newbury Park, CA: Sage.

Blumer, H. (1969). *Symbolic interactionism.* Englewood Cliffs, NJ: Prentice Hall.

Bode, B. (1989). *No bells to toll: Destruction and creation in the Andes.* New York: Scribners.

Bolton, P. (2001). Local perception of the mental health effects of the Rwandan genocide. *Journal of Nervous and Mental Disease, 189,* 243–248.

Bolton, P., & Tang, A. M. (2004). Using ethnographic methods in the selection of postdisaster mental health interventions. *Prehospital and Disaster Medicine, 19,* 97–101.

Creswell, J. W., Clark, V. L., Gutmann, M. L., & Hanson, W. E. (2003). Advanced mixed methods research designs. In A. Tashakkori & C. Teddlie (Eds.), *Handbook of mixed methods in the social and behavioral sciences* (pp. 209–240). Thousand Oaks, CA: Sage.

Deren, S., Shedlin, M., Hamilton, T., & Hagen, H. (2002). Impact of the September 11th attacks in New York City on drug users: A preliminary assessment. *Journal of Urban Health, 79,* 409–412.

Eisenbruch, M. (1991). From posttraumatic stress disorder to cultural bereavement: Diagnosis of Southeast Asian refugees. *Social Science and Medicine, 33,* 673–680.

Fraser, D. (2000). *QSR NVivo NUD*IST Vivo reference guide.* Melbourne: QSR International.

Geertz, C. (1973). *The interpretation of cultures.* New York: Basic Books.

Glaser, B. G., & Strauss, A. L. (1967). *The discovery of grounded theory: Strategies for qualitative research.* New York: Aldine de Gruyter.

Harris, K. J., Jerome, N. W., & Fawcett, S. B. (1997). Rapid assessment procedures: A review and critique. *Human Organization, 56,* 375–378.

Husserl, E. (1931). *Ideas: A general introduction to pure phenomenology.* New York: Humanities Press.

Johnson, J. C., & Weller, S. (2002). Elicitation techniques in interviewing. In J. Gubrium & J. Holstein (Eds.), *Handbook of interview research* (pp. 491–514). Newbury Park, CA: Sage.

Kleinman, A. (1995). *Writing at the margin: Discourse between anthropology and medicine.* Berkeley, CA: University of California Press.

LeCompte, M. D., & Schensul, J. J. (1999). *Designing and conducting ethnographic research.* Walnut Creek, CA: Altamira Press.

Lincoln, Y. S., & Guba, E. G. (1985). *Naturalistic inquiry.* Beverly Hills, CA: Sage.

Marsella, A. J., & Christopher, M. A. (2004). Ethnocultural considerations in disasters: An overview of research, issues, and directions. *Psychiatric Clinics of North America, 27,* 521–539.

Miller, W. L., & Crabtree, B. F. (1992). Primary care research: A multimethod typology and qualitative read map. In B. F. Crabtree & W. L. Miller (Eds.), *Doing qualitative research* (pp. 3–30). Newbury Park, CA: Sage.

Morgan, D. L. (1988). *Focus groups as qualitative research.* Newbury Park, CA: Sage.

Norris, F. H., Weisshar, D. L., Conrad, M. L., Diaz, E. M., Murphy, A. D., & Ibañez, G. E. (2001). A qualitative analysis of posttraumatic stress among Mexican victims of disaster. *Journal of Traumatic Stress, 14,* 741–756.

Oliver-Smith, A. (1992). *The martyred city: Death and rebirth in the Peruvian Andes.* Prospect Heights, IL: Waveland.

Oliver–Smith, A. (1996). Anthropological research on hazards and disasters. *Annual Review of Anthropology, 25,* 303–328.

Palinkas, L. A., Downs, M. A., Petterson, J. S., & Russell, J. (1993). Social, cultural and psychological impacts of the *Exxon Valdez* oil spill. *Human Organization, 52,* 1–13.

Palinkas, L. A., Petterson, J. S., Downs, M. A., & Russell, J. (2004). Ethnic differences in symptoms of posttraumatic stress after the *Exxon Valdez* oil spill. *Prehospital and Disaster Medicine, 19,* 102–112.

Palinkas, L. A., Prussing, E., Landsverk, J., & Reznik, V. M. (2003). Youth violence prevention in the aftermath of the San Diego East County school shootings: A qualitative assessment of community explanatory models. *Ambulatory Pediatrics, 3,* 246–252.

Palinkas, L. A., Prussing, E., Reznik, V. M., & Landsverk J. A. (2004). The San Diego East County school shootings: A qualitative study of community level posttraumatic stress. *Prehospital and Disaster Medicine, 19,* 113–121.

Patton, M. Q. (2002). *Qualitative evaluation and research methods* (3rd ed.). Thousand Oaks, CA: Sage.

Ricouer, P. (1981). *Hermeneutics and the human sciences.* Cambridge, UK: Cambridge University Press.

Scrimshaw, S. C. M., & Hurtado, E. (1987). *Rapid assessment procedures for nutrition and primary health care.* Los Angeles: UCLA Latin American Center Publications.

Sofaer, S. (1999). Qualitative methods: What are they and why use them? *Health Services Research, 34,* 1101–1118.

Spradley, J. P. (1979). *The ethnographic interview.* New York: Holt, Rinehart & Winston.

Stallings, R. A. (1997). Methods of disaster research: Unique or not? *International Journal of Mass Emergencies and Disasters, 15,* 7–19.

Teddlie, C., & Tashakkori, A. (2003). Major issues and controversies in the use of mixed methods in the social and behavioral sciences. In A. Tashakkori, & C. Teddlie (Eds.),

Handbook of mixed methods in the social and behavioral sciences (pp. 3–50). Thousand Oaks, CA: Sage.

Tobin, G. A., & Whiteford, L. M. (2002). Community resilience and volcano hazard: The eruption of Tungurahua and evacuation of the faldas in Ecuador. *Disasters, 26,* 28–48.

Weller, S. C., & Romney, A. K. (1988). *Systematic data collection.* Newbury Park, CA: Sage.

Young, A. (1995). *The harmony of illusions: Inventing post-traumatic stress disorder.* Princeton, NJ: Princeton University Press.

PART IV

Research for Planning, Policy, and Service Delivery

CHAPTER 11

Public Mental Health Surveillance and Monitoring

SANDRO GALEA and FRAN H. NORRIS

Public health surveillance is "the ongoing, systematic collection, analysis, interpretation, and dissemination of data about a health-related event for use in public health action to reduce morbidity and mortality and to improve health" (Centers for Disease Control and Prevention [CDC], 2001a, p. 1). A public health surveillance system should include the capacity for systematically collecting data, its analysis, and dissemination of results to persons who can implement effective interventions. Historically, most surveillance efforts and systems have focused on communicable disease detection, and it is only recently that the notion of surveillance has been broadened to include surveillance for chronic diseases and, potentially, mental disorders. It is the purpose of this chapter to frame the key issues surrounding public health surveillance as they might apply to mental health. To do so, first we will summarize the history of and key concepts underlying public health surveillance. Second, we will discuss key issues in the collection and analysis of surveillance data with particular reference to the relevance of these issues to public mental health surveillance. Third, we will discuss the central role that public mental health surveillance can play in mitigating the mental health consequences of disasters. We will conclude with a discussion of the potential features of a national public mental health surveillance system.

PUBLIC HEALTH SURVEILLANCE: HISTORY AND KEY CONCEPTS

Evolution of Public Health Surveillance

The notion of systematically collecting data for public health purposes is not new, and dates back to Hippocrates (Eylenbosch & Noah, 1998). Formal efforts at public health surveillance probably began in the Middle Ages, when public health officials in Italy systematically assessed persons onboard ships, screening for bubonic plague, with the intention of quarantining such persons and preventing them from spreading disease in the general population (Moro & McCormick, 1988). In the 18th century, governments in western Europe increasingly assumed responsibility for the health of their populations and established regulations about the handling of food, burial, and the pollution of public water. The evolution of public health as a formal profession followed soon. For example, in France, rapidly changing demographics and the economic situation in urban areas contributed to *hygiene publique*, or public health, becoming formally constituted as a science (Coleman, 1982). During the first half of the 19th century, Louis René Villermé and other *hygienistes* implemented programs aimed at monitoring disease conditions in France. Contemporaneously, in London, William Farr, one of the founders of the modern concept of surveillance, in his capacity as the superintendent of the statistical department of the Registrar General's office of England and Wales, developed systems for collecting vital statistics and disseminating those data to policymakers and to the general public (Langmuir, 1976).

Systematic collection and reporting of disease data in the United States began in 1874 in Massachusetts; in 1878, Congress authorized the collection of morbidity data for use in quarantine against infectious diseases such as yellow fever (Trask, 1915). The poliomyelitis epidemic of 1916 and the influenza pandemic of 1918–1919 prompted participation in national morbidity reporting by all U.S. states by 1925 (National Office of Vital Statistics, 1953). The use of survey data as a means of surveillance is relatively new, with the first national health survey in the United States being conducted in 1935 (Thacker, 2000).

Prerequisites to Public Health Surveillance

As the historic examples suggest, there are several key prerequisites to the development and functioning of a public health system in general, and to surveillance systems in particular. Perhaps most fundamentally, a public health surveillance system needs to be grounded on a functioning and organized health care system within a stable government. Although, at this writing, countries in the Western world have developed such systems, public health surveillance remains rudimentary or simply absent in many parts of the world where national governments function poorly if at all. Second, public health surveillance rests on clear classification of illness and disease (Thacker, 2000). As we shall discuss further on in this chapter, this continues to be a particular challenge in the context of developing effective and practicable public mental health surveillance. Third, public health surveillance fundamentally relies on accurate, replicable measurement systems that incorporate both the collection of data systematically as well as its timely analysis and consistent interpretation. The development of statistics and epidemiology as viable disciplines during the past 150 years has provided public health professionals with the tools needed to collect and evaluate surveillance data.

Evolving Concepts of Surveillance

Coincident with the evolution of systematic data collection for the purpose of public health monitoring, the notion of what constitutes surveillance has also been evolving, particularly in the past 50 years. There are three concepts worth mentioning in this regard. First is the question of whether surveillance functions include public health intervention. Early concepts of surveillance incorporated both the monitoring of disease as well as implementation of public health intervention to address the detected disease, but now the term *surveillance* is limited to the collection and dissemination of data, thus separating public health *intervention* (i.e., disease control) functions from disease monitoring (Langmuir, 1963; Thacker, 2000).

The historic, and growing, role of infectious disease monitoring at the heart of surveillance also merits comment. Much of our thinking about surveillance has evolved from public health systems aimed at monitoring communicable disease transmission. Therefore, earlier concepts of surveillance were rooted in infectious disease concepts and paradigms. Although modern surveillance has expanded substantially beyond these paradigms, in many respects monitoring infectious diseases remains at the core of surveillance functions in the United States and in much of the world. In the wake of recent fears about bioterrorism, substantial investment has been made in infrastructural development for the purposes of enhancing infectious disease surveillance throughout the country. However, development of surveillance for less traditional diseases, including psychiatric disorders, has not kept pace. As we will discuss below, there are particular considerations relevant to mental health surveillance that require advancing beyond notions of surveillance centered on infectious diseases.

A final note is about the relationship between surveillance and research. Public health surveillance has traditionally been a public health function that is primarily concerned with the description of diseases in the population. However, integral to public health surveillance is the interpretation of patterns and an effort to understand why diseases are occurring in a specific manner. Research is typically considered to be original investigation undertaken to gain knowledge or understanding. Therefore, research would exclude the routine data collection and analysis that is typical of surveillance systems. However, the line between the two often blurs. Data that are collected primarily for surveillance purposes can lead, and frequently have led, to the advancement of knowledge. Also, surveillance systems have amassed tremendous amounts of data that have contributed to etiological insights about behaviors and chronic disease. For the purposes of this chapter we consider surveillance to be the collection of data for the express purpose of monitoring population health and disease. We consider surveillance to be a function of public health practice, not research, but recognize that data collected for surveillance purposes also can contribute to the advancement of knowledge when it is called upon to serve as a foundation for biomedical and behavioral research.

Types of Public Health Surveillance Systems

One can classify surveillance systems in several ways. We adopted a functionalist perspective based on mode of data gathering: (1) intensive disease-specific monitoring, (2) syndromic surveillance, and (3) systematic data collection and monitoring.

Disease-Specific Monitoring

The earliest form of surveillance, and probably the dominant and most common form of surveillance in place today, involves the focused and intensive monitoring of potentially worrisome diseases, typically infectious diseases. During the Middle Ages, Venetian public health officials who boarded ships in an attempt to stop passengers with the bubonic plague from disembarking were practicing a form of disease-based monitoring. Disease-specific monitoring may be *passive* or *active*. Passive systems are initiated by providers, in which health care practitioners who observe an unusual disease pattern notify local health authorities, who then investigate. The 1999 outbreak of West Nile virus in New York City was a classic case of provider-initiated surveillance where a local physician, noting an unusual disease manifestation, notified the New York Department of Health and Mental Hygiene, which subsequently conducted an investigation (Nash et al., 2001). Active surveillance systems are generally initiated or supervised by public health authorities. Mandatory reporting is in place for many infectious diseases in the United States, and local and state public health authorities monitor these reports for unusually high rates of particular diseases and launch investigations where appropriate. Both active and passive forms of disease-specific surveillance thus rest on disease case-finding and the subsequent investigation of detected anomalies.

Syndromic Surveillance Systems

Syndromic surveillance is the monitoring of key health events or symptoms through specific sites, events, health providers, or laboratories. Syndromic surveillance systems use data that are not necessarily diagnostic of a disease, but rather suggest early stages of a disease in the community. A manual form of syndromic surveillance was used to detect additional anthrax cases in the fall of 2001 in New York City after the recognition of the initial anthrax case (Tan et al., 2002). The key characteristic of syndromic surveillance is the use of both symptom and indicator data, such as chief complaints in emergency departments, retail drug purchases, and work absenteeism. Therefore, syndromic surveillance extends the traditional unit of analytic interest in surveillance beyond the typical infectious disease outcomes to other proxy outcomes using new data types.

Systematic Data Collection and Monitoring

Systematic monitoring of health, risk behavior, and disease is a cornerstone of public health surveillance in the United States. These systems collect data on a regular basis expressly for the purposes of monitoring health and behavior. Several such formal systematic surveillance systems are currently in place. Key among these are (1) the Behavioral Risk Factor Surveillance System (BRFSS), a monthly telephone interview of U.S. adult residents that focuses on assessing changes in risk behavior over time; (2) the National Health and Nutrition Examination Survey (NHANES), which conducts in-person interviews and collects biometric data from a nationally representative sample; and (3) the National Health Interview Survey (NHIS), an annual in-person interview with a representative sample of U.S. residents. Information from these surveys and systematic collections of biometric data has been invaluable to monitor disease trends in the United States over time and to guide national policy and interventions. For example, the recent concern about the rising prevalence of obesity nationwide arose in response to BRFSS and NHIS results. Although there is currently no formal surveillance system dedicated to mental health surveillance, the National Comorbidity Survey, fielded from the fall of 1990 to the spring of 1992, was the first nationally representative mental health survey in the United States to use a fully structured research diagnostic interview to assess the prevalence and correlates of DSM-III-R disorders (Kessler et al., 1994). The recent replication of this study, fielded in 2001 and 2002, has allowed us a glimpse into the potential of such monitoring, documenting the patterns and predictors of the course of mental and substance use disorders and evaluating the effects of primary mental disorders in predicting the onset and course of secondary substance disorders (Kessler et al, 2005).

KEY ISSUES IN THE SURVEILLANCE OF MENTAL HEALTH

Mental health has not historically been, nor is it currently, a focus of surveillance in the United States. It probably should be. Mental and behavioral disorders affect more than 25% of people during their lifetime and are estimated to be present in 10% of the adult population at any given time (World Health Organization, 2001). The *Global Burden of Disease* report for 2000 (Murray & Lopez, 1996) estimated that mental health problems accounted for 12% of the total Disability Adjusted Life Years (DALYs) lost worldwide and for 31% of the years of life lived with a disability. Beyond their impact on the individual, mental health and behavioral problems are frequently accompanied by social and economic impact on families and society. For example, it is estimated that anxiety and depression account for up to a third of all presentations in primary care settings (Goldberg & Lecubrier, 1995; Katon, Kleinman, & Rosen, 1982; Marks, 1986).

Of the challenges that will be faced in the implementation of mental health surveillance, three are particularly noteworthy: (1) establishing case definitions of "disease" and disorders; (2) linking syndromic data on symptoms to morbidity, dysfunction, and needs; and (3) deriving models appropriate for analyzing and interpreting mental health surveillance data.

Establishing Case Definitions

Public health surveillance depends upon the extant definitions of what constitutes health and disease and an appreciation of the baseline prevalence of disease. The definitions of diseases that are commonly subject to surveillance, particularly infectious diseases, are well established. The definition of disease, however, is potentially more complicated when considering mental health outcomes. Although the establishment of the *Diagnostic and Statistical Manual of Mental Disorders* (DSM) has systematized psychiatric definitions, and the science of psychiatric nosology is advancing rapidly, the ongoing revisions of psychiatric definitions through subsequent versions of the DSM suggest that this challenge will continue to dog public mental health surveillance efforts for years to come. There is also tremendous interpractitioner variability in the diagnosis of psychiatric disorders, suggesting that passive surveillance of mental health may be particularly challenging.

There are several promising developments that may help overcome this challenge. Standardized diagnostic instruments, such as the Composite International Diagnostic Interview (CIDI; World Health Organization, 1997), that have been used in national and international prevalence estimate surveys (Andrade et al., 2003) provide a common point of reference that could be used as the building block of active surveillance. Yet, the time and training required to administer diagnostic interview schedules would make this a costly approach that may not be practical in many situations.

Linking Symptoms to Morbidity and Needs

Syndromic surveillance methods hold particular promise for effective monitoring of the public's mental health. Surveillance of self-reported psychological symptoms (e.g., posttraumatic stress, depression, general distress) or other indicators (e.g., psychiatric presentations to emergency departments) may transcend some of the definitional and implementation challenges associated with a disease-specific approach. However, an issue of particular importance for syndromic mental health surveillance is the meaning of distress in the absence of reports of impaired functioning. If surveillance systems identify symptoms that do not reflect morbidity, the link between surveillance and attendant action may be tenuous. Thus, it is advisable to measure both distress and dysfunction in mental health surveillance.

A related concern is the utility of surveillance data for community needs assessment. Population surveys have long been held to be superior to most other approaches to needs assessment in terms of the scientific quality of the data they provide (Bell, Warheit, & Schwab, 1977). As defined by McKillup (1998, p. 261), a need is a *value judgment* that a particular group in a particular circumstance has a problem that can be solved by appropriate action. This definition implies that data on the prevalence of disorder, distress, and dysfunction are most useful if they lead to conclusions about needs/problems and actions/solutions. For this to be true, information about the extent to which distress and dysfunction are elevated (presumably meaning that need for services is elevated) must be coupled with information on barriers to use of services, especially key elements of availability, awareness, acceptability, and accessibility. Moreover, it is advisable to balance assessment of needs or deficits with assessment of resources or strengths that community members can draw upon to address those needs.

Deriving Analytic Models

An additional challenge for mental health surveillance is the need for further development of appropriate models for analyzing and interpreting the data. The absence of longitudinal mental health data collected from population-based samples limits our understanding of the natural course of mental disorders. Underlying patterns (e.g., seasonal variations) and systematic errors (e.g., climate changes that influence reporting of depressive disorders) may complicate the interpretation of cross-sectional data on mental health (Strup, Brookmeyer, & Kalsbeek, 2004).

In addition, well-established models for infectious disease surveillance may not be directly applicable to mental health surveillance. For example, models of spatiotemporal analysis that take into account the spread of infectious disease through interpersonal contact may not be relevant for the analysis of mental health surveillance where social contagion may have substantially different implications. Similarly, well-documented ecological inference problems in the analysis of surveillance data (i.e., drawing conclusions about the individual likelihood of disease from observed population rates of disease) may be less of a concern in the context of mental health surveillance that is intended to guide the implementation of community-level (ecological) interventions. None of these problems is insurmountable, and with the growing systematization of public mental health assessments and the potential implementation of surveillance systems, these problems will be tackled and solved. However, in the short term, they represent important considerations in the development and analysis of public mental health surveillance.

PUBLIC MENTAL HEALTH SURVEILLANCE IN THE CONTEXT OF DISASTERS

Estimating Mental Health Burden after a Disaster

We see three contributions of mental health surveillance in the aftermath of disasters. First, most importantly, public mental health surveillance can play a key role in helping to monitor the morbidity associated with postdisaster distress and disorder. One of the primary challenges faced by public health planners in the aftermath of a disaster is to accurately document the scope of the potential mental health consequences of the event. Our ability to do this is limited, and recent events have provided ample examples of the misestimation of the consequences of disasters. Most notably, after the September 11, 2001, terrorist attacks, predictions of incident psychopathology in New York City were substantially higher than was subsequently borne out in empirical study. Such questions will continue to be difficult to answer unless comparable data are collected at regular intervals across major disasters. Such documentation will, over time, establish a much clearer understanding of the natural history of psychopathology after disasters.

Although surveillance of disaster-related morbidity may well begin in the immediate aftermath of the event, ideally postdisaster surveillance is embedded within a system of ongoing mental health surveillance that has provided normative (predisaster or baseline) data on a local, regional, or national level. The larger mental health surveillance system could convincingly establish norms for the population and subpopulations, making the interpretation of estimates of the mental health burden after a disaster easier. One of the key limitations of current postdisaster estimates of psychopathology is that public heath practitioners cannot be certain of the extent to which documented psychosocial problems are higher than they might have been anyway, regardless of the disaster. For example, Norris and colleagues' (Norris, Murphy, Baker, & Kaniasty, 2005) ability to show that their sample of displaced Mexican disaster victims had strikingly low social support was enhanced by the availability of concurrent Mexican norms for their measures of social support. Unless the surveillance is undertaken on a very large scale, only rarely can surveillance samples themselves be studied prospectively in the aftermath of disaster, but it would happen occasionally. Two sites in the Epidemiologic Catchment Area Survey (St. Louis and Puerto Rico), for example, experienced major disasters within a year or two and were reassessed (Bravo, Rubio-Stipec, Canino, Woodbury, & Ribera, 1990; Robins et al., 1986).

Evaluating Effects of Policies and Interventions and Facilitating Planning

Second, an early understanding of the potential mental health consequences of disasters can guide the implementation of programs that may alleviate some of the burden of psychopathology. Returning to the earlier point about the translation of surveillance data to value judgments about community needs is also important. A question that in our minds remains unanswered is whether the symptoms documented in postdisaster studies constitute psychopathology or whether they are simply normal and transient reactions to mass traumatic events. The two alternatives have different implications for postdisaster intervention, with the former implying the need for expanded clinical services, the latter implying the need for psychosocial programs that provide support, educate that public about expected reactions to trauma, and identify the minority of persons who are at risk for longer-term adverse reactions.

The evidence base for interventions aimed at improving population mental health in the aftermath of disasters is nascent (Gibson, Hamlden, Zvolensky, & Vujanovich, Chapter 13, this volume; Marshall, Amsel, Neria, & Suh, Chapter 14, this volume). Similarly, very few empirical studies have successfully demonstrated a link between public health policies and mental health in select groups after disaster. What we do know about what may or may not work after a disaster stems from two sources: (1) findings of studies aimed at assessing specific interventions that may not be generalizable to other postdisaster contexts; and (2) studies that have assessed proxy markers of mental health status, such as emergency department or hospital ward presentations. Not surprisingly, results from the latter type of studies have frequently been inconclusive as investigators are forced to draw inference from insufficient or suboptimal data.

Unfortunately, until we can determine with some degree of certainty whether specific interventions are efficacious in reducing the burden of psychopathology after a disaster, it will remain difficult for public health practitioners and policymakers to devote resources to novel interventions aimed at minimizing this psychopathology. Definitive assessments of crisis counseling programs and other forms of postdisaster intervention are hampered by the absence of baseline data and by our limited understanding of what the course of psychopathology in the population after these disasters may have been had these programs not been implemented. Therefore, a public mental health surveillance system, through establishing baseline prevalence and natural history of psychopathology, will lend itself to assessing how this excess prevalence may be reduced, or recovery hastened, by social experimentation. Moreover, such surveillance could tap achievement of key public health intervention goals, such as the public's understanding of program messages, awareness of services, and reduction of stigma. This clearly lies at the heart of what a postdisaster mental health surveillance system could achieve and how it would ultimately improve the health of the population. Policymakers may be more willing to invest in bold public mental health interventions within the context of a surveillance system that can systematically evaluate the impact of such interventions.

Generating Hypotheses and Stimulating Research

Third, a program of postdisaster surveillance could advance the research agenda in this field. One of the major criticisms of current research assessing the mental health consequences of disasters is that far too often disaster research concerns itself with documenting the prevalence of psychopathology after a disaster at the expense of tackling more challenging, and in the long-term more rewarding, etiological research questions (see Benight, McFarlane, & Norris, Chapter 4, this volume). Although we concur that this criticism is valid, absent an appreciation of the scope of the consequences of a given disaster, and given concerns about generalizability of results stemming from studies that were designed only to assess the consequences of a disaster in a particular context, it is unavoidable that researchers and public health practitioners will first and foremost be concerned with the magnitude of the mental health consequences of the disaster that has stricken their community. The presence of an effective public mental health surveillance system would obviate such research. More important than rendering these basic prevalence questions unnecessary, a public mental health surveillance system can stimulate etiological research that asks *why* we may observe specific consequences in certain groups. Analogously, very little research today concerns itself with assessing the prevalence of infectious diseases in the United States; much of those estimates are available through health departments and their surveillance systems. This has both freed up researchers to pursue questions pertaining to the etiology of infectious diseases and their transmission and has provided data that has guided inquiry into the full range of potential risk factors from genetic factors, to individual behaviors, to contextual determinants.

A STRATEGY FOR NATIONAL PUBLIC MENTAL HEALTH SURVEILLANCE IN THE UNITED STATES

We make no attempt here at specific prescription regarding implementation of a public mental health surveillance system, recognizing that such prescription is far beyond the scope of a book chapter. We offer instead a brief discussion of the central tenets of such a system that might overcome the challenges it could face and maximize its potential. Below, we describe the purposes, stakeholders, and essential features of the proposed system and conclude by describing a tiered system under development by a federally sponsored working group.

Purposes

Any public mental health surveillance system needs to have a clearly defined purpose that is conservative enough to be achievable but bold enough to make such a system truly effective. We make three primary recommendations. First, we recommend a functionally hybrid system to maximize cost-effectiveness. Because frequent disease-specific surveillance of psychological disorders (diagnoses) would be prohibitively expensive, we recommend ongoing syndromic surveillance focusing on key indicators of current depression, posttraumatic stress, dysfunction, anxieties/fears, and psychosocial resources, punctuated with occasional disease-specific surveys that provide reliable estimates of current psychological disorders and more in-depth assessment of risk/protective factors. The periodic combination of the two types of data (indicators and diagnoses) would facilitate interpretation of the indicator data, which would be collected more frequently and regularly.

Second, we recommend that surveillance be implemented on a large enough scale as to provide hybrid data for specific racial, ethnic, and socioeconomic groups. This information would increase understanding of the differences in the need for and use of mental health services. In light of the threat of terrorism, the surveillance system should overrepresent large urban centers, such as New York City and Los Angeles.

Third, we recommend that public mental health surveillance aim to educate major stakeholders, including the general public. The fact that relatively fewer resources are devoted to mental health as compared to physical health stems largely from lack of understanding of the nature of mental health problems, the stigma that remains associated with mental health problems, and misconceptions about the burden of psychopathology in the general population. The early efforts by public health practitioners such as William Farr to document health status and to use such documentation to guide public health intervention were instrumental in educating the public about health measurement and, indirectly, in making physical disease a subject worthy of governmental attention and intervention. Public mental health surveillance needs to make a similar contribution today.

Stakeholders

A public mental health surveillance system needs to be responsive to a wide range of stakeholders without bogging such a system down with competing demands from disparate groups' interests. As medical care becomes increasingly sophisticated and complicated, the implementation of public mental health surveillance would have important implications for diverse entities. Clearly, such a system needs to be developed in concert with national and local public health authorities. Most of the surveillance efforts in the United States are conducted by the Centers for Disease Control and Prevention (CDC) or by local health authorities. Federal leadership in developing such a system would then be natural, with the inclusion of representatives from local health authorities being critical both to system implementation and to acceptance of system results. Apart from federal and local public health authorities, it is likely that SAMHSA, NIMH, the medical–industrial complex, medical practitioners, mental health professionals, and patient (client) groups would also be key stakeholders in such a system. Clearly, multiple stakeholders run the risk of grounding any effort at developing public mental health surveillance. A clear and committed vision about the usefulness of the task at hand as a high priority for national public health would be essential to transcend the sectarian differences that one might expect in any such process.

Essential Features

The exact form that public mental health surveillance could take would depend, of necessity, on a balance between desired system purpose, resources available, and political compromise. Regardless of the specific mechanisms of its implementation, four features of any such system would be preeminent: usefulness, acceptability, stability, and flexibility.

First and foremost, public mental health surveillance needs to be *useful*. Keeping this feature in mind may avoid many of the potential pitfalls in its development. Surveillance certainly should be good enough to generate hypotheses and stimulate research, but its primary purpose is to provide data to inform public mental health efforts. Therefore, public mental health surveillance needs to be useful to its primary consumers—public health practitioners.

A viable public mental health surveillance system must be *acceptable* to all key stakeholders. There can be several barriers to acceptability of a public mental health system. For example, nosological issues and assessment controversies may jeopardize the extent to which surveillance data are accepted and used. Similarly, developers of mental health surveillance must grapple early with the concept of what truly constitutes "need" in mental health. A system that produces data without clear guidelines for practitioners as to what might constitute grounds for intervention would likely quickly be unacceptable, in addition to not being useful.

A public mental health surveillance system must also be *stable*. Some of the most useful surveillance systems currently in place are made all the more useful by virtue of their longevity, having provided data over time that allows policymakers to see trends emerge and consider their actions. For example, it is the *rise* in obesity nationwide, as documented through ongoing surveillance such as the BRFSS and NHANES, more than the current absolute prevalence of obesity itself that is driving national concern about the issue and attendant public health interventions. Similarly, efforts to ban smoking in public spaces are buttressed by assessments of surveillance data over time that suggest that these efforts may indeed decrease the prevalence of smoking in the population. Therefore, maximizing the utility of mental health surveillance will require a long-term commitment to stable funding for such a system. Implementation of a system that meets its intended goals but is affordable is probably better than the development of an overly sophisticated but unsustainable system. The addition of mental health surveillance to ongoing health surveillance efforts may prove, in the long term, to be more cost-effective than the *de novo* development and implementation of a national mental health surveillance system.

Much as a public mental health surveillance system needs to be stable and robust to changing political pressures, it must also be *flexible*, able to be adapted to provide policymakers and public health practitioners with useful information. This may be most readily apparent in considering how such a system must contribute to the disaster relief effort. Any public mental health surveillance in the United States should be scalable to heightened surveillance during periods of particular concern, such as after disasters. Therefore, resources and reserves should be built into the system such that it can provide different, or more, data if necessary.

Work in Progress

Our proposal is largely consistent with that of a national "needs assessment working group" whose work is in progress as of this writing (personal communication, Patricia Watson, May 22, 2005). In August 2003, an international panel of experts was convened in Bethesda, Maryland, to discuss screening, assessment, outreach, and intervention for mental health and substance abuse needs following disasters and mass violence. The meeting was sponsored by the U.S. Department of Veterans Affairs and the U.S. Department of Health and Human Services, including representatives of the National Institute of Mental Health, CDC, and SAMHSA's Center for Mental Health Services, the agency responsible for administering the federal crisis counseling program after presidentially declared disasters. Several working groups were formed by the panel. One of these working groups focused on needs assessment and surveillance and organized its recommendations using the concept of tiers.

Tier 1 was composed of a 5- to 10-minute set of surveillance items assessing functioning, exposure to traumatic stress, distress, behavior change, and perceptions of risk, to be included within an existing ongoing national health survey. Tier 2 involved a more in-depth assessment that would be implemented after a critical event in a community, the purpose of which would be to gather information that would inform intervention. In Tier 2, a 20- to 25-minute set of surveillance items would be administered via a phone survey to separate samples drawn randomly on a weekly or monthly basis following a disaster or terrorist incident. Tier 2 would track several topics of potential policy relevance, including distress, functioning, and continued needs of the community; media habits and how people receive information; perceptions of risk and recovery; perceived barriers to services and trusted sources of information; and the reach and impact of screening, outreach, and intervention efforts. Tier 3 would mark a shift of purposes from surveillance to research by supporting in-depth studies on predictors of resilience to posttraumatic psychopathology; genetic and environmental interactions that increase risk for posttraumatic disorders; biomarkers, behavioral assessments, and phenotypic characterizations of posttraumatic disorders; neurohormonal, physiological, and behavioral parameters in disease development; and the success/failure of current and new interventions.

CONCLUSIONS

There is little question in our minds that the health of the public would be well served by the development of a program of comprehensive public mental health surveillance. Many factors have slowed the evolution of mental health surveillance, but none is insurmountable. The science of surveillance is rapidly evolving, as is the science of mental health in general. With suitable political will, public mental health surveillance is achievable and has the potential to immeasurably add to our knowledge of the general population's mental health, improve our responses to disasters, and integrate mental health concerns into the mainstream of medicine and public health.

ACKNOWLEDGMENTS

Preparation of this chapter was supported by Grant Nos. R25 MH070552, R01 DA 017642, R01 MH 66081, and R01 MH 066391 and by Grant No. R25 MH068298 from the National Institutes of Health.

REFERENCES

Andrade, L., Caraveo-Anduaga, J., Berglund, P., Bijl, R., De Graaf, R., & Vollebergh, W. (2003). The epidemiology of major depressive episodes: Results from the International Consortium of Psychiatric Epidemiology (ICPE) Surveys. *International Journal of Methods Psychiatry Research, 12,* 3–21.

Bell, R., Warheit, G., & Schwab, J. (1977). Needs assessment: A strategy for structuring change. In R. Coursey, G. Specter, S. Murrell, & B. Hunt (Eds.), *Program evaluation in mental health: Methods, strategies, and participants* (pp. 67–76). New York: Grune & Stratton.

Bravo, M., Rubio-Stipec, M., Canino, G., Woodbury, M., & Ribera, J. (1990). The psychological sequelae of disaster stress prospectively and retrospectively evaluated. *American Journal of Community Psychology, 18,* 661–680.

Centers for Disease Control and Prevention. (2001a). Updated guidelines for evaluating public health surveillance systems: Recommendations from the guidelines working group. *Morbidity and Mortality Weekly Report 2001, 50*(No. RR–13), 1–35.

Coleman, C. (1982). *Death is a social disease: Public health and political economy in early industrial France.* Madison, WI: University of Wisconsin Press.

Eylenbosch, W. J., & Noah, N. D. (1998). Historical aspects. In W. J. Eylenbosch & N. D. Noah (Eds.), *Surveillance in health and disease* (pp. 3–8). Oxford, UK: Oxford University Press.

Goldberg, D. P., & Lecubrier, Y. (1995). Form and frequency of mental disorders across centers. In T. B. Ostun & N. Sartorius (Eds.), *Mental illness in general health care: An international study* (pp. 323–334). Chichester, UK: Wiley (on behalf of the World Health Organization).

Katon, W., Kleinman, A., & Rosen, G. (1982). Depression and somatization: Part I. A review. *American Journal of Medicine, 72,* 127–135.

Kessler, R. C., McGonagle, K. A., Zhao, S., Nelson, C. B, Hughes, M., Eshleman, S., et al. (1994). Lifetime and 12-month prevalence of DSM-III-R psychiatric disorders in the United States: Results from the National Comorbidity Survey. *Archives of General Psychiatry, 51*(1), 8–19.

Kessler, R. C., Demler, O., Frank, R. G., Olfson, M., Pincus, H. A., Walters, E. E, et al. (2005). Prevalence and treatment of mental disorders, 1990 to 2003. *New England Journal of Medicine, 16,* 2515–2523.

Langmuir, A. D. (1963). The surveillance of communicable diseases of national importance. *New England Journal of Medicine, 268,* 182–192.

Langmuir, A. D. (1976). William Farr: Founder of modern concepts of surveillance. *International Journal of Epidemiology, 5,* 13–18.

Marks, I. M. (1986). Epidemiology of anxiety. *Social Psychiatry, 21,* 167–171.

McKillip, J. (1998). Need analysis: Process and techniques. In L. Bickman & D. Rog (Eds.), *Handbook of applied social research methods* (pp. 261–284). Thousand Oaks, CA: Sage.

Murray, C. J. L., & Lopez, A. D. (Eds.). (1996). *The global burden of disease: A comprehensive assessment of mortality and disability from diseases, injuries and risk factors from 1990 and projected to 2020* (report, Global Burden of Disease and Injury Series, Vol. I). Cambridge, MA: Harvard School of Public Health (on behalf of the World Health Organization and the World Bank).

Moro, M. L., & McCormick, A. (1998). Surveillance for communicable disease. In W. J. Eylenbosch & D. Noahh (Eds.), *Surveillance in health and disease* (pp. 166–182). Oxford, UK: Oxford University Press.

Nash, D., Mostashari, F., Fine, A., Miller, J., O'Leary, D., & Murray, K. (2001). The outbreak of West Nile virus infection in the New York City area in 1999. *New England Journal of Medicine, 344,* 1807–1814.

National Office of Vital Statistics. (1953). Reported incidence of selected notifiable disease: United States, each division and state, 1920–1950. *Vital Statistics Select Reports* (National Summaries), *37,* 1180–1181.

Norris, F., Baker, C., Murphy, A., & Kaniasty, K. (2005). Social support mobilization and deterioration after Mexico's 1999 flood: Effects of context, gender, and time. *American Journal of Community Psychology, 36* (1–2), 15–28.

Robins, L., Fischbach, R., Smith, E., Cottler, L., Solomon, S., & Goldring, E. (1986). Impact of disaster on previously assessed mental health. In J. Shore (Ed.), *Disaster stress studies: New methods and findings* (pp. 22–48). Washington, DC: American Psychiatric Press.

Stroup, D. F., Brookmeyer, R., & Kalsbeek, W. D. (2004). Public health surveillance in action: A framework. In R. Brookmeyer & D. Stroup (Eds.), *Monitoring the health of populations: Statistical principles and methods for public health surveillance* (pp. 1–36). Oxford, UK: Oxford University Press.

Tan, C. G., Sandhu, H. S., Crawford, D. C., Redd, S. C., Beach, M. J., & Buehler, J. W. (2002). Surveillance for anthrax cases associated with contaminated letters, New Jersey, Delaware, and Pennsylvania, 2001. *Emerging Infectious Disease, 8,* 1073–1076.

Thacker, S. B. (2000). Historical development. In S. M. Teutsch & R. E. Churchill (Eds.), *Principles and practice of public health surveillance* (2nd ed., pp. 1–16). Oxford, UK: Oxford University Press, 2000.

Trask, J. W. (1915). Vital statistics: A discussion of what they are and their uses in public health administration. *Public Health Report 1915, 30*–34.

World Bank. (1993). *World Development report 1993: Investing in health.* New York: Oxford University Press (for the World Bank).

World Health Organization. (1997). *Composite International Diagnostic Interview (CIDI). Version 2.1.* Geneva, Switzerland: Author.

World Health Organization. (2001). *Mental health: New understanding, new hope.* Geneva, Switzerland: Author.

CHAPTER 12

Mental Health Services and Evaluation Research
Precepts, Pragmatics, and Politics

CRAIG S. ROSEN and HELENA E. YOUNG

Research on the psychological effects of disasters and terrorist acts has expanded greatly over the past several years. A growing body of experimental research has also examined the efficacy of different psychosocial interventions in aiding recovery from traumatic events. Yet, the organization and delivery of disaster mental health services remain largely guided by tradition and clinical judgment (Litz & Gray, 2002). There are few empirical data on the amount, type, and quality of services disaster survivors typically receive; even less is known about how helpful these services are in facilitating recovery.

In this chapter, we consider the use of program evaluation in mental health services research that examines the reach, quality, and outcomes of disaster-driven service programs. We focus on three major themes. The *precepts*, or core principles and research questions in health services research and program evaluation, are discussed, emphasizing the use of theoretical frameworks to generate and test hypotheses about program operation and service delivery. The *pragmatics* of data gathering are explored, emphasizing the use of archival data sources. We also discuss the *politics* of evaluation, particularly the importance of engaging stakeholders in the design, implementation, interpretation, and reporting of evaluation research.

PRECEPTS: WHAT IS HEALTH
SERVICES RESEARCH?

Program evaluation is a discipline involving the assessment of activities and outcomes of defined social programs or policy initiatives; in medicine, this province is often referred to as health services research. Investigations in the health services research domain consider how social factors, financing systems, organizational structures, technology, and human behavior influence health care delivery, quality, cost, access, and outcomes (Agency for Healthcare Research and Quality, 2001). Health services research focuses on studying "what is" under naturalistic field conditions, rather than "what is possible" in controlled environments.

Typical research problems relevant to disaster mental health include: What resources are available for providing services after disasters or terrorist attacks? Who is in the greatest need of services? Who seeks out and obtains access to services? What kinds and quantities of services do survivors receive? Is care delivered in accordance with best practices? What client, setting, or context factors influence access to and quality of services? Is receipt of services associated with improved functioning?

Using Program Theory to Generate and Clarify Research Questions

The program theory, or logic model, is the set of hypotheses and causal assumptions about how the program works (Weiss, 1997). An explicit program theory enables stakeholders to determine not only what a program is accomplishing but also why a program is successful in meeting its goals. If programs fail to deliver expected results, the logic model can be used to disentangle whether these effects arise from features of program delivery, unreliable data, or basic flaws in the program theory (Scheirer, 1987).

Elements of the Logic Model

Logic models specify a program's inputs, activities, outputs, and outcomes. Figure 12.1 illustrates a theoretical model for a postdisaster counseling program. Event characteristics, such as the type of event or the estimated number of people needing services, can influence the various elements of the logic model. Disaster mental health services may also be influenced by the demographics of the affected community.

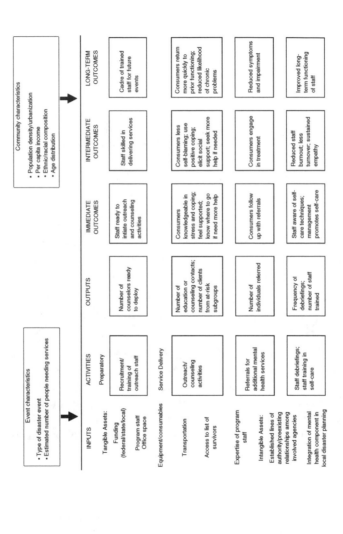

FIGURE 12.1. Logic model for a crisis counseling program.

196

Inputs include the tangible and intangible assets available to the program. *Activities*, the ways in resources are deployed to effect programmatic objectives, include preparatory activities (e.g., hiring staff and interagency networking) and direct service delivery (psychoeducation, public relations and outreach, crisis or intensive counseling, and referral coordination). *Outputs* are quantified with respect to "how much" service was rendered (the number of staff trained in a program's preparatory phase, or the number of outreach visits or counseling contacts in a crisis counseling program). *Outcomes* refer to "how much good" (actual benefits) consumers derive from receipt of services, and can be measured in the short, intermediate, and/or long term. Desired immediate outcomes of education in a crisis counseling program, for example, may be increased understanding on the part of consumers about disaster-related stress reactions and awareness of positive coping mechanisms that can be used to reduce level of distress; intermediate outcomes might be reflected in reduced psychiatric symptoms and substance use, and long-term outcomes might include institution of an emergency preparedness infrastructure and community unity and resilience in dealing with subsequent crisis events.

Using the Logic Model: An Example

Let us suppose an evaluation team wished to calculate whether services are penetrating all ethnic groups in an affected region. Census data could be used to determine the racial makeup in each affected county (a community variable), and then the proportion of various minorities among the program's clients in each county (an output variable) could be compared to the community profile. Evaluators could also assess whether representation of clients from particular subgroups increased after initiation of new program activities, such as targeted outreach efforts or the hiring of additional indigenous staff.

PRAGMATICS: HOW DO YOU GET THE DATA?

Evaluation data can be obtained from a variety of sources: from the material record (the correspondence trail, information logs, and report narratives); from program staff, via qualitative interviews, focus groups, and staff surveys; from the recipients of services; and from the community at large.

Archival Quantitative Data

Valuable quantitative information can be extracted from existing archival data sources. Census data provide information on background characteristics of the affected community (population density, per capita income, racial/ethnic distribution) that may influence service needs and service delivery. Tangible inputs (particularly budget information) can often be determined from notifications of grant awards or other financial records. The types and amounts of services delivered (program outputs) are best determined from contact logs or from summary reports based on such logs. Contact records can also provide basic information about the types of clinical activities undertaken by a program and, in some cases, can capture client characteristics (e.g., age, gender, ethnicity, primary language, geographic location).

There are inherent difficulties in working with existing data. First, records may be incomplete, which is problematic because information is often not missing at random; simply excluding projects lacking data, then, may produce biased results. For example, if projects that are inadequately administered have poorer documentation and poorer results, ignoring projects with missing data may positively skew the findings. Further, even if the records seem to be complete, program projects may use different definitions and procedures for generating those records; in a crisis counseling program, for example, one project might code a 30-second conversation between a consumer and an outreach worker who is handing out a brochure as "materials distribution," whereas another project might code it as an "educational contact."

In the ideal case, evaluators are involved at the outset in establishing data collection and quality-monitoring procedures to ensure data completeness and consistency—this was the case for Project Liberty (Felton, 2002). Where health services researchers must work with existing information of unknown quality, they must approach the data skeptically, maintaining an awareness that observed differences across sites or projects might reflect differences in record keeping as well as differences in services.

In a retrospective analysis of archival data from federal disaster programs (Rosen & Young, 2005), we employed several procedures to distinguish meaningful from irrelevant data. We inventoried quantitative variables for completeness and consistency. We checked data quality by testing whether expected axiomatic relationships were observed (e.g., whether "total people served" was strongly correlated with "total number of service contacts"). We sought alternative sources for missing information; for example, we obtained community demographics data from census records where grantee documentation was unavailable. Missing information was sometimes imputed as an alternative to removing cases from analysis (e.g., if projects did not report total expenditures, a regression equation was used to estimate likely expenditures from the total budget awarded). We examined outliers carefully and, in several instances, repeated analyses with outliers removed to confirm that our overall pattern of findings was not distorted by one or two discrepant cases. Finally, we noted inherent limitations that could not be ameliorated by the above techniques.

Content Analyses of Archival Narrative Records

Whereas quantitative investigations address questions about the amounts and types of services provided by a program, and about the characteristics of customers served, qualitative analyses provide complementary detail on what programs experience and generate hypotheses about why certain patterns identified in the quantitative findings might occur. Content analysis can elucidate program experience in such areas as sustainable infrastructure created by programs, approaches that programs reported as being innovative, and lessons learned by staff over the course of the project (Young & Rosen, 2005). Themes identified in the content analysis can suggest directions to pursue in reanalyzing the quantitative material or issues to be addressed in further studies.

Content analysis is accomplished by reading program documentation narratives in their entirety, in order to develop general categories of concepts and themes emerging from the data that reflect specified topics of interest to stakeholders, and to identify subcategories and their properties (e.g., administrative organization and access might be subcategories of "lessons learned," and intra- and interorganizational communication, turf issues, and multiple roles and responsibilities might be properties of "administrative organization"). Coding is also performed with a view toward providing a theory of relationship between categories, to detect theoretical source or causal conditions for certain phenomena. Data are reduced by coding the content of the narrative record, using variables that have been summarized in a "coding tree," a tool that defines these categories. This task can be accomplished via manual, nonautomated analysis or by using commercially available software, such as "N6" or "Ethnograph."

Qualitative analysis can be limited by factual inconsistencies and imprecision in the text and by incomplete narrative information. It is important, therefore, to identify references to coding tree descriptors throughout the text rather than coding only those sections labeled by authors as pertaining to the category of interest. Also, narrative analysis is inherently subjective. Several safeguards, however, can be built into the process, such as reviewing coding tree themes with other project investigators or evaluating coded narratives relative to other sources of project data.

Information from Program Staff

Workforce members are easily identified and often motivated to provide their perspectives on the subject of program operations. Semistructured interviews are useful devices in initial evaluation studies when investigators have not yet clearly identified key issues and dynamics or wish to obtain interactive feedback from staff vis-à-vis specific evaluation directions (e.g., Norris et al., 2006). Staff interviews also shed light on intangible inputs to the program and on outcomes for staff, such as stress or growth.

When planning qualitative research with staff, it is important to consider the respondent's place within the program hierarchy. Program directors or managers can provide a comprehensive project overview, particularly with regard to organizational issues, such as challenges encountered during the initial response, applying for funding, or interagency collaboration (Elrod & Hamblen, 2005). Frontline outreach and counseling staff can provide detail on the actual conduct of outreach and clinical activities and on their reception by consumers.

Focus groups are helpful in eliciting a wide range of ideas and diverse perspectives, but participants must feel comfortable talking freely in front of colleagues; individual interviews may be preferable to focus groups if there is tension within the work group or if the interview topic is controversial. Managers should be interviewed separately from staff.

Surveys, used to elicit staff feedback once key questions have been identified, should employ reliable quantitative measures, allowing statistical comparison of results across sites or against historical norms. Measures of job satisfaction, job stress (Boudreaux, Mandry, & Brantley, 1997), burnout or compassion fatigue (Arthur, 1990; Maslach, 1982) and posttraumatic growth (Tedeschi & Calhoun, 1996) developed for other helping professions can be modified for use with disaster mental health workers. Procedures to maintain the confidentiality of results and nondisclosure to administrators are critical (questionnaires might be distributed in staff meetings and returned to an independent analyst via postage-paid envelopes). In small projects, even aggregate results might compromise the privacy of participants.

Information from Clients

Information on outcomes must be drawn directly from clients—it cannot be obtained from program staff or archival records. Methods for assessing consumer satisfaction and clinical outcomes in mental health settings generally are well established, but there are several unique challenges in eliciting information from recipients of disaster mental health services. These clients often have limited contact with the project and therefore little investment in providing detailed feedback. Further, crisis counseling programs typically do not keep formal records on individual clients to ensure anonymity, and requesting clients to complete a written survey may raise concerns about adequate protection of privacy. Another concern is respondent and staff burden; completing a lengthy questionnaire may be daunting in the aftermath of a disaster. The least intrusive approach to collecting information from clients is the brief (i.e., one-page) satisfaction survey, which can be administered to unidentified respondents. Successive iterations of anonymous cross-sectional studies can monitor trends over the lifespan of a project.

Measures developed for mental health settings (e.g., Attkisson & Greenfield, 1996) can be supplemented with relevant questions about client perceptions of perceived benefits and ease of access to program services. Questions about perceived value should reflect the types of outcomes that a program can realistically be expected to produce (for example, asking survivors whether crisis counseling resulted in symptom reduction may be less appropriate than inquiring whether services provided useful information about coping strategies, afforded reassurance, reduced stigma, or were informative about accessing additional aid). Client satisfaction measures tend to be positively biased (Davies & Ware, 1988), and so survey instruments should allow a wide range of response options to avoid ceiling effects. Establishing normative data across different events would also aid interpretation of satisfaction results. Another value of consumer surveys is in their elicitation of systematic information on the clients themselves, such as the nature of disaster exposure to the traumatic event and the amount of life disruption experienced—information that can help programs to determine how well they are reaching individuals who are at highest risk.

Several strategies can improve survey response rates and reduce nonresponse bias. The sampling frame should be limited to service recipients who have had enough contact with the program to induce participation. If the program is large, sampling from the client population (i.e., surveying some individuals during several specified time periods rather than surveying all clients) can reduce respondent and staff overload. Small incentives might be offered to survey participants. Finally, outreach workers must be trained in presenting the survey to clients and explaining its purpose and anonymity. Surveys should be framed as an expected element of program operations, and staff members appreciated as necessary to the effort.

The collection of longitudinal data on client outcomes in disaster mental health settings is encumbered by several issues. Monitoring changes in consumer functioning may require recontacting individuals after they are no longer receiving services. Following people over time requires that consumers agree to confidentiality ("we know who you are but promise we won't tell anyone else") rather than anonymity ("even *we* don't know who you are"). Although standards for maintaining confidentiality in research are well established, it is unclear whether consumers of disaster mental health services would have adequate confidence in these procedures (Jones, 2003). Another complication is identifying measures that fit a program's intended outcomes. Client perceptions of the helpfulness of services, a proxy for measuring outcomes, do not always correspond with actual changes in functioning (Berman, Rosen, Hurt, & Kolarz, 1998). Although there are numerous well-validated measures of changes in psychiatric symptoms, measures of remoralization, reduced stigma, and increased coping efficacy (e.g., Benight, Ironson, & Durham, 1999) are less well established, and their sensitivity to change is less certain. After disasters, most people return to normal functioning. Demonstrating that an intervention produces faster-than-normal recovery requires comparing the improvements shown by individuals who did and did not receive that intercession. It is probably unrealistic to expect most disaster mental health programs to routinely track longitudinal changes in client outcomes over time; however, some experimental or quasi-experimental research studies have assessed innovations in care after disasters (e.g., Chemtob, Nakashima, & Hamada, 2002; Goenjian et al., 1997). These efforts required additional resources for research and were often conducted one or more years after the event rather than during the initial crisis period. Developing strategies for conducting research on community-based interventions should be a high priority for this field.

Community Surveys

Some aspects of service delivery require input from the community at large. For example, assessing barriers to access requires information from affected individuals who did not engage in services. Community studies are not standard in program operations, but they may be worthwhile after large-scale disasters. Community surveys conducted after the terrorist attacks in New York assessed influences on service penetration (Rudenstine, Galea, Ahern, Felton, & Vlahov, 2003) and compared the course of recovery among individuals who did and did not receive program services (Boscarino, Adams, & Figley, 2005). Because service recipients are self-selected, analyses must control for potential confounds of help-seeking before interpreting the results.

POLITICS: HOW DO YOU GET BUY-IN?

An important aspect of health services research evaluation is the political dimension. Analysts internal to the organization have a deep understanding of its goals and procedures, but may be unable to highlight problems with impunity; external evaluators, on the other hand, may have insufficient understanding of the realities with which a program is faced. One solution to the insider–outsider dynamic is a collaborative analysis, responsive to the requirements of its manifold stakeholders.

Getting Input into the Evaluation Design

An evaluation is apt to be credible and to influence policy if it is sensitive to different cultural, spiritual, or local perspectives. Judgments about values are context-dependent (Scriven, 1998) and may reflect different participants' ethical, scientific, or political philosophies. The strength of a programmatic activity is enhanced if all participants are working on a shared set of assumptions and if stakeholders at all levels are able to communicate their own assumptions about what works about what they do.

Program sponsors are likely to be concerned about workability of the program management structure, timeliness of infrastructure development and service delivery, adequacy of resources, service access by targeted groups, legislative mandates, and cost of care. Project directors and team leaders are likely to be concerned about resource availability and the timeliness of service delivery, effectual staffing and directed-access outcomes, and consumer and staff satisfaction. Clients, program partners, and advocacy groups may be concerned with confidentiality, the ability of the program to address consumer needs, service satisfaction, and the sustainability of community linkages after program closure (see Rosen, Young, & Norris, 2006).

Engaging Stakeholders to Provide Usable Data

Obtaining useful data for disaster mental health services research requires top-down support; it requires developing an "evaluation culture" that engages program sponsors, service providers, and the intended and actual consumers of services. Without concrete guidance from senior managers and detailed training support on the mechanics of data collection, the quality and completeness of the information may suffer. If program assessment is viewed as onerous by field supervisors and support staff, if the data collection toolkit is difficult to use, or if the process is viewed as threatening, evaluation activities will be unsystematic, and the data will not be instructive for real-time monitoring activities. This prospect underscores the importance of obtaining user input on means to make the evaluation user friendly.

An evaluation component for disaster events might be crafted in a continuing discourse, enlisting stakeholder consensus at the federal and then local levels, folding in concerns about what is experienced as meaningful to measure by the various stakeholder factions. Government sponsors of disaster mental health programs might consider assembling a durable working group of state-based emergency personnel to share lessons learned from previous events and to articulate evaluation needs; members of emergency task forces in the disaster preparedness start-up phase could consult with colleagues from more mature and previously evaluated programs to duplicate those features that were found to be beneficial.

Program staff experience ownership of the evaluation process when their counsel is acknowledged and acted upon. Not only can data collection be enhanced by this dialectic, but also programmatic guidelines can evolve in the service of improved product delivery.

Program feedback can be invaluable in addressing delays in the allocation and/or processing of grant funds, adjusting project duration, and working out algorithms to estimate staffing levels. Their suggestions can speak to the need to upgrade information transfer across agencies and between national, regional, and local activities, or to better delineate lines of administrative influence and accountability. Outreach staff may voice ideas about what kinds of services should be offered that differ from those specified by the theoretical program model, and evaluators may then have to question some premises of the initial model.

Analyzing and Communicating Results

At the inception of the evaluation process it is important to make explicit who will "own" and analyze the data and who will put the "slant" on findings. Consensus about the evaluation design and the implementation procedure and about the means by which results will be communicated should be achieved at the start of the process, always attempting to reconcile client needs with those of other stakeholders.

The analysis and the conclusions drawn from the data by the evaluator must be methodologically sound, face valid for the decision makers (Patton, 1978), and actionable statistical analyses may not be meaningful to some stakeholders; others may dismiss qualitative data as merely anecdotal. Evaluators may find their results are most credible if they function as narrative storytellers (Greene, 2000), using a combination of quantitative and case study or focus group results to shed light on the program. The most effective communication of results employs simple, nontechnical language, includes vivid examples, and conveys clear conclusions and recommendations (Rosen et al., 2006).

Evaluation results should be shared in a climate that is sympathetic and inquisitive rather than penalizing. Sharing interim results with sponsors and other stakeholders (such as members of a program's advisory unmet needs committee) prior to issuing a final report is a powerful way to foster buy-in of the results and affords an occasion for the listeners to stipulate concerns that the evaluation team may have overlooked. The disclosure of findings to all stakeholders also permits conflicts of interest and value differences to be dealt with openly. Project directors should be encouraged to communicate results of program monitoring efforts via regular staff meetings and ongoing updates to elicit reactions on ways to improve program product (for example, by sharing innovative outreach techniques).

CONCLUSIONS: INCREASING TECHNICAL RIGOR

Mental health interventions are ideally assessed in randomized clinical trials, which are often not feasible in fast-paced disaster environments. What kinds of research, then, can be done? We propose four directions for expanding evidence-based knowledge about disaster mental health interventions.

First, we should aim to obtain accurate data to assess whether services reach those who are most vulnerable. Consistent recording of client demographics and inclusion of queries about disaster exposure in consumer surveys are needed to determine whether those who have sustained the greatest exposure and other individuals at high risk—such as children and mothers of young children (Norris et al., 2002)—and are being served.

Second, we should aim to capture the practical experience developed by program administrators and staff. Program directors often are in the position of "reinventing the wheel" with respect to solving common problems because they have no way of accessing prior knowledge and experience (Elrod & Hamblen, 2005; Young & Rosen, 2005). Conducting qualitative exit interviews with key program staff at program closure and disseminating those findings online or in training venues provides a means of sharing lessons learned.

Third, we should aim to systematically monitor coping outcomes for program staff. Stress and vicarious traumatization, sometimes coupled with direct trauma exposure, are common challenges for disaster mental health workers. Project administrators are increasingly aware of this issue but lack effective methods for regular assessment of staff coping strategies. Confidential or anonymous surveys are a potentially valuable mechanism for assessing the success with which staff cope with (or mature in response to) work-related stressors.

Fourth, we should aim to incorporate questions about awareness, access, and use of disaster mental health services in epidemiological studies conducted after large-scale disasters. Studies conducted following the terrorist attacks of September 11, 2001, demonstrated the utility of community surveillance methods in providing feedback about public awareness of (Rudenstine et al., 2003) and access to services (Fairbrother, Stuber, Galea, Pfefferbaum, & Fleischman, 2004) and clinical outcomes (Boscarino et al., 2005).

One of the hallmarks of disaster mental health programs is their flexibility. In the wake of disasters or terrorism, mental health services are not offered in structured clinical settings; they are delivered through proactive and innovative means that adapt to evolving community needs. The investigation of disaster mental health services must be equally flexible, in the service of advancing methodological rigor.

REFERENCES

Agency for Healthcare Research and Quality (2001). AHRQ profile: Quality research for quality healthcare. AHRQ Publication No. 00-P005, March 2001. Agency for Healthcare Research and Quality, Rockville, MD. Available at ahrq.gov\about\profile.htm

Arthur, N. M. (1990). The assessment of burnout: A review of three inventories for research and counseling. *Journal of Counseling and Development, 69,* 186–189.

Attkisson, C. C., & Greenfield, T. K. (1996). The Client Satisfaction Questionnaire (CSQ) Scales and the Service Satisfaction Scale-30 (SSS-30). In L. I. Sederer & B. Dickey (Eds.), *Outcomes assessment in clinical practice* (pp. 120–127). Baltimore, MD: Williams & Wilkins.

Benight, C. C., Ironson, G., & Durham, R. I. (1999). Psychometric properties of a hurricane coping self-efficacy scale. *Journal of Traumatic Stress, 12,* 379–386.

Berman, W. H., Rosen, C. S., Hurt, S. W., & Kolarz, C. M. (1998). Toto, we're not in Kansas anymore: Measuring and using outcomes in behavioral health care. *Clinical Psychology: Science and Practice, 5,* 115–133.

Boscarino, J. A., Adams, R. E., & Figley, C. R. (2005). A prospective cohort study of the effectiveness of employer-sponsored crisis interventions after a major disaster. *International Journal of Emergency Mental Health, 7,* 9–22.

Boudreaux, E., Mandry, C., & Brantley, P. J. (1997). Stress, job satisfaction, coping, and psychological distress among emergency medical technicians. *Prehospital and Disaster Medicine, 12,* 242–249.

Chemtob, C. M., Nakashima, J. P., & Hamada, R. S. (2002). Psychosocial intervention for postdisaster trauma symptoms in elementary school children: A controlled community field study. *Archives of Pediatrics and Adolescent Medicine, 156,* 211–216.

Davies, A. R., & Ware, J. E., Jr. (1988). Involving consumers in quality of care assessment. *Health Affairs, 7,* 33–48.

Elrod, C. L., & Hamblen, J. L. (2005). Directors' perspectives on disaster mental health services. In F. H. Norris, C. S. Rosen, C. L. Elrod, H. E. Young, L. E. Gibson, & J. L. Hamblen, *Retrospective 5-year evaluation of the crisis counseling program* (pp. C5–C81). White River Junction, VT: U.S. Department of Veterans Affairs, National Center for Posttraumatic Stress Disorder.

Fairbrother, G., Stuber, J., Galea, S., Pfefferbaum, B., & Fleischman, A. R. (2004). Unmet need for counseling services by children in New York City after the September 11th attacks on the World Trade Center: Implications for pediatricians. *Pediatrics, 113,* 1367–1374.

Felton, C. J. (2002). Project Liberty: A public health response to New Yorkers' mental health needs arising from the World Trade Center terrorist attacks. *Journal of Urban Health: Bulletin of the New York Academy of Medicine, 79,* 429–433.

Goenjian, A. K., Karayan, I., Pynoos, R. S., Minassian, D., Najarian, L. M., Streinberg, A. M., et al. (1997). Outcome of psychotherapy among early adolescents after trauma. *American Journal of Psychiatry, 154,* 536–542.

Greene, J. C. (2000). Understanding social programs through evaluation. In N. K. Denzin & Y. S. Lincoln (Eds.), *Handbook of qualitative research* (pp. 981–999). Thousand Oaks, CA: Sage.

Jones, G. E. (2003). Crisis intervention, crisis counseling, confidentiality, and privilege. *International Journal of Emergency Mental Health, 5,* 137–140.

Litz, B., & Gray, M. (2002). Early intervention for mass violence: What is the evidence, what should be done? *Cognitive and Behavioral Practice, 9,* 266–272.

Maslach, C. (1982). *Burnout: The cost of caring.* Englewood Cliffs, NJ: Prentice Hall.

Norris, F. H., Friedman, M. J., Watson, P. J., Byrne, C. M., Diaz, E., & Kaniasty, K. (2002). 60,000 disaster victims speak: Part I. An empirical review of the empirical literature, 1981–2001. *Psychiatry. 65,* 207–239.

Norris, F. H., Hamblen, J. L., Watson, P. J., Ruzek, J., Gibson, L. E., Price, J. L., et al. (2006). Toward understanding and creating systems of postdisaster care: A case study of New York's response to the World Trade Center disaster. In E. C. Ritchie, P. J. Watson, & M. J. Friedman (Eds.), *Interventions following mass violence and disaster: Strategies for mental health practice* (pp. 343–364). New York: Guilford Press.

Patton, M. Q. (1978). *Utilization-focused evaluation.* Beverly Hills, CA: Sage.

Rosen, C. S., & Young, H. E. (2005). Quantitative analysis of archival data from crisis counseling grants. In F. H. Norris, C. S. Rosen, C. L. Elrod, H. E. Young, L. E. Gibson, & J. L. Hamblen, *Retrospective 5-year evaluation of the crisis counseling program* (pp. B9–B42) White River Junction, VT: U.S. Department of Veterans Affairs, National Center for Posttraumatic Stress Disorder.

Rosen, C. S., Young, H. E., & Norris, F. H. (2006). On a road paved with good intentions, you still need a compass: Monitoring and evaluating disaster mental health services. In E. C. Ritchie, P. J. Watson, & M. J. Friedman (Eds.), *Interventions following mass violence and disasters: Strategies for mental health practice* (pp. 206–224). New York: Guilford Press.

Rudenstine, S., Galea, S., Ahern, J., Felton, C., & Vlahov, D. (2003). Awareness of perceptions of a communitywide mental health program in New York City after September 11. *Psychiatric Services, 54,* 1404–1406.

Scheirer, M. A. (1987). Program theory and implementation theory: Implications for evaluators. In L. Bickman (Ed.), *Using program theory in evaluation: Vol. 33. New Directions for Program Evaluation* (pp. 59–76). San Francisco: Jossey-Bass.

Scriven, M. (1998). The least theory that practice requires. *The American Journal of Evaluation, 19,* 57–70.

Tedeschi, R. G., & Calhoun, L. G. (1996). The Posttraumatic Growth Inventory: Measuring the positive legacy of trauma. *Journal of Traumatic Stress, 9,* 455–471.

Young, H. E., & Rosen, C. S. (2005). Qualitative analysis of archival data from crisis counseling grants. In F. H. Norris, C. S. Rosen, C. L. Elrod, H. E. Young, L. E. Gibson, & J. L. Hamblen, *Retrospective 5-year evaluation of the crisis counseling program* (pp. B43–B88). White River Junction, VT: U.S. Department of Veterans Affairs, National Center for Posttraumatic Stress Disorder.

Weiss, C. H. (1997). How can theory-based evaluation make greater headway? *Evaluation Review, 21,* 501–524.

CHAPTER 13

Evidence-Based Treatments for Traumatic Stress

An Overview of the Research Literature with an Emphasis on Disaster Settings

LAURA E. GIBSON, JESSICA L. HAMBLEN,
MICHAEL J. ZVOLENSKY, and ANKA A. VUJANOVIC

Major disasters have brought worldwide attention to the need for effective interventions for survivors of trauma. Left untreated, many individuals who have been directly exposed to disasters will suffer enduring psychological effects such as posttraumatic stress disorder (PTSD), panic disorder, and major depressive disorder (Norris et al., 2002). These conditions can result in substantial impairment across the lifespan (Ferdinand & Verhulst, 1995), with 40–60% of individuals with anxiety and mood disorder diagnoses reporting moderate to severe occupational role dysfunction and disability (Ormel et al., 1994). These data underscore the public health relevance of effectively assessing and intervening with psychological vulnerability factors following traumatic life events like disasters.

The disaster intervention literature is hampered by many methodological problems related to the challenging circumstances under which disaster and mass violence research takes place. Before reviewing the relevant intervention literature, we want to highlight some common problems and challenges that interfere with the implementation of carefully controlled clinical trials in the disaster intervention field. For example, early intervention research implemented after disasters typically takes place in rushed and chaotic conditions. Because disasters generally occur without warning, intervention research is usually not extensively preplanned in anticipation of a given event. Even if researchers have a general research model in place prior to a specific disaster, it typically takes several months (at best) to secure funding. Furthermore, researchers may need to network with local community groups and providers, obtain permission from institutional review boards, address cultural or regional barriers, and overcome the logistical issues inherent in applying their intervention to the specific disaster setting under study (e.g. traveling to the disaster site, locating and training local clinicians to participate in the trial).

Early intervention researchers face the additional complication that, even *without* intervention, the majority of individuals experience a decline in symptoms over time following exposure to a traumatic event (Rothbaum, Foa, Riggs, Murdock, & Walsh, 1992; Valentiner, Foa, Riggs, & Gershuny, 1996). Ideally, participants in clinical trials are randomly assigned to experimental or control groups to ensure that symptom reduction occurring in the first few months of an intervention trial is due to the intervention under study rather than the passage of time or some other methodological confound (e.g. self-selection for treatment). Methodological flaws present in much early intervention research include a lack of randomization, lack of standardized assessment measures, lack of treatment adherence measures, lack of clear target symptoms, and/or lack of blind raters.

Although tightly controlled randomized clinical trials (RCTs) are the gold standard for intervention research, the unique and often chaotic conditions that accompany disasters render RCTs extremely difficult to undertake in these settings (Litz & Gibson, 2006). Potentially more practical alternatives to RCTs are experimental and quasi-experimental research designs that may be easier to introduce into disaster-stricken communities. One such design is a balanced design, which would entail providing an intervention at Site A but not at Site B (Yule, 1992). Block random assignment is another option that may be more acceptable to some policymakers, clinicians, and consumers who object to the notion of individual random assignment to interventions. Randomized block design entails the use of random assignment at the group level (e.g. schools, neighborhoods, classes) rather than at the individual level (Hardin et al., 2002). These alternative methodologies can be implemented with high levels of internal control and external validity, and they might represent more feasible designs than RCTs for intervention research in disaster settings.

Translational research also plays an important role in terms of evaluating interventions that may be appropriate after disasters. Given the multiple challenges of conducting research in the disaster setting, it is critical that interventions that have been shown to be efficacious in other settings be considered for importation into communities affected by disasters. For example, it may be much more feasible to implement early intervention trials in hospital settings than in disaster settings. Although the psychological needs of disaster survivors will inevitably differ from those of other survivors in some respects, there is no theoretical reason to believe that symptom-specific interventions (e.g., for PTSD, major depressive disorder) would not be transportable from one group of survivors to another.

In order to better understand the state of the science in disaster intervention research, we conducted a systematic review of the extant literature on evidence-based interventions for traumatic stress. Below, we summarize this literature under the major categories of early and later-stage interventions. Methodological strengths and weaknesses of this literature are described throughout, and attention is given to challenges that may be encountered when conducting intervention research in disaster settings. Interventions for both youths and adults are reviewed.

Clinical trials conducted with mass violence or disaster survivors were included in the review whenever possible. Due to the dearth of methodologically sound RCTs with disaster survivors, strong studies conducted with other groups of trauma-exposed individuals are included when the interventions under study were theoretically translatable to disasters. Studies included in the review were identified through a search of the PsycINFO and PILOTS databases, spanning the years from 1967 through May 2005. Some additional manuscripts were identified through personal communication with key workers in the field. All studies included in the review were classified using a system forwarded by the International Society for Traumatic Stress Studies (Foa, Keane, & Friedman, 2000), based on a general system of evidence classification developed by the Agency for Healthcare Research and Quality (AHRQ; formerly the Agency for Health Care Policy and Research). Only studies that met Level A, B, or C criteria are included in this review, but Level A evidence (RCTs) is highlighted. Throughout the review, methodological strengths and limitations beyond the levels of evidence are noted, with reference to Foa and Meadows's (1997) gold standards for clinical research (Table 13.1).

EARLY INTERVENTIONS FOR TRAUMATIC STRESS

For purposes of this review, early interventions refer to those that are introduced within the first month after a traumatic event. This section focuses primarily on psychological debriefing and cognitive-behavioral interven-

TABLE 13.1. The Agency for Healthcare Research and Quality's Levels of Evidence and Foa and Meadows's Gold Standards for Clinical Research

AHRQ levels of evidence (Foa et al., 2000)

- *Level A:* Evidence is based upon randomized, well-controlled clinical trials for individuals with PTSD.
- *Level B:* Evidence is based upon well-designed clinical studies, without randomization or placebo comparison for individuals with PTSD.
- *Level C:* Evidence is based on service and naturalistic clinical studies, combined with clinical observations that are sufficiently compelling to warrant use of the treatment technique or that follow the specific recommendation.

Gold standards for clinical research (Foa & Meadows, 1997)

- Clearly defined target symptoms
- Reliable and valid measures
- Blind evaluators
- Assessor training
- Manualized, replicable, specific treatment programs
- Unbiased (random) assignment to treatment
- Treatment adherence measures

tions, given that they are the interventions that have been most extensively empirically examined. Although the literature base regarding early pharmacotherapy and early interventions for children is in its infancy, we have noted significant studies in these areas. Eye movement desensitization and reprocessing (EMDR) is not included in this section because it has not yet been examined in well-designed RCTs for use within the first month after a trauma. It is included in the review of later-stage interventions.

Psychological Debriefing

Psychological debriefing became the standard of care for disaster response in the 1980s and 1990s, although there was little empirical support for this approach. It is a semistructured intervention that can be implemented in either an individual or a group format, originally designed to facilitate emotional processing and promote normal recovery among first responders exposed to traumatic events. It consists of a semistructured review of a traumatic event or "critical incident." The majority of interventions introduced and studied in the first month posttrauma have been classified in the literature as "debriefing" interventions, although the interventions contained in such studies are not uniform. Although some debriefing studies have been conducted within the first 48 hours of an incident (e.g., Bunn & Clarke, 1979; Hobbs, Mayou, Harrison, & Worlock, 1996; Lavender & Walkinshaw, 1998; Small, Lumley, Donohue, Potter, & Waldenstroem, 2000), most began at least 1 week posttrauma.

Recent reviews of the early intervention literature (e.g., Bisson, 2003; Litz, Gray, Bryant, & Adler, 2002; Watson et al., 2003), a Cochrane review (Rose, Bisson, & Wessely, 2002), and a meta-analysis of early single-session interventions (Van Emmerick, Kamphuis, Hulsbosch, & Emmelkamp, 2002) have all concluded that psychological debriefing is inadequate in terms of preventing long-term psychological sequelae, and that it is potentially detrimental in terms of psychological recovery from trauma. In a review of 13 single-session RCTs that have been included in many reviews of the debriefing literature, Bisson (2003) observed that the only three RCTs that yielded positive outcomes (Bordow & Porritt, 1979; Bunn & Clarke, 1979; Lavender & Walkinshaw, 1998) "did not adhere to a formal psychological debriefing intervention" (p. 495). It would probably be most accurate to refer to this research base as "single-session" early psychological interventions, as opposed to "debriefing" interventions per se, given the lack of treatment adherence measures and the variability of the interventions studied.

Litz, Adler, et al. (2004) recently undertook a large-scale RCT of a group debriefing intervention that significantly improved upon the extant debriefing research literature. These researchers randomized 1,050 soldiers deployed on peacekeeping missions to one of three groups: critical incident stress debriefing (CISD), a stress education condition, or a survey-only condition. Unlike most debriefing trials, this one included measures of treatment adherence and utilized a formal CISD protocol administered by trained CISD personnel. This trial also was prospective, including an evaluation of soldiers prior to deployment as well as at two postintervention follow-up periods. The authors found no differences among the CISD, stress education, and survey-only conditions on any behavioral health outcome, including PTSD, depression, general well-being, aggressive behavior, marital satisfaction, perceived organizational support, or morale. There was no evidence that the intervention caused harm. Specifically, heart rate and blood pressure readings before and after the sessions did not indicate a change in physiological stress; subjective ratings of distress did not change pre- to postsession; soldiers rated their satisfaction with CISD as high; and mental health outcomes at follow-up did not worsen as a result of CISD.

In sum, although the debriefing literature indicates that individuals seem to regard these interventions positively, they appear to be ineffective in terms of preventing significant psychological sequelae.

Cognitive-Behavioral Therapy

The other major approach to early intervention that has been empirically examined in acutely traumatized adults is cognitive-behavioral therapy (CBT). Studies of CBT generally contain the common elements of psychoeducation, anxiety management techniques, exposure techniques, and cognitive restructuring. CBT has been examined as an intervention introduced within the first month after a trauma, with most studies of CBT being implemented at least 10 days posttrauma. Early intervention studies utilizing CBT have tended to be more methodologically sound than studies of debriefing, and the outcomes have been more promising (for recent reviews, see Ehlers & Clark, 2003; Litz et al., 2002; Watson et al., 2003). Of the six published CBT RCTs identified, five (Bryant, Harvey, Dang, Sackville, & Basten, 1998; Bryant, Moulds, Guthrie, & Nixon, 2005; Bryant, Sackville, Dang, Moulds, & Guthrie, 1999; Echeburua, deCorral, Sarasua, & Zubizarreta, 1996; Gidron et al., 2001) found superiority of the CBT group in reducing PTSD symptomatology as compared to a control group, whereas one (Brom, Kleber, & Hofman, 1993) did not. The studies by Bryant and colleagues (1998, 1999, 2005) of individuals with acute stress disorder (ASD) indicated that a structured CBT intervention administered approximately 2 weeks after serious trauma reduces the likelihood that participants will develop PTSD. These particular studies deserve note, as they meet all of Foa and Meadows's (1997) gold standards for clinical research. Because they serve as good models for future research, these studies are described in more detail below.

At a mean of 10 days posttrauma, Bryant and colleagues randomly assigned adult motor vehicle accident (MVA), industrial accident, or nonsexual assault survivors to five individual 1.5-hour sessions of either CBT or a supportive counseling control condition. In the 1998 study, Bryant and colleagues found that fewer individuals in the CBT group than in the control group met criteria for PTSD at posttreatment and 6 months later. They also showed greater reductions in intrusive, avoidance, and depressive symptoms than those in the supportive counseling condition. In their 1999 study, Bryant et al. compared two different individual CBT interventions (prolonged exposure plus anxiety management and prolonged exposure) to supportive counseling. Both CBT groups showed superior reductions in PTSD symptoms as compared to the supportive counseling group. This finding was evident both at posttreatment and at the 6-month follow-up. A recent trial suggests that the addition of a hypnotic induction prior to the imaginal exposure component of this CBT approach further increased its potency (Bryant et al., 2005).

A final study (Bryant, Moulds, & Nixon, 2003) reported on the long-term functioning of participants in two earlier studies conducted by Bryant and colleagues. Four years after receiving treatment, participants from the 1998 and 1999 CBT experimental groups showed less intense (although not less frequent) PTSD symptoms than participants who had received supportive counseling alone in those trials. The results provide preliminary evidence that an early CBT intervention for ASD is associated with long-term benefits in psychological functioning.

Although these studies provide the strongest literature base from which to draw conclusions about early interventions, none was conducted with disaster-affected populations. The multitude of challenges associated with conducting early intervention research in the acute aftermath of disasters highlights the need for translating findings derived from intervention research with other acutely traumatized individuals (e.g. motor vehicle accident survivors) to disaster-affected populations. Nonetheless, the feasibility and appropriateness of introducing CBT interventions into the acute aftermath of disaster or mass violence-affected settings remains untested.

Pharmacotherapy

A few studies investigating the effects of pharmacotherapy in the acute aftermath of trauma suggest early intervention might have a preventative effect on the development of posttraumatic symptomatology. Pilot RCTs of imipramine in children and adolescents (Robert, Blakeney, Villarreal, Rosenberg, & Meyer, 1999), and propranolol and hydrocortisone in adults have shown promising results (Pitman et al., 2002; Schelling et al., 2001). In each study, the administration of medication was associated with improved trauma-related symptoms relative to the controls.

Psychosocial Interventions for Children and Adolescents

The research literature regarding early psychosocial interventions for children and adolescents is in its infancy. To our knowledge, no well-designed RCTs of acute interventions for children or adolescents have been published, either within or outside of disaster settings. Early intervention research with children and adolescents is difficult to implement, as researchers face enumerable obstacles, including passing child- and adolescent-relevant protocols through institutional review boards, gaining informed consent from children and parents/guardians, and establishing access to potential child participants.

To illustrate the type of acute intervention research that has been undertaken thus far with children, one especially relevant postdisaster early intervention for children is described below. Although the study was a critical first step in attempting to document the effectiveness of treatment for youth after a disaster, it had many shortcomings. Yule (1992) conducted a naturalistic comparison of children from two different schools who had been involved in a large-scale shipping disaster. One school had offered an early group intervention (termed "debriefing"), but the other school had offered no early intervention. Yule found that those children who had received the intervention showed fewer intrusive PTSD symptoms and fear symptoms 5–9 months after the disaster. Unfortunately, the intervention that was offered was not standardized or monitored, so there is no way of evaluating its content. Furthermore, children in the two schools may have differed in any number of ways (e.g., exposure, prior mental health problems, socioeconomic status) that could have potentially confounded their psychological functioning postintervention. Future studies could improve upon this design by using a quasi-experimental design in which randomization is used at the class or school level. In addition, standardized pretests and posttests, treatments, and treatment adherence measures are needed.

LATER-STAGE INTERVENTIONS FOR TRAUMATIC STRESS

The literature on treatment of chronic PTSD is much more extensive and methodologically sound than is the literature on early interventions. This section focuses on the two major behavioral health interventions, CBT and EMDR, with the most extensive research base for treatment of PTSD. Promising pharmacological interventions for PTSD are also discussed. There are anecdotal and case study reports of numerous other psychological interventions (e.g., thought-field therapy, traumatic incident reduction) that may or may not ultimately prove to be effective in the treatment of chronic PTSD. Although there is at least one RCT that examined psychodynamic therapy for the treatment of PTSD symptoms (Brom, Kleber, & Defares, 1989), it was marked by substantial methodological limitations that hinder a meaningful interpretation of the findings (e.g., lack of treatment adherence measures, unclear distinctions between treatment conditions, use of different therapists in different conditions). Despite the fact that the majority of the RCTs reviewed in this section were not conducted with disaster survivors, these interventions may be generalizable to this population, as demonstrated in the first study described below (Başoğlu, Şalcioğlu, Livanou, Kalendar, & Acar, 2005).

Cognitive-Behavioral Therapy

One recent and methodologically strong RCT of CBT directly relates to disaster survivors. Başoğlu, and colleagues (2005) randomly assigned 59 earthquake survivors in Turkey to either a single-session behavioral treatment or a waiting-list control condition. The intervention was offered approximately 3 years after the earthquake. The authors chose to utilize a one-session intervention due to pragmatic and logistical issues involving engaging survivors in longer-term treatment. The treatment session consisted of (1) identifying the presenting problems, (2) providing a treatment rationale, and (3) setting behavioral targets and providing instruction in self-exposure. Systematic cognitive restructuring was not used in the treatment. Follow-up assessments were conducted at weeks 6, 12, 24, and 1–2 years posttreatment. Improvements were significant at all time points on all measures. Using the criterion of 2 standard deviations or more improvement since baseline (Jacobson & Truax, 1991), the percentage of improvement on the Clinician Administered PTSD Scale (CAPS) total scores was 29% at week 6, 64% at week 12, 75% at week 24, and 71% at 1–2 year follow-up. The results of this RCT are very promising and in need of further replication, as the findings suggest that a very brief (i.e., one-session) cost-effective treatment can lead to significant clinical gains for disaster survivors with PTSD.

Most of the RCTs to date on CBT have compared component parts of CBT with one another, with waiting-list control conditions, and with supportive counseling conditions. Studies cited in this section are of high methodological quality, with most of them meeting all of Foa and Meadows's (1997) criteria. Further work is needed to determine the CBT components that are best tolerated, work most quickly, and are most efficacious. To date, the components of CBT that have been associated with the largest effects in the treatment of PTSD are cognitive restructuring (CR) and exposure therapy (e.g., Bryant, Moulds, Guthrie, Dang, & Nixon, 2003 et al., 1999; Foa, Rothbaum, Riggs, & Murdock, 1991; Resick, Nishith, Weaver, Astin, & Feuer, 2002). Currently researchers are exploring whether exposure alone or cognitive restructuring alone is as effective in reducing PTSD as the two CBT components in combination.

Several studies have now compared the effects of CR to the effects of exposure, with fairly consistent results. In four RCTs comparing CR to exposure, similar decreases were seen in PTSD symptoms between the CR and exposure-based groups (Foa et al., 1999; Marks, Lovell, Noshirvani, Livanou, & Thrasher, 1998; Resick et al., 2002; Tarrier et al., 1999). However, Tarrier and Sommerfield (2004) recently found surprising results in a 5-year follow-up to the Tarrier et al. (1999) study. Five years after treatment, participants who had been randomized to the CR condition were less likely to meet criteria for PTSD and showed fewer PTSD symptoms on the CAPS than participants in the exposure condition. In contrast to studies that found equivalent reductions in PTSD between CR and exposure groups at posttreatment, but consistent with Tarrier and Sommerfield's 5-year follow-up findings, Bryant, Moulds, Guthrie et al. (2003) found that participants who received a combined treatment of imaginal exposure–cognitive restructuring (IE-CR) demonstrated greater reductions in PTSD symptoms than participants in the IE-alone condition, at posttreatment.

Although the studies cited above are tightly controlled with good internal and external validity, differences in the implementation of exposure techniques and CR suggest that further controlled clinical research is needed before firm conclusions can be drawn regarding the optimal delivery of CBT for the treatment of PTSD. For example, the exposure conditions in two of the studies above (Bryant, Moulds, Guthrie et al., 2003; Tarrier et al., 1999) used imaginal exposure only (i.e., they omitted *in vivo*) in the exposure condition, which potentially decreased the potency of the exposure condition.

Eye Movement Desensitization and Reprocessing

Although there is research support for EMDR, it remains a somewhat controversial intervention, as questions remain regarding the change mechanisms underlying EMDR and whether these mechanisms are different from traditional exposure treatment. Several RCTs have been published over the past few years that suggest that EMDR is effective in reducing PTSD symptoms (Devilly & Spence, 1999; Ironson, Freund, Strauss, & Williams, 2002; Lee, Gavriel, Drummond, Richards, & Greenwald, 2002; Power et al., 2002; Rothbaum, 1997; Taylor et al., 2003). However, these studies have generally not been of the same methodological quality as the RCTs of CBT cited above (Hertlein & Ricci, 2004). Common problems found in EMDR studies include a lack of blind raters and lack of strict treatment adherence measures. Of the five RCTs comparing EMDR and CBT, all found that both treatments were efficacious in reducing PTSD symptoms and found minimal differences in treatment outcome between the treatments. Although some authors found a slight superiority of EMDR (Ironson et al., 2002; Lee et al., 2002; Power et al., 2002), others found a slight superiority of CBT (Devilly & Spence, 1999; Taylor et al., 2003). In two of the three studies that found a slight superiority of EMDR, however, interviewers were not blind to the conditions and were not always independent of the treating therapist (Lee et al., 2002; Power et al., 2002). This introduces the problem of possible bias or allegiance effects, insofar as ratings may have been affected by the theoretical orientation of the raters.

Pharmacotherapy

Although the primary focus of this review is on psychosocial interventions, there is a growing literature regarding the psychopharmacological treatment of PTSD that deserves mention. The interested reader is referred to Friedman (2005) for a more extensive review of this literature. Over the past 10 years there have been significant advances in the area of pharmacotherapy for PTSD, perhaps most significantly U.S. Food and Drug Administration (FDA) approval for two selective serotonin reuptake inhibitors (SSRIs): sertraline and paroxetine. Two clinical practice guidelines (American Psychiatric Association, in press; Veterans Health Administration,

2004) report that SSRIs should serve as the first-line medications in the treatment of PTSD.

Although SSRIs are favored because of their broad spectrum effects against all PTSD symptoms, other psychopharmacological agents also have shown promise (Friedman, 2005). Preliminary findings with venlafaxine have been especially promising. Monoamine oxidase inhibitors (MAOIs) and tricyclic antidepressants (TCAs) have proven efficacy in PTSD, although the side effects are greater than those for the SSRIs. Antiadrenergic agents, such as prazosin, have been shown to improve nightmares and overall symptom severity. Other antiadrenergic agents such as propranolol, clonidine, and guanfacine are in the early stages of study. Finally, preliminary results suggest that atypical antipsychotics and anticonvulsants may be useful. Other medications have proven less effective. Benzodiazepines, conventional antipsychotics, and lithium are not recommended for PTSD patients.

Interventions for Children and Adolescents with PTSD

The literature on treatment of chronic PTSD among youths is quite limited, compared to the literature on adult treatments. Nonetheless, a variety of types of interventions for traumatized children and adolescents have shown promising results in recent RCTs. Replication is needed before any particular intervention can be recommended. Chemtob, Nakashima, and Carlson (2002) reported encouraging results from an RCT of EMDR for children exposed to a hurricane. The intervention consisted of three individual sessions of EMDR introduced approximately 3.5 years after the hurricane. The authors reported reductions in PTSD symptoms, anxiety, and depressive symptoms among the children who had received EMDR. Chemtob, Nakashima, and Hamada (2002) also reported promising results from a well-designed RCT of a psychosocial intervention for hurricane-exposed children that was offered 2 years posthurricane. The authors indicated that this four-session intervention entailed a combination of structured play therapy and cognitive interventions, and was offered in both individual and group formats. After treatment, children in both the individual and group interventions showed fewer traumatic stress symptoms than children assigned to the waiting-list control group.

In a nonrandomized but controlled study, Goenjian and colleagues (1997) examined the outcome of therapy among early adolescents who had been exposed to a severe earthquake in Armenia. All sixth- and seventh-grade students from four schools participated in the trial. Students at two schools received a combination of "trauma-grief focused" brief individual therapy and group therapy, while students at the other two schools were not offered treatment. Damage to the four schools and their surrounding areas was reportedly equivalent, and there were no pretreatment differences between the groups in terms of PTSD symptomatology. The intervention consisted of 4 half-hour group sessions and an average of two 1-hour individual sessions conducted over a 3-week period. The posttest, conducted 3 years after the earthquake, indicated that students who had participated in the treatment showed a reduction in PTSD scores as compared to their pretest, whereas students who had received no treatment actually showed an increase in PTSD symptoms. PTSD symptoms were lower in the treated group than in the nontreated group. In addition, while there was no change in depressive symptoms in the treated group, depressive symptoms worsened in the nontreated group.

A recent RCT of a school-based intervention for sixth-grade students directly exposed to violence in Los Angeles provides highly relevant information regarding the treatment of youth exposed to disasters or mass violence (Stein et al., 2003). In this study, sixth-graders with PTSD who had personally witnessed or been exposed to violence were randomly assigned to either a group CBT condition or a waiting-list delayed intervention comparison group. The intervention was delivered by school counselors in a 10-week group format. PTSD, depressive symptoms, and psychosocial dysfunction were all lower in the treated group. After the control group received the CBT protocol, these differences disappeared. This study demonstrates that the children suffering from violence-related PTSD appear to respond to a time-limited CBT protocol that can be offered within the school setting. Such interventions could prove an extremely useful means of reaching large numbers of children after disasters.

In addition, several high-quality RCTs, supporting the efficacy of CBT interventions, exist regarding the treatment of abused youth (e.g. Berliner & Saunders, 1996; Cohen & Mannarino, 1996; Deblinger, Lippmann, & Steer, 1996). Further work is needed to determine whether these CBT protocols would be generalizable to youths exposed to disasters.

PRIORITIES FOR FUTURE DISASTER INTERVENTION RESEARCH

As this chapter reveals, there is much yet to learn regarding the effective implementation of psychosocial and psychopharmacological interventions after disasters. Overall, the psychosocial intervention with the best evidence base for the treatment of PTSD in both children and adults is CBT. This holds true for both early and later-stage interventions. However, very few treatment outcome studies have actually utilized disaster survivors as participants. Such studies are critically needed in order to have an empirically based knowledge of whether CBT interventions are appropriate for disaster-exposed populations. In terms of psychopharmacological interventions, SSRIs have the most empirical support for treatment of chronic PTSD. However, research is lacking regarding psychiatric treatment for acute trauma and for the treatment of traumatized children and adolescents.

Numerous issues would benefit from further empirical examination. For example, it remains unclear whether CBT would be a viable early intervention after disaster in terms of the availability of appropriately trained therapists. One possibility would be to develop "just-in-time" training programs that could be transported into disaster-affected communities to teach CBT skills to therapists in an affected area (Marshall, Amsel, Neria, & Suh, Chapter 14, this volume). There is some indication that such an approach may be feasible and that such training may result in effective and efficacious service delivery (Gillespie, Duffy, Hackmann, & Clark, 2002). Gillespie and colleagues (2002) used such a model to train individuals with minimal background in CBT to deliver a cognitive restructuring intervention after a bombing in northern Ireland, yielding positive results for the reduction of PTSD symptoms.

Because CBT requires a high level of therapist resources, some researchers are examining the possibility of using Internet applications of CBT protocols to make it more accessible. A therapist-assisted Internet self-help program for traumatic stress symptoms is currently being studied in an RCT with survivors of the attack on the Pentagon on 9/11 (Litz, Williams, Wang, Bryant, & Engel, 2004). The intervention uses a modified version of stress inoculation training (SIT) that is implemented through a combination of an initial face-to-face therapy session followed by 8 weeks of structured Internet-based intervention. The authors argue that SIT is a good intervention model for enhancing coping abilities because of its emphasis on "acquiring stress-reduction habits through practice and applying these skills to situations that trigger trauma memories in vivo" (p. 629). After the first face-to-face session, the patient is asked to log onto a treatment website daily for 8 weeks. Their therapist monitors symptom reports and homework assignments over this time period and can serve as a resource via telephone calls or electronic mail, if needed. Outcome data regarding this intervention are pending, but preliminary results indicate that no participants to date have experienced symptom exacerbation, and there have been no treatment dropouts (Litz, Williams et al., 2004).

There are debates regarding the appropriateness of treating ASD in the early aftermath of disasters. Given the unique and profound challenges typically associated with disasters (e.g., losing one's home, loved ones, cherished possessions, etc.), many, if not most, individuals may be forced to attend to more immediate needs in the initial days or weeks after a disaster. For example, many survivors will spend the initial days after a disaster securing food and shelter or searching for loved ones. Once these needs have been met, many disaster-impacted individuals will be left with still more unfinished business. They may be required to put tremendous amounts of time into life-rebuilding tasks such as securing insurance payments, planning funerals or memorial services, tending to physical injuries, rebuilding damaged homes, or securing new housing altogether. While treating ASD may be a reasonable goal for some disaster survivors in the first month after the trauma, it may be lower on the hierarchy of needs for many other survivors. Questions remain regarding which survivors should be targeted for early treatment and when such treatment should be offered. The appropriate format of such interventions (e.g. group, individual, Internet-based, etc.) also would benefit from further study. Further research into the needs of disaster-affected populations will help these questions continue to become clarified and should help inform the timing and dissemination of both early and later-stage interventions for ASD and PTSD after disasters.

Dismantling research is needed to parse out the active components of interventions that appear to be effective, such as CBT. It would be useful to compare the efficacy, speed of response, and tolerability (i.e., dropout rate) associated with different CBT components (e.g., exposure and cognitive restructuring) offered after disasters.

Research is also needed regarding interventions that address a broad array of outcomes across a diversity of populations. For example, future studies should examine outcomes other than (or in addition to) PTSD, such as depression, substance abuse, and panic disorder. Furthermore, little is known about how to best handle the needs of individuals who suffer traumatic bereavement. Research is also critically needed regarding how to best address the needs of children and adolescents who survive disasters.

Another priority for future intervention research involves how to make services most accessible and acceptable to an international body of potential consumers. Related to this issue are questions about how to best minimize the stigma of seeking mental health services and how to best disseminate services to large numbers of people. These are particularly salient issues when disasters occur on a massive scale or in areas that do not have adequate therapist resources, such as in Asia after the recent tsunami. An international perspective is needed when planning for the implementation of psychological interventions around the world.

It will also be important for researchers to further examine the impact of survivor education and support rather than structured psychological interventions per se. The dissemination of self-help or psychoeducational materials and brochures is widely practiced after disasters but has yet to be evaluated to determine whether this practice aids in recovery. The provision of support and education may be more feasible than structured clinical interventions on a large scale, but it is unknown whether such interventions are associated with true improvements in functioning. Similarly, although social support is widely acknowledged to be important in postdisaster recovery, interventions designed to improve support among family members, friends, and work colleagues have yet to be developed and evaluated. While much has been learned from large-scale events such as the terrorist attacks on September 11, 2001, and the Asian tsunami, these events also highlight the many areas in need of additional research support and attention.

REFERENCES

American Psychiatric Association (in press). Practice guidelines for the treatment of patients with acute stress disorder and posttraumatic stress disorder. *American Journal of Psychiatry.*

Başoğlu, M., Şalcioğlu, E., Livanou, M., Kalender, D., & Acar, G. (2005). Single-session behavioral treatment of earthquake-related posttraumatic stress disorder: A randomized waitlist controlled trial. *Journal of Traumatic Stress, 18,* 1–12.

Berliner, L., & Saunders, B. E. (1996). Treating fear and anxiety in sexually abused children: Results of a controlled 2-year follow-up study. *Child Maltreatment, 1,* 294–309.

Bisson, J. I. (2003). Single-session early psychological interventions following traumatic events. *Clinical Psychology Review, 23,* 481–499.

Bordow, S., & Porritt, D. (1979). An experimental evaluation of crisis intervention. *Social Science and Medicine, 13A,* 251–256.

Brom, D., Kleber, R. J., & Defares, P. B. (1989). Brief psychotherapy for posttraumatic stress disorders. *Journal of Consulting and Clinical Psychology, 57,* 607–612.

Brom, D., Kleber, R. J., & Hofman, M. C. (1993). Victims of traffic accidents: Incidence and prevention of post-traumatic stress disorder. *Journal of Clinical Psychology, 49,* 131–140.

Bryant, R. A., Harvey, A. G., Dang, S. T., Sackville, T., & Basten, C. (1998).Treatment of acute stress disorder: A comparison of cognitive-behavioral therapy and supportive counseling. *Journal of Consulting and Clinical Psychology, 66,* 862–866.

Bryant, R. A., Moulds, M. L., Guthrie, R. M., Dang, S. T., & Nixon, R. V. D. (2003). Imaginal exposure alone and imaginal exposure with cognitive restructuring in treatment of posttraumatic stress disorder. *Journal of Consulting and Clinical Psychology, 71,* 706–712.

Bryant, R. A., Moulds, M. L., Guthrie, R. M., & Nixon, R. V. D. (2005). The additive benefit of hypnosis and cognitive-behavioral therapy in treating Acute Stress Disorder. *Journal of Consulting and Clinical Psychology, 73,* 334–340.

Bryant, R. A., Moulds, M. L., & Nixon, R. V. D. (2003). Cognitive behaviour therapy of acute stress disorder: A four-year follow-up. *Behaviour Research and Therapy, 41,* 489–494.

Bryant, R. A., Sackville, T., Dang, S. T., Moulds, M., & Guthrie, R. (1999). Treating acute stress disorder: An evaluation of cognitive behavior therapy and supportive counseling techniques. *American Journal of Psychiatry, 156,* 1780–1786.

Bunn, T., & Clarke, A. (1979). Crisis intervention: An experimental study of the effects of a brief period of counseling on the anxiety of relatives of seriously injured or ill hospitalized patients. *British Journal of Medical Psychology, 52,* 191–195.

Chemtob, C. M., Nakashima, J., & Carlson, J. G. (2002). Brief treatment for elementary school children with disaster-related posttraumatic stress disorder: A field study. *Journal of Clinical Psychology, 58,* 99–112.

Chemtob, C. M., Nakashima, J. P., & Hamada, R. S. (2002). Psychosocial intervention for postdisaster trauma symptoms in elementary school children: A controlled community field study. *Archives of Pediatric and Adolescent Medicine, 156,* 211–216.

Cohen, J. A., & Mannarino, A. P. (1996). A treatment outcome study for sexually abused preschool children: Initial findings. *Journal of the American Academy of Child and Adolescent Psychiatry, 3,* 42–50.

Deblinger, E., Lippmann, J., & Steer, R. (1996). Sexually abused children suffering posttraumatic stress symptoms: Initial treatment outcome findings. *Child Maltreatment, 1,* 310–321.

Devilly, G. J., & Spence, S. H. (1999). The relative efficacy and treatment distress of EMDR and a cognitive-behavior trauma treatment protocol in the amelioration of posttraumatic stress disorder. *Journal of Anxiety Disorders, 13,* 131–157.

Echeburua, E., deCorral, P., Sarasua, B., & Zubizarreta, I. (1996). Treatment of acute posttraumatic stress disorder in rape victims: An experimental study. *Journal of Anxiety Disorders, 10,* 185–199.

Ehlers, A., & Clark, D. M. (2003). Early psychological interventions for adult survivors of trauma: A review. *Biological Psychiatry, 53,* 817–826.

Ferdinand, R., & Verhulst, F. (1995). Psychopathology from adolescence into young adulthood: An 8-year follow-up study. *American Journal of Psychiatry, 152,* 586-594.

Foa, E. B., Dancu, C. V., Hembree, E. A., Jaycox, L. H., Meadows, E. A., & Street, G. P. (1999). A comparison of exposure therapy, stress inoculation training, and their combination for reducing posttraumatic stress disorder in female assault victims. *Journal of Consulting and Clinical Psychology, 67,* 194–200.

Foa, E. B., Keane, T. M., & Friedman, M. J. (Eds.). (2000). *Effective treatments for PTSD: Practice guidelines from the International Society for Traumatic Stress Studies.* New York: Guilford Press.

Foa, E. B., & Meadows, E. A. (1997). Psychosocial treatments for post-traumatic stress disorder: A critical review. In J. Spence, J. M. Darley, & D. J. Foss (Eds.), *Annual review of psychology* (Vol. 48, pp. 449–480). Palo Alto, CA: Annual Reviews.

Foa, E. B., Rothbaum, B. O., Riggs, D. S., & Murdock, T. B. (1991). Treatment of posttraumatic stress disorder in rape victims: A comparison between cognitive-behavioral procedures and counseling. *Journal of Consulting and Clinical Psychology, 59,* 715–723.

Friedman, M. J. (2005). PTSD and acute post-traumatic reactions. Kansas City, MO: Compact Clinicals.

Gidron, Y., Gal, R., Freedman, S. A., Twiser, I., Lauden, A., Snir, Y., et al. (2001). Translating research findings to PTSD prevention: Results of a randomized-controlled pilot study. *Journal of Traumatic Stress, 14,* 773–780.

Gillespie, K., Duffy, M., Hackmann, A., & Clark, D. M. (2002). Community based cognitive therapy in the treatment of post-traumatic stress disorder following the Omagh bomb. *Behaviour Research and Therapy, 40*(4), 345–357.

Goenjian, A. K., Karayan, I., Pynoos, R. S., Minassian, D., Najarian, L. M., Steinberg, A. M., et al. (1997). Outcome of psychotherapy among early adolescents after trauma. *American Journal of Psychiatry, 154,* 536–542.

Hardin, S. B., Weinrich, S., Weinrich, M., Garrison, C., Addy, C., & Hardin, T. L. (2002).

Effects of a long-term psychosocial nursing intervention on adolescents exposed to catastrophic stress. *Issues in Mental Health Nursing, 23,* 537–551.

Hertlein, K. M., & Ricci, R. J. (2004). A systematic research synthesis of EMDR studies: Implementation of the platinum standard. *Trauma, Violence, and Abuse, 5,* 285–300.

Hobbs, M., Mayou, R., Harrison, B., & Worlock, P. (1996). A randomized trial of psychological debriefing for victims of road traffic accidents. *British Medical Journal, 313,* 1438–1439.

Ironson, G., Freund, B., Strauss, J. L., & Williams, J. (2002). Comparison of two treatments for traumatic stress: A community-based study of EMDR and prolonged exposure. *Journal of Clinical Psychology, 58,* 113–128.

Jacobson, N. S., & Truax, P. (1991). Clinical significance: A statistical approach to defining meaningful change in psychotherapy research. *Journal of Consulting and Clinical Psychology, 59,* 12–19.

Lavender, T., & Walkinshaw, S. A. (1998). Can midwives reduce postpartum psychological morbidity? A randomized trial. *Birth, 25*(4), 215–219.

Lee, C., Gavriel, H., Drummond, P., Richards, J., & Greenwald, R. (2002). Treatment of PTSD: Stress inoculation training with prolonged exposure compared to EMDR. *Journal of Clinical Psychology, 58,* 1071–1089.

Litz, B. T., Adler, A. B., Castro, C. A., Wright, K., Thomas, J., & Suvak, M. K. (2004, November). A controlled trial of group debriefing. In M. Friedman (Chair), *Military psychiatry, then and now.* Plenary session presented at the 20th annual meeting of the International Society for Traumatic Stress Studies, New Orleans, LA.

Litz, B. T., & Gibson, L. E. (2006). Conducting research on mental health interventions. In M. Friedman, C. Ritchie, & P. Watson (Eds.), *Interventions following mass violence and disaster: Strategies for mental health practice* (pp. 387–904). New York: Guilford Press.

Litz, B. T., Gray, M. J., Bryant, R. A., & Adler, A. B. (2002). Early intervention for trauma: Current status and future directions. *Clinical Psychology: Science and Practice, 9,* 112–134.

Litz, B. T., Williams, L., Wang, J., Bryant, R., & Engel, C. C. (2004). A therapist-assisted internet self-help program for traumatic stress. *Professional Psychology: Research and Practice, 35,* 628–634.

Marks, I., Lovell, K., Noshirvani, H., Livanou, M., & Thrasher, S. (1998). Treatment of posttraumatic stress disorder by exposure and/or cognitive restructuring: A controlled study. *Archives of General Psychiatry, 55,* 317–325.

Norris, F. H., Friedman, M. J., Watson, P. J., Byrne, C. M., Diaz, E., & Kaniasty, K. (2002). 60,000 disaster victims speak: Part I. An empirical review of the empirical literature, 1981–2001. *Psychiatry, 65,* 207–239.

Ormel, J., VonKorff, M., Ustun, B., Pini, S., Korten, A., & Oldehinkel, T. (1994). Common mental disorders and disability across cultures. *Journal of the American Medical Association, 272,* 1741–1748.

Pitman, R, K., Sanders, K. M., Zusman, R. M., Healy, A. R., Cheema, F., Lasko, N.B., et al. (2002). Pilot study of secondary prevention of posttraumatic stress disorder with propranolol. *Biological Psychiatry, 51,* 189–192.

Power, K., McGoldrick, T., Brown, K., Buchanan, R., Sharp, D., Swanson, V., et al. (2002). A controlled comparison of eye movement desensitization and reprocessing versus exposure plus cognitive restructuring versus waiting list in the treatment of post-traumatic stress disorder. *Clinical Psychology and Psychotherapy, 9,* 299–318.

Resick, P. A., Nishith, P., Weaver, T. L., Astin, M. C., & Feuer, C. A. (2002). A comparison of cognitive-processing therapy with prolonged exposure and a waiting condition for the treatment of chronic posttraumatic stress disorder in female rape victims. *Journal of Consulting and Clinical Psychology, 70,* 867–879.

Robert, R., Blakeney, P. E., Villarreal, C., Rosenberg. L., & Meyer, W. (1999). Imipramine treatment in pediatric burn patients with symptoms of acute stress disorder: A pilot study. *Journal of the American Academy of Child and Adolescent Psychiatry, 38,* 873–882.

Rose, S., Bisson, J., & Wessely, S. (2002). Psychological debriefing for preventing posttraumatic stress disorder (PTSD). (Cochrane Review). In *The Cochrane Library, 2.* Oxford: Update Software.

Rothbaum, B. O. (1997). A controlled study of eye movement desensitization and reprocessing in the treatment of posttraumatic stress disordered sexual assault victims. *Bulletin of the Menninger Clinic, 61,* 317–334.

Rothbaum, B., Foa, E., Riggs, D., Murdock, T., & Walsh, W. (1992). A prospective examination of post-traumatic stress disorder in rape victims. *Journal of Traumatic Stress, 5,* 455–475.

Schelling, G., Briegel, J., Roozendale, B., Stroll, C., Rothenhausler, H., & Kapfhammer, H. (2001). The effect of stress doses of hydrocortisone during septic shock on posttraumatic stress disorder in survivors. *Biological Psychiatry, 50,* 978–985.

Small, R., Lumley, J., Donohue, L., Potter, A., & Waldenstroem, U. (2000). Randomised controlled trial of midwife led debriefing to reduce maternal depression after operative childbirth. *British Medical Journal, 321,* 1043–1047.

Stein, B. D., Jaycox, L. H., Kataoka, S. H., Wong, M., Tu, W., Elliott, M. N., et al. (2003). A mental health intervention for school children exposed to violence: A randomized controlled trial. *Journal of the American Medical Association, 290,* 603–611.

Tarrier, N., Pilgrim, H., Sommerfield, C., Faragher, B., Reynolds, M., Graham, E., et al. (1999). A randomized trial of cognitive therapy and imaginal exposure in the treatment of chronic post traumatic stress disorder. *Journal of Consulting and Clinical Psychology, 67,* 13–18.

Tarrier, N., & Sommerfield, C. (2004). Treatment of chronic PTSD by cognitive therapy and exposure: A 5-year follow-up. *Behavior Therapy, 35,* 231–246.

Taylor, S., Thordarson, D. S., Maxfield, L., Fedoroff, I. C., Lovell, K., & Ogrodniczuk, J. (2003). Comparative efficacy, speed, and adverse effects of three PTSD treatments: Exposure therapy, EMDR, and relaxation training. *Journal of Consulting and Clinical Psychology, 71,* 330–338.

Veterans Health Administration, (2004). VA/DoD clinical practice guidelines for management of post-traumatic stress. Retrieved June 14, 2005, from www.oqp.med.va.gov/cpg/PTSD/PTSD_Base.htm

Valentiner, D. P., Foa, E. B., Riggs, D. S., & Gershuny, B. S. (1996). Coping strategies and posttraumatic stress disorder in female victims of sexual and nonsexual assault. *Journal of Abnormal Psychology, 105,* 455–458.

Van Emmerick, A. A. P., Kamphuis, J. H., Hulsbosch, A. M., & Emmelkamp, P. M. G. (2002). Single session debriefing after psychological trauma: A meta-analysis. *Lancet, 360,* 766–771.

Watson, P. J., Friedman, M. J., Gibson, L. E., Ruzek, J. I., Norris, F. H., & Ritchie, E. C. (2003). Early intervention for trauma-related problems. *Review of Psychiatry, 22,* 97–124.

Yule, W. (1992). Post-traumatic stress disorder in child survivors of shipping disasters: The sinking of the 'Jupiter.' *Psychotherapy and Psychosomatics, 57,* 200–205.

CHAPTER 14

Strategies for Dissemination of Evidence-Based Treatments

Training Clinicians after Large-Scale Disasters

RANDALL D. MARSHALL, LAWRENCE AMSEL,
YUVAL NERIA, and EUN JUNG SUH

A core assumption in disaster response models is that there will be a sudden increase in health problems that will exceed the community's existing services infrastructure, sometimes referred to as its "surge capacity," and that the community will therefore require humanitarian aid in the form of funding, personnel, and interventions. Models for postdisaster mental health services in the United States traditionally have emphasized crisis counseling interventions that aim to promote resilience and recovery in the community. However, the terrorist attacks on the World Trade Center on September 11, 2001, sharply raised awareness that it is sometimes necessary to increase local capacity to provide specialized treatment for serious or chronic mental health problems and disorders (Herman, Felton, & Suzzer, 2002). Thus, the core question addressed by this chapter is this: After large-scale disasters, when it is reasonable to anticipate a high incidence of psychological disorders, how can capacity be increased to meet the needs of seriously affected disaster victims? In other words, is it possible to train clinicians to implement evidence-based treatments (EBTs) on a large enough scale so as to have a meaningful public health impact on rates of disorder in the community?

Rapid dissemination of EBTs is a very recent area of investigation. We do not attempt to provide a comprehensive examination of all approaches that are presently under investigation. For example, Litz, Williams, Wang, Bryant, and Engel (2004) developed a therapist-assisted Internet-based self-help program to allow treatment of large numbers of traumatized individuals with limited clinical resources. We focus on one particular strategy that may have widespread applicability—the development of rapidly deployable training that can increase skill level in relatively large numbers of mental health providers quickly, efficiently, and effectively. We draw heavily upon our efforts after the September 11th attacks to develop a training program that eventually trained approximately 1,500 licensed clinicians in two EBTs, specifically prolonged exposure therapy (Foa & Rothbaum, 1998) and complicated grief therapy (Shear, Frank, Houck, & Reynolds, 2005).

We have organized this chapter around five key questions that dissemination programs should address. First, is there a need to disseminate EBTs at all? (Is there a surge-capacity problem?) Second, what disorders will require increased availability of EBTs? Third, which EBTs should be disseminated to improve outcomes for the disorders in question? Fourth, what is the most efficient, effective way of disseminating these EBTs? And, fifth, to what degree were the objectives accomplished? After discussing these five questions and illustrating them with our own thinking and experiences after the attacks on September 11, we briefly summarize the research we conducted to evaluate the effectiveness of training as a strategy for dissemination. We conclude by describing additional research strategies that might be employed for this purpose in the future.

IS THERE A NEED TO DISSEMINATE EBTs?

The answer to this question depends upon (1) the anticipated incidence of psychological disorders and (2) the skill level of local mental health providers to diagnose and treat those disorders. Prior research does indeed show that after major disasters, especially those involving mass violence or numerous fatalities, there is a predictable sudden increase in rates of serious but treatable mental disorders in the affected community (see Norris & Elrod, Chapter 2, this volume). Consistent with this body of research, epidemiological studies of the mental health consequences of the September 11th terrorist attacks found significant rates of new-onset posttraumatic stress disorder (PTSD) in those directly and indirectly exposed in New York (Galea et al., 2002; Hoven et al., 2005) and, surprisingly, also in persons across the United States (e.g., Silver, Holman, McIntosh, Poulin, & Gil-Rivas, 2002). In interpreting epidemiological data, small percentages can translate into large absolute numbers (e.g., a rate of 1% in the New York metropolitan area = 158,000 persons). It was correctly predicted that there would be a sudden, increased need for EBTs in greater New York (Herman et al., 2002).

A high incidence of new-onset disorders would not necessarily be a problem if the health care system were prepared for diasters. Little is known about actual practices in the community in treating serious mental disorders, including PTSD. However, everything we do know suggests that PTSD is seldom diagnosed and is therefore almost certainly inadequately treated (see Marshall, in press). Moreover, research on practice patterns in the United States suggests that most clinicians are either unaware of EBTs for PTSD or simply do not practice them because of lack of training (60%), resistance to manualized treatments (25%), or fears of retraumatizing patients (22%)(Becker, Zayfert, & Anderson, 2004). Ideally, a capacity to provide EBTs in response to disaster should predate the experience of a disaster, but at present, ad hoc training and treatment programs will be needed whenever there is a sudden surge in serious mental disorders. Certainly, in our case, the attacks on September 11, 2001, provoked an urgent awareness of the lack of expert evidence-based care in New York.

WHAT DISORDERS REQUIRE INCREASED AVAILABILITY OF EBTS?

Research to date suggests that PTSD and major depressive disorder (MDD) are the two most likely new-onset disorders to occur in the aftermath of disasters (Norris & Elrod, Chapter 12, this volume). These are highest among direct victims (people who experience actual loss or harm) but occur with lower frequency among indirect victims (Galea & Resnick, 2005). Subthreshold PTSD was three to four times as common as full PTSD in the greater New York area after the terrorist attacks (Galea et al., 2002). Subthreshhold PTSD is also associated with clinical and functional impairment (e.g., Marshall et al., 2001; Stein et al, 1997) and, we believe, should be targeted for treatment when associated with impairment.

The importance of PTSD and MDD relative to other potential outcomes appears to hold across different disaster types (Norris & Elrod, Chapter 2, this volume), although the prevalence may vary with disaster severity. Although it has been studied less often, complicated grief, often comorbid with PTSD, appears to be another important outcome in the aftermath of disasters involving mass fatalities (Neria et al., in press; Shear et al., 2005). At this time, there is little research to guide judgments regarding the disorders most likely to follow a bioterrorist attack, but if the media broadcast dramatically frightening scenes of persons falling ill, being trapped in quarantines, or dying, it seems possible that the phenomenon seen in New York would recur—that of large numbers of PTSD and subthreshold PTSD cases in the community at large, in part through media exposure.

How can simply *being confronted with* a terrorist attack through the media precipitate a subjective response (criterion A2) severe enough to cause PTSD among persons who were not threatened with death or physical injury? Drawing upon the New York case, we believe that the scale, unpredictability, and potential threat of terrorist attacks created a perception of meaningful, imminent, ongoing threat. In vulnerable individuals, this reaction can be consolidated and intensified through hours of additional media viewing and multiple warnings. Finally, the ongoing stresses of the postattack environment may tax and deplete coping strategies that would, under less severe circumstances, lead to successful processing of the disaster-related trauma.

In summary, the evidence to date suggests that PTSD, subtheshhold PTSD, MDD, and complicated grief are the most likely postdisaster disorders and all have exposure-related treatments. After terrorist attacks, it appears especially likely that psychopathology will not be confined to direct victims but will extend to others who were indirectly exposed.

WHICH EBTs SHOULD BE DISSEMINATED?

There are several convincing single-site studies that demonstrate the utility of brief trauma-focused cognitive-behavioral therapy (CBT) for persons with acute stress disorder and acute PTSD (see Gibson, Hamblen, Zvolensky, & Vujanovic, Chapter 13, this volume). However, it is extremely difficult to disseminate EBTs quickly enough to treat acute disaster-related disorders. These skills must be developed in the community through professional training and preparedness efforts *prior* to the event. Our discussion therefore focuses on dissemination of EBTs provided 6 months to 5 years after a disaster.

Foa and colleagues have recently conducted a series of dissemination projects that increased the capacity of a community-based outpatient program to provide prolonged exposure therapy to victims of sexual assault (Cahill, Hembree, & Foa, in press). These dissemination efforts demonstrate that community treatment clinics can be trained to deliver specialized treatment with intensive supervision. Unfortunately these programs typically are not feasible in the postdisaster context, because they are slow, expensive, and time-intensive. The next phase of dissemination research will need to extract the essential components of these efforts to create more efficient models of dissemination (Barlow, Levitt, & Bufka, 1999; Corrigan, Steiner, McCracken, Blaser, & Barr, 2001; Wells et al., 2002). Fortunately, for most serious mental disorders that are caused by large-scale disasters, there are at least two distinctly different treatment options with a strong evidence base. For PTSD and MDD, there are several pharmacological treatments and several time-limited, manualized treatments that can provide the content for a dissemination program.

A particularly lucid model of the evidence-based approach has been outlined as a five-step procedure by Sackett, Rosenberg, Gray, Haynes, and Richardson (1996; see also Amsel, Neria, Suh, & Marshall 2005). The first step is to clarify a dissemination problem by reframing it in the form of an empirically answerable question. For example, we decided, based on clinical instincts and early needs assessments, to focus on increasing practitioner capacity to provide psychotherapy for chronic PTSD. This seemingly simple step is fundamental to the subsequent success of the dissemination effort. It forces a clear focus on well-defined diagnostic or clinical problems and a single-treatment approach or at most a few comparable approaches.

The second and third steps in the evidence-based approach are to evaluate relevant clinical trials in terms of their validity (quality and lack of biases), impact (the effect size or clinical significance of a positive finding), and applicability (the relevance of participants and their clinical problems to the current situation). It is beyond the scope of this chapter to review evidence supporting various CBTs for PTSD (see Gibson et al., Chapter 13, this volume). However, a key finding is that all empirically validated CBTs incorporate some form of exposure to the traumatic memory—that is, a clinician-guided remembering and retelling of the traumatic event.

The fourth step in the EB approach is using clinical expertise to adapt the treatment to suit the patient's values, circumstances, and physiology. Some researchers have insisted that a proven treatment must be applied with a high degree of adherence to its original formulation in order to be useful (Waltz, Addis, Koerner, & Jacobson, 1993). In direct contradiction, others have focused on the need to adapt the proven treatment to a variety of situations and explicitly recognize the need to modify the techniques accordingly (Schulte, 1996). We refer to this debate as the *adopt versus adapt* controversy. The final step is to evaluate the outcome of this whole process and make ongoing adjustments.

Evidence-based psychotherapy may also be controversial because it touches on questions of professional autonomy and the role of the professional's individuality as a therapeutic tool. The very notion of standardization in psychotherapy can be the most difficult adjustment for psychotherapists without prior CBT training. Adopting CBT-based skills will require a fundamental attitudinal shift as well as significant behavior change on the part of the clinician-trainees. It is therefore crucial that the training model address these issues.

WHAT IS THE MOST EFFICIENT, EFFECTIVE WAY OF DISSEMINATING THESE EBTs?

Training programs to teach professionals EBTs universally consist of (1) didactic training and (2) supervision of the trainee by more senior and experienced professionals. Because the processes of diagnosis and treatment mostly involve operational learning (skills) and not informational learning (facts), the mental health tradition has depended heavily on supervision to pass on skills from master to apprentice (medieval metaphor intended). Reliance on this mode of teaching unfortunately creates a bottleneck in the postdisaster setting because it is entirely dependent on a highly scarce resource—gifted and experienced teachers with enough time (assuming there is funding) to supervise trainees in time-intensive review of their ongoing cases. It was thus immediately clear to us after September 11th that we had to find an alternative to this time-honored tradition and "gold standard" for psychotherapy training.

When extensive supervision is not feasible, the challenge is to frame the active components of an EBT in a way that that can be easily applied by individual practitioners. In our work, we first identified aspects of prolonged exposure therapy that were both central to the therapy and that distinguished it from psychodynamic psychotherapy as widely practiced in the community. We recognized that the educational experience would be very different for a psychodynamic-oriented therapist and a CBT-oriented therapist, even if neither had experience with PTSD. Blagys and Hilsenroth (2002) identified six activities distinctive to CBTs. These were: (1) the use of homework and outside-of-session activities; (2) the direction of session activity through manualized guidelines; (3) the teaching of skills to patients to cope with symptoms; (4) the emphasis on patients' future experiences rather than past experiences; (5) providing patients with information about their treatment, disorder, or symptoms; and (6) an intrapersonal cognitive focus, that is, cognitive restructuring. For PTSD, the ability to conduct exposures to traumatic memories (*in vivo*) are an additional distinctive component.

HOW WILL WE KNOW IF WE HAVE
ACCOMPLISHED OUR OBJECTIVES?

The goal of any dissemination effort is to change clinician behavior. A number of theoretical models are applicable here, ranging from adult education theories (Jaccard, 1975) to stages-of-change models (Prochaska & Velicer, 1997). We found new work in the basic sciences of decision making and motivation to be most compelling as a template for our trainings. These models build upon the simple common-sense proposition that intentions precede and direct actions (Fishbein & Ajzen, 1975). Such intentions (e.g., the intention to conduct an exposure exercise with a patient) are called behavioral intentions. The stronger the behavioral intention, the greater the likelihood that a person will enact the behavior.

Three key factors predict the strength of such behavioral intentions (Jaccard, 1975). The first factor is the *expected value of the outcome*, that is, the positive consequences that are expected to result from the behavior. In the clinical situation this would involve a clinician's expectations and beliefs about whether a treatment will benefit the patient. These expectations may be based on prior training or experience, on published literature or on a training program experience.

The second factor is one's *belief about existing norms*. Even when we believe that an action would benefit us, we are less likely to act if it is inconsistent with the norms of behavior in our environment. Thus, a clinician's belief about what peers and thought leaders are using as treatments may affect practice more than the available evidence in the given clinical field.

The third key factor is *self-efficacy*, the belief that one can successfully and effectively perform the behavior. Training must take into account the relative difficulty of adopting a recommendation among trainers. Finally, a wide range of other factors, especially unanticipated barriers, may prevent a behavioral intention from effectively becoming an actual behavior. The nearly universal failure to carry out one's New Year's resolutions makes the point.

We used these three principles in designing both the trainings and the evaluations of their effectiveness. Two-day trainings were structured to influence expected values, beliefs about existing norms, and self-efficacy in order to maximize the behavioral intention to implement the new skills and framework. Trainings made use of three educational modalities (used in this order): lectures, demonstrations, and small group role play, in which trainees alternated playing the therapist and the patient in pairs. Discussion was encouraged throughout the training, particularly of trainee reservations, doubts, and fears about the new techniques.

Lectures followed by discussion were created to give brief, specific instructions about a technique, as well as a clear and convincing clinical rationale for using it. We hypothesized that lectures would primarily influence expected values and norms. Trainers conducted demonstrations (with one playing the patient, modeling the later role-play exercise) of a particular technique that had just been presented in the lecture-for example, the first exposure exercise in prolonged exposure therapy. Demonstrations were intended primarily to influence norms (by showing an expert successfully conducting a treatment), and also self-efficacy through contributing to skill acquisition. In later trainings, the demonstrations were shown on videotape. This allowed both for standardization and for greater flexibility (by decreasing the need for several trainers), but whether it is as compelling as a live demonstration is an empirical question.

Both lectures and clinical demonstration are passive teaching modalities for the participants. Because active practice is required to alter skill levels (Amsel et al., 2005) we conducted multiple role-play sessions during the 2-day training. By allowing the practice of unfamiliar techniques in a supportive setting, this training modality was expected to have the strongest impact on skill acquisition. We also hoped it could help clinicians to anticipate and overcome barriers via an experiential process.

In summary, by building on previous empirical findings and introducing theory from the basic behavioral sciences, we developed an initial workshop design that was aimed at having maximum impact on those factors that influence behavior change. To test these assumptions, we asked participants to complete questionnaires on the training experience and on changes in attitudes resulting from the training.

PILOT FINDINGS

To illustrate these various points, we present data from our training of licensed community practitioners in the use of prolonged exposure therapy. A group of 104 clinicians, who each averaged 17 years in practice, participated in the training workshops and completed questionnaires at the start and the close of the training (Amsel et al., 2005).

Our assumption was that trainee behavior could be predicted in part by three metrics: *overall favorability* ratings collapsing values and norms; *self-efficacy* with regard to implementing that component; and the difference between the two, which we refer to as the *implementation gap*. The ideal situation is for both favorability and self-efficacy ratings to be high with an implementation gap near zero. Table 14.1 gives the pretraining rating results from our pilot study with respect to core components of prolonged exposure therapy. Several different patterns are evident, with different implications for training.

TABLE 14.1. Pretraining Attitudes Toward Components of Prolonged Exposure Therapy

Prolonged exposure therapy component	Favorability		Self-efficacy		Implementation gap
	M	(SD)	M	(SD)	
Psychoeducation	4.6	(0.7)	3.8	(1.8)	0.8
Prolonged (imaginal) exposure	2.5*	(2.2)	0.3*	(2.8)	2.2**
In vivo exposure	2.6*	(2.2)	0.1*	(3.0)	2.4**
Use of manual	1.5*	(2.6)	0.3*	(2.9)	1.1
Structured instruments	2.9*	(2.0)	1.8*	(2.7)	1.1
Homework	3.0*	(2.1)	0.7*	(3.0)	2.3**
Cognitive restructuring	3.0*	(2.3)	1.2*	(2.9)	1.8*
Assessment	3.8	(1.9)	1.9*	(2.8)	1.9*
Subjective Units of Discomfort awareness	3.4	(1.7)	2.1*	(2.6)	1.3
Breathing training	4.1	(1.3)	3.2	(2.2)	0.9

Note. Favorability and self-efficacy were both rated on a scale from -5 to +5. The implementation gap is the difference between favorability and self-efficacy.

* Rating or gap different from that for psychoeducation tested, tested with paired t-test, $p < .01$.

The mean favorability ratings for psychoeducation and for breathing retraining, were close to the maximum possible values, making the implementation gap minimal.

At the other extreme, the CBT practice of using a manual had the lowest favorability rating, and the second-lowest self-efficacy rating. Therapists did not approve of the recommendation and had poor skills to apply it. This pretraining status indicates a general lack of motivation to change skills or practice with respect to using manuals. This is the most difficult starting point vis à vis changing behavior in a training. Interestingly, this finding is reflected in the psychotherapy research literature, where the "adopt versus adapt" controversy is being actively debated. Garfield (1998) has argued that strict adherence to a manual (i.e., adopting an EBT directly as used in the research literature) can reduce the efficacy of psychotherapy, because therapists are not able to respond to patients' individual and unique needs. Castonguay, Goldfried, Wiser, Raue, and Hayes (1996) found that, in treatment for depression, an overly rigid adherence to the CBT manual correlated negatively with treatment outcome. Gibbon et al. (2002) took an intermediate position. While she argued for the usefulness of manuals, she believed they need to be applied with flexibility. Her study demonstrated that highly trained therapists applied the manuals with considerable flexibility and sensitivity to patients' needs (i.e., they adapted the principles and techniques).

Another pattern that emerged from the trainees' responses involved a high (or moderate) favorability rating but a low self-efficacy rating. Recommendations with these patterns should respond most robustly to skill-based trainings. Notably, both imaginal exposure and *in vivo* exposure fell into this category.

The favorability scores for recommendations regarding careful assessment, cognitive restructuring, assigning therapeutic homework, and the use of structured assessment instruments were close to one another but higher than for prolonged exposure, thus falling somewhere in the middle of all recommendations. These recommendations were probably seen as the workhorse components of the treatment—not well understood but not particularly controversial. Again, skill-building training could be expected to influence adoption of this group of recommendations.

To evaluate the effectiveness of the core training modalities (lectures, demonstration, role play), trainees rated each with respect to accomplishing seven educational objectives we developed from the motivation science literature: conveying theoretical principles, conveying procedures and details of the therapy, changing beliefs about the treatment, changing initial objections, helping them overcome barriers to implementation, promoting skill acquisition, and motivating to change their practice. Objectives were rated on a Likert scale of −5 (highly ineffective) to +5 (highly effective). We had hypothesized, based on the literature, that (1) lectures would be rated the most effective for conveying theory, but less effective for all other objectives (as the most passive modality); and (2) role play (as the most active modality) would be rated the most effective by trainees for most objectives.

To our surprise, our initial findings were that trainees rated demonstrations as the most effective educational modality for all seven objectives. Role play was rated the second most effective modality for most objectives, and lectures were rated least effective for most educational objectives, especially skills training and helping to overcome barriers. Contrary to expectation, lectures had little effect in changing beliefs about the treatment or in reducing initial objections to it. As expected, role play was rated most effective in promoting skill acquisition and motivation.

These tentative findings await confirmation. If the findings are replicated in larger samples, there are several important implications for postdisaster trainings and perhaps for psychotherapy training in general:

1. *Lectures* are minimally useful for imparting skills or other forms of procedural knowledge, and are best used to convey theory and basic information. At best, they should motivate trainees to learn more.

2. *Demonstration* was rated highly effective and broadly successful as an educational tool. There are many implications for this finding if it is replicated. It suggests that expert demonstration of skills should be a core component of psychotherapy training in general, and postdisaster training

in particular. This might include live demonstrations, videotapes of patients, videotapes of simulated patient encounters, or new ways of demonstrating skills yet to be developed.

3. *Role play* is particularly useful to impart skills and motivation, but it is not as effective in this setting as theory would predict. Perhaps role play, as the most active and demanding modality, is too difficult for introductory trainings but becomes more useful at a later stage of training and skill acquisition.

Finally, clinicians did not perceive that the training effectively addressed perceived barriers to implementation. Overcoming barriers may require an entirely new and dedicated training modality (Gollwitzer, 1999).

STUDYING POSTDISASTER SERVICE DELIVERY AFTER LARGE-SCALE DISASTER

This field is in its infancy, such that basic methodologies that would allow feasible study of services delivery after large-scale disaster, with measurement of clinical outcomes, still need to be developed. Successful services research models that accomplish this (e.g., Lieberman et al., 2005) might be adapted for the postdisaster setting, and ideally should be developed as a preparedness objective. The train-the-trainers model that includes regular supervision for psychotherapy training is extremely difficult to implement on a large scale unless many experts are available; this is the rate-limiting factor for this dissemination model. We believe that more efficient forms of supervision (e.g., periodic group supervision, internet-based supervision, etc.) should also be studied in comparison to the gold standard set by Foa and colleagues (Foa et al., 2005) with intensive supervision and in comparison to a well-conceptualized training.

There are many issues to consider in researching services outcome after postdisaster trainings. Presumably only the highly motivated therapists would enroll in training and supervision programs, since attending such training events requires significant sacrifices in time and often income. This might bias outcome and limit generalizability. Convincing institutions (hospitals, outpatient clinics) to allow staff to attend trainings can be a major barrier in itself. A number of sampling methodologies might be applicable, but the decentralized nature of some service delivery systems (like the United States) makes this particularly difficult.

Educational models deserve much more study, given their central role in improving the quality of care provided in the community and in disseminating new research findings. The vast resources devoted to lecture-based continuing professional education (CPE) trainings (which are ineffective in imparting new skills) could be used instead to develop and evaluate educational programs that are actually effective and efficient.

CONCLUSIONS

There have been an extraordinary number of lost opportunities for serious research after every major disaster that would have involved no sacrifice at all, only better planning. Even minimal program evaluation methodologies are typically eschewed as yet another obstacle to program implementation. In other words, the inevitable resistance to research that is encountered within any service delivery system is framed after a disaster as a life-and-death race against time. This is a difficult objection to overcome in the postdisaster setting. It must be overcome before disaster strikes. For this to occur, services researchers will have to form partnerships with governmental and philanthropic agencies that are mandated to respond to community disasters. Researchers can play important direct and indirect roles in trying to influence service providers toward greater accountability (i.e., program evaluation) and inspire all stakeholders to want to contribute to humanitarian knowledge that can benefit future disaster victims.

ACKNOWLEDGMENTS

This work was supported in part by National Institute of Mental Health (Grant Nos. MH01412 and MH 66081), National Institute on Drug Abuse (Grant No. DA14219-01S1), The New York Times Foundation, The Atlantic Philanthropies, United Way of New York City and The New York Community Trust, the Spunk Fund, and The Commonwealth Fund.

REFERENCES

Amsel, L. V., Neria, Y., Suh, E. J., & Marshall, R. D. (2005). Training Therapists to treat the psychological consequences of terrorism: Disseminating psychotherapy research and researching psychotherapy dissemination. *Journal of Aggression, Maltreatment and Trauma, 10*, 633–647.

Barlow, D. H., Levitt, J. T., & Bufka, L. F. (1999). The dissemination of empirically supported treatments: A view to the future. *Behavior Research and Therapy, 37*, 147–162.

Becker, C. B., Zayfert, C., & Anderson, E. (2004). A survey of psychologists' attitudes towards and utilization of exposure therapy for PTSD. *Behaviour Research and Therapy, 42*(3), 277–292.

Blagys, M. D., & Hilsenroth, M. J. (2002). Distinctive activities of cognitive-behavioral therapy: A review of the comparative psychotherapy process literature. *Clinical Psychology Review, 22,* 671–706.

Cahill, S. P., Hembree, E. A, & Foa, E. B. (in press). Dissemination of prolonged exposure therapy for posttraumatic stress disorder: Successes and challenges. In Y. Neria, R. Gross, R. Marshall, & E. Susser (Eds.), *September 11, 2001: Treatment, research and public mental health in the wake of a terrorist attack.* New York: Cambridge University Press.

Castonguay, L. G., Goldfried, M. R., Wiser, S., Raue, P. J., & Hayes, A.M. (1996). Predicting the effect of cognitive therapy for depression: A study of unique and common factors. *Journal of Consulting and Clinical Psychology, 64,* 497–504.

Corrigan, P. W., Steiner, L., McCracken, S. G., Blaser, B., & Barr, M. (2001). Strategies for disseminating evidence-based practices to staff who treat people with serious mental illness. *Psychiatric Services, 52,* 1598–1606.

Fishbein, M., & Ajzen, I. (1975). *Belief, attitude, intention and behavior: An introduction to theory and research.* Reading, MA: Addison-Wesley.

Foa, E. B., & Rothbaum, B. O. (1998). *Treating the trauma of rape: Cognitive-behavioral therapy for PTSD.* New York: Guilford Press.

Foa, E. B., Hembree, E. A., Cahill, S. P., Rauch, S. A., Riggs, D. S., Feeny, N. C., et al. (2005). Randomized trial of prolonged exposure for posttraumatic stress disorder with and without cognitive restructuring: Outcome at academic and community clinics. *Journal of Consulting and Clinical Psychology, 73,* 953–964.

Galea, S., & Resnick, H. (2005). Posttraumatic stress disorder in the general population after mass terrorist incidents: Considerations about the nature of exposure. *CNS Spectrums, 10,* 107–115.

Galea, S., Ahern, J., Resnick, H., Kilpatrick, D., Bucuvalas, M., Gold, J., et al. (2002). Psychological sequelae of the September 11 terrorist attacks in New York City. *New England Journal of Medicine, 346,* 982–987.

Garfield, S. L. (1998). Some comments on empirically supported treatments. *Journal of Consulting and Clinical Psychology, 66,* 121–125.

Gibbon, M. B., Crits-Christoph, P., Levinson, J., Gladis, M., Siqueland, L., Barber, J. P., et al. (2002). Therapist interventions in the interpersonal and cognitive therapy sessions of the Treatment of Depression Collaborative Research Program. *American Journal of Psychotherapy, 56,* 3–26.

Gollwitzer, P. M. (1999). Implementation intentions: Strong effects of simple plans. *American Psychologist, 54,* 493–503.

Herman, D., Felton, C., & Susser, E. (2002). Mental health needs in New York State following the September 11th attacks. *Journal of Urban Health, 79,* 322–331.

Hoven, C. W., Duarte, C. S., Lucas, C. P., Wu, P., Mandell, D. J., Goodwin, R. D., et al. (2005). Psychopathology among New York City school children 6 months after September 11. *Archives of General Psychiatry, 62,* 545–552.

Jaccard, J. (1975). A theoretical analysis of selected factors important to health education strategies. *Health Education Monographs, 3,* 152–167.

Litz, B., Williams, L., Wang, J., Bryant, R., & Engel, C. (2004). A therapist-assisted internet self-help program for traumatic stress. *Professional Psychology: Research and Practice, 35,* 628–634.

Marshall, R. D., Olfson, M., Hellman, F., Blanco, C., Guardino, M., Struening, E. (2001). Comorbidity, impairment, and suicidality in subthreshold PTSD. *American Journal of Psychiatry, 158,* 1467–1473.

Marshall, R. D. (in press). Science for the community after 9/11: Introduction to Treatment

Section. In Y. Neria, R. Gross, R. Marshall, & E. Susser (Eds.), *September 11, 2001: Treatment, research and public mental health in the wake of a terrorist attack*. New York: Cambridge University Press.

Neria, Y., Gross, R., Litz, B., Insel, B., Maguen, S., Seirmarco, G., et al. (in press). Complicated grief, comorbidity, and suicidal ideation in persons experiencing loss in the 9/11 attacks. *Journal of Traumatic Stress*.

Prochaska, J. O., & Velicer, W. F. (1997). The transtheoretical model of health behavior change. *American Journal of Health Promotion, 12*, 38–48.

Schulte, D. (1996). Tailor-made and standardized therapy: Complementary tasks in behavior therapy. A contrarian view. *Journal of Behavior Therapy and Experimental Psychiatry, 27*, 119–126.

Shear, K., Frank, E., Houck, P. R., & Reynolds, C. F. (2005). Treatment of complicated grief: A randomized controlled trial. *Journal of the American Medical Association, 293*, 2601–2608.

Silver, R. C., Holman, E. A., McIntosh, D. N., Poulin, M., & Gil-Rivas, V. (2002). Nationwide longitudinal study of psychological responses to September 11. *Journal of the American Medical Association, 288*, 1235–1244.

Stein, M. B., Walker, J. R., Hazen, A. L., & Forde, D. R. (1997). Full and partial posttraumatic stress disorder: Findings from a community survey. *American Journal of Psychiatry, 154*, 1114–1119.

Waltz, J., Addis, M. E., Koerner, K., & Jacobson, N. S. (1993). Testing the integrity of a psychotherapy protocol: Assessment of adherence and competence. *Journal of Consulting and Clinical Psychology, 61*, 620–630.

Wells, K. B., Miranda, J., Bauer, M. S., Bruce, M. L., Durham, M., Escobar, J., et al. (2002). Overcoming barriers to reducing the burden of affective disorders. *Biological Psychiatry, 52*, 655–675.

PART V

Special Challenges in Disaster Research

CHAPTER 15

Conducting Research on Children and Adolescents after Disaster

ALAN M. STEINBERG, MELISSA J. BRYMER,
JESSE R. STEINBERG, and BETTY PFEFFERBAUM

Studies of the biological, psychological, and behavioral impact of natural disasters on children and adolescents have been growing steadily over the past two decades, with earthquakes and hurricanes being the most widely investigated disasters. More recently, there has been a growing body of scientific literature concerning the adverse effects of political violence and terrorism. Such research is imperative if we are to better understand the full range of consequences of catastrophic events on this vulnerable population and put in place effective preparedness and response programs to foster resilience and promote recovery.

Despite this body of work, there remains much to be learned. As a result of the development of psychometrically sound assessment instruments for children and adolescents, most studies to date have focused primarily on symptomatic response, including posttraumatic stress, depressive, somatic, grief, and anxiety reactions. For adolescents, substance abuse and engagement in high-risk behaviors have also been observed. As a result, it is now well documented that both acute and persistent psychological reactions occur among youths, and that the severity of these reactions is highly associated with the degree of exposure to trauma, loss, and postdisaster adversity. However, studies of children and adolescents often have lacked representative samples, adequate control/comparison groups, and longitudinal designs. More information is especially needed regarding diverse cultural and socioeconomic groups, and the impact of disaster on family systems and community-level processes (Norris et al., 2002).

This chapter provides a selected review of issues that have been prominent in our national and international research with children, adolescents, and families after disasters and terrorism. These include methodological issues in research design and selection of instruments, coordination of research efforts among research groups, a variety of ethical issues, and special considerations in regard to intervention outcome studies. The last section of the chapter focuses on recommendations for important areas of future research, including the evaluation of early interventions that can be provided to children, adolescents, and families in the acute aftermath of catastrophic events.

METHODOLOGICAL ISSUES
IN DESIGNING RESEARCH

Study Design

Because of the unpredictable nature of disaster and terrorism, and the chaos that typically permeates the postevent environment, mental health research in the acute aftermath has often been conducted with hasty planning in regard to a variety of design issues, including sampling strategies, methodology and metrics, and careful consideration of research questions and hypotheses. To some extent this is understandable, as research needs to be integrated into the postevent ecology. In addition, as community systems, including schools, mental health and health care, are focusing on responding, it is often difficult to utilize optimal research strategies while integrating research efforts within these response activities.

In general, studies after disaster have had difficulty in interpreting findings due to lack of baseline information about rates of distress and impairment in the general population. Often, convenience samples drawn for the purpose of obtaining a nonaffected comparison group do not provide real baseline data. For example, in our studies after earthquakes in Armenia (Goenjian et al., 1995) and Greece (Roussos et al., 2005), we used a "dose of exposure" design to demonstrate that the high-exposure group at the epicenter showed more distress and impairment as compared with the group at the periphery of the earthquake zone. However, it was doubtful that the comparison group provided accurate baseline data, as many of these children had regularly gone to the earthquake zone after the earthquake to help family members, had family members come to live with them after the earthquake, and had viewed images of the destruction and death in newspapers and on television. Pfefferbaum and colleagues (2000) after the bombing of the Murrah federal building noted that children from an area geographically remote from Oklahoma City endorsed posttraumatic stress reactions related to media viewing. Often comparison groups may differ in many respects, including community resources, preevent levels of community violence, religion, and socioeconomic status. Ongoing surveillance would provide much needed information on incidence and prevalence rates of disorders and functional impairment to allow for clearer interpretation of observed postevent findings (Galea & Norris, Chapter 11, this volume).

Developing and Selecting Appropriate Instruments

In our experience in providing consultation to researchers after mass trauma, we have consistently confronted several important psychometric issues. First, issues arise in the development of instruments to assess the type and level of exposure to trauma, which are key variables that need to be controlled for in many subsequent data analyses. Exposure screens need to be tailored to the ecology of the event, so as to include an event-specific typology of objective and subjective features of exposure, loss, and adversity. These vary by type of disaster and need to be developed with thorough information about what occurred. We recommend that interviews with key informants be initially conducted to more fully and accurately characterize the ecology of the event and to identify important features of exposure, loss, and adversity that need to be included in screening. The Terrorism and Disaster Branch of the National Child Traumatic Stress Network (NCTSN; at www.nctsn.org) has developed models of exposure screens for hurricanes, tornadoes, tsunamis, and wildfires.

Second, there are invariably questions about selection of appropriate instruments, including from among several that assess the same domain. Indeed, a difficulty in comparing findings in regard to levels of distress across disaster studies has been the use of different instruments to assess PTSD, depression, anxiety, and behavioral consequences. A recent review (Balaban et al., 2005) evaluated the most commonly used instruments among children and adolescents after mass trauma, and proposed guidelines to promote more psychometric uniformity in order to permit comparisons across studies. The most widely used PTSD instrument for children and adolescents after natural disasters is the UCLA PTSD Reaction Index for DSM-IV (Steinberg, Brymer, Decker, & Pynoos, 2004). This instrument has proved useful in comparing findings across a number of hurricanes (Goenjian et al., 2001). More recently there has been increased interest in the use of abbreviated scales. Where sensitivity and specificity are high, abbreviated distress measures provide an efficient means for carrying out needs assessment, screening, and surveillance (Steinberg et al., 2004). A number of studies have advanced the literature by reporting on the severity of PTSD intrusion, avoidance, and arousal subscales, and have broadened the domains of assessment to include traumatic grief, separation anxiety, and reactivity to trauma and loss reminders (Goenjian et al., 1995; Layne et al., 2001).

PRACTICAL AND LOGISTICAL ISSUES IN CONDUCTING RESEARCH

Researcher Communication

An important overarching issue in implementing postdisaster research among youths is related to the need to coordinate research efforts across different groups of researchers. For example, after the war in Kosovo, a large number of international research groups independently conducted studies among affected children and adolescents. Some schools were inundated with research, with no way of evaluating research credentials, while other schools were completely neglected. The Education Department of the provisional government was encouraged to set up a mechanism for review of research proposals to coordinate research throughout the school system to reduce burden and redundancy. However, with no authority to enforce compliance, this effort was minimally successful (Brymer, Stuvland, & Medway, 2005). In contrast, as discussed by Fleischman, Collogan, and Tuma (Chapter 5, this volume), such a strategy was more effective in Oklahoma City after the bombing of the Murrah Federal Building, where a procedure was established for pairing investigators from outside Oklahoma City with local clinicians to assess acute clinical issues requiring intervention (North, Pfefferbaum, & Tucker, 2002).

Conversely, where schools wish to undertake research to collect data, it is important that they be paired with academic researchers to enhance their capacity to undertake systematic investigations. The Los Angeles Unified School District was interested in collecting systematic needs assessment data to inform a school-based mental health recovery program after the 1994 Northridge earthquake. In collaboration with the UCLA Trauma Psychiatry Program, school mental health teams were able to conduct school-wide screenings of students, parents, and teachers to identify those who had been most affected, and plan needed resources to assist in the recovery of school communities. Lessons learned from this collaboration led the U.S. Department of Education to deploy a team of experienced clinicians, administrators, and researchers to help the Oklahoma City public school district organize a response. The team recommended that a local clinician be involved in program design and implementation, setting the stage for a close partnership between the school district and University of

Oklahoma. This partnership had several advantages. It placed the school district firmly in control of its own programming, brought in local clinical support from those who were familiar with the community and would be there to help over the course of recovery, and established mentorship from the U.S. Department of Education team for developing and implementing child disaster mental health research (Pfefferbaum, Call, & Sconzo, 1999).

Research in Schools

Schools represent a major setting for conducting research among children and adolescents after mass trauma. We have consistently encountered a common set of administrative and logistical obstacles. There is often an initial resistance on the part of teachers and school administrators to conducting classroom screenings. Often we have heard, "The students have already lost too much time," "Talking about what happened will upset them and make them worse," and "The students seem to be over it because they are not talking about it anymore." From our experience, it is important to first engage school personnel in understanding their own experiences and current levels of distress, to help them better appreciate the effects on students, and realize the importance of identifying those who may need additional assistance. We also explain that students often welcome the opportunity to talk about and understand what they are experiencing, and that our past research has indicated that very few students will need extra support after having completed a classroom survey (Saltzman, Steinberg, Layne, Aisenberg, & Pynoos, 2002).

This issue of whether research participants need extra support remains an important area for study (Fleischman et al., Chapter 5, this volume). Future studies conducted among children and adolescents after mass trauma should include a component to collect empirical data on children's perceptions regarding their research participation. This will contribute to the evidence base regarding the question of whether, and in what respects, disaster research affects children. The data would be extremely important for researchers to help them clarify the type and extent of risk involved in youth participation in research. The Response to Research Participation Questionnaire would be useful for this purpose (Kassam-Adams & Newman, 2005). In our experience in conducting research among youths after mass trauma, we have consistently observed that participation in research can serve an important psychoeducational function. In responding to items on distress measures, students have often expressed relief in learning that their reactions were known to us, and that these reactions were normal, expectable reactions after trauma and loss. In such a case, participation in research may be quite beneficial.

In regard to taking up classroom time, we have found it helpful to explain that classroom screening can be conducted efficiently during one class period, and that research has shown that providing services to those who need assistance can improve the school milieu, enhance academic performance, and reduce absenteeism (Layne et al., 2001; Stein et al., 2003). It is often helpful to schedule screening of a classroom of students during their gym period, so as to reduce the impact on academic learning.

Informed Consent

Issues of informed consent are paramount and can represent a challenge in obtaining a representative sample and adequate sample size. Research with children requires both parental consent and child assent. In school settings, many researchers have faced difficulties in obtaining parental consent through sending consent forms by mail or by having students take them home and return them to the classroom. In the past, it has been possible to get passive consent from parents in the United States, where parents need only return the consent form to indicate that they do not wish their child to participate in research. Currently, active consent is required within schools (U.S. Department of Education, 2000). Some strategies we have used to increase return rates of consent forms have included attending parent meetings to reinforce the importance of the research and to obtain parental/caretaker consent at that time. It is also helpful to have the request for consent come from the school board.

Child Abuse Reporting

Another important issue facing researchers generally, and of special note in school settings, relates to mandatory reporting of child abuse. All states specify categories of mandated reporters that are legally bound to file good-faith reports of suspected child abuse. To date, researchers are not specifically designated as mandated reporters in any state statute, although most Human Subject Protection Committees across the United States interpret state laws as applying to researchers, especially when researchers are health and mental health professionals (Steinberg, Pynoos, Goenjian, Sossanabadi, & Sherr, 1999). We have adopted this position, and in our work with schools have consistently informed the school administration of this requirement. In several instances, this has prompted concern among school officials, and on occasion has led to our having to remove some items from our instruments that specifically ask about exposure to physical abuse, sexual abuse, neglect, and domestic violence. Despite limiting our instrumentation, there have been numerous occasions in conducting in-depth research interviews with students that we have uncovered information that required us to file a report. We recommend that researchers be completely transparent with school officials about this requirement. There may be both civil and criminal liability for failure to file such a report.

Evaluating Interventions

In both school and community settings, special issues arise in investigating the effectiveness of acute psychosocial interventions for children and adolescents. These include: (1) difficulty in obtaining IRB approval in a timely manner; (2) apprehensiveness about placing an additional research burden on survivors so soon after a tragic event; (3) difficulty in obtaining follow-up data from a population that may be mobile and hard to track; and (4) difficulty in designing research with adequate control groups. Research teams should work with Institutional Review Boards prior to the occurrence of a disaster or terrorist event to obtain advance approval of a general research protocol, along with an assessment battery, that could then be modified to fit a specific event in order to expedite implementation of rapid response research. In regard to the potential additional burden of research, evaluation of satisfaction with the intervention, if obtained through brief questions postintervention, does not constitute an excessive burden. Follow-up evaluation interviews, when embedded in a comprehensive disaster system of care, should not be objectionable. Mental health service delivery after disasters that includes registries would then allow for tracking and recontact for follow-up research.

Taking Care of Researchers

An overlooked aspect of conducting research among youths after mass trauma, especially in nonindustrialized countries, involves the impact on the researchers themselves of working under harsh conditions while being exposed daily to the plight of so many affected children and families. This was an important feature of our work in the earthquake zone in Armenia after the 1988 Spitak earthquake. Our research team, including research staff from the United States and local research and translator staff, often felt overwhelmed by their poor living conditions and daily exposure to severely distressed children who were living under extremely adverse postearthquake circumstances. We would recommend that research procedures include strategies to support research staff under these types of conditions. First, especially for the local researchers who strongly identified with the victims, it was necessary to establish criteria for determining when a researcher should be relieved of field research responsibility.

Second, we found it important to work with research staff to determine their limitations, so that they could be assigned appropriate research tasks. For example, some researchers expressed a preference for not being involved in that part of the research that included children who had been severely physically injured or those living in orphanages. Third, we paired two researchers together so that no researcher ever worked in the affected areas alone. Finally, we made it a practice to hold weekly meetings of the research team to discuss our field experiences, how we were affected, and strategies for positive coping, including taking time to relax and avoiding excessive work (Goenjian, 1993).

FUTURE DIRECTIONS

The next decade of research should expand the focus on symptoms to better characterize protective and risk factors that moderate or mediate a variety of adverse outcomes. Outcome domains need to be broadened to include biological alterations and physical health; developmental disruptions, including moral development (Goenjian et al., 1999); disturbances in peer and social relationships; family conflict; impairments in academic functioning; effects on prosocial behavior, citizenship, and motivation for learning and career; and disruption of the school and community milieu. Factors that need to be studied include the severity of exposure to trauma and loss; physical injury and disability; the severity of postevent adversities; the frequency of exposure to trauma and loss reminders, and associated reactivity and avoidance; age; sex; prior traumatic experiences and losses; history of psychopathology; self-esteem and self-efficacy; coping repertoire and style; and the level of peer, family, school, and social support. Research is also needed to evaluate the effectiveness of mitigation, preparedness, response, and recovery strategies in schools, communities and nationally, and the effectiveness of acute, intermediate, and long-term interventions in promoting resilience and the long-term recovery of children and adolescents.

An important area for research that has immediate practical implications is research on the impact of the media, especially television viewing, on the recovery of children and adolescents (Pfefferbaum et al., 2001). This information would enhance our ability to help parents, who have often expressed concern about how to limit their children's exposure to media, and how to talk to them afterward. In addition, research on the effectiveness of risk communication and emergency public information is especially needed in regard to scenarios involving weapons of mass destruction. Potential differences in response to natural disaster as opposed to human perpetrated violence have still to be better characterized (Goenjian et al., 1994). There is also a need for more research among special populations, including orphans, unaccompanied minors, street children, children with special needs, and refugees and displaced children. Animal studies have the potential to inform issues related to fear acquisition and extinction with significant clinical implications (Pynoos, Ritzmann, Steinberg, Goenjian, & Prisecaru, 1996). As an overarching principle, future studies need to be conducted from within a sound developmental, cultural, and ecological framework (Steinberg & Ritzmann, 1990; Pynoos, Steinberg, & Wraith, 1995; Pynoos, Steinberg, & Piacentini, 1999).

To meet the need for some of this critical information, the National Institute of Mental Health (NIMH), the Substance Abuse and Mental Health Services Administration, and the National Institute for Nursing Research have funded a number of programs across the United States to develop rapid response disaster research training curricula and to provide training and resources for career development in order to enhance our national capacity to conduct state-of-the-art rapid response research in the aftermath of disasters and terrorism. The Terrorism and Disaster Branch of the UCLA/Duke University National Center for Child Traumatic Stress is currently developing a research training curriculum related to special issues involved in research with children and families after mass trauma. The curriculum includes modules on (1) the current state of knowledge and gaps in research; (2) the National Response Plan; (3) special issues in research design, methodology, and analysis; (4) assessment instruments; (5) risk communication and risk management; (6) ethical issues; and (7) applying research findings to planning and delivering mental health services for children and families. The training also includes discussion of methods for establishing linkages with response systems to gain access to study populations and methods for assisting key community leaders (education, health, mental health, public health, first-responder, faith-based sectors, and government agencies) to appreciate the critical importance of research, the ways that research can help inform a recovery program, and ways that these systems can coordinate and integrate their response activities in collaboration with research.

ACKNOWLEDGMENTS

The authors are from the Terrorism and Disaster Branch, UCLA/Duke University National Center for Child Traumatic Stress, University of California, Los Angeles, which is funded through the Center for Mental Health Services, Substance Abuse and Mental Health Services Administration), U.S. Department of Health and Human Services.

REFERENCES

Balaban, V. F., Steinberg, A. M., Brymer, M. J., Layne, C. M., Jones, R. T., & Fairbank, J. A. (2005). Screening and assessment for children's psychosocial needs following war and terrorism. In M. J. Friedman & A. Mikus-Kos (Eds.), *Promoting the psychosocial well-being of children following war and terrorism* (pp. 121–161). Brussels, Belgium: NATO.

Brymer, M. J., Stuvland, R., & Medway, P. J. (2005). Issues in the development of psychosocial programs for children, adolescents and families in Kosovo. In M. J.

Friedman & A. Mikus-Kos (Eds.), *Promoting the psychosocial well-being of children following war and terrorism* (pp. 73–88). Brussels, Belgium: NATO.

Goenjian, A. K. (1993). A mental health relief programme in Armenia after the 1988 earthquake. Implementation and clinical observations. *British Journal of Psychiatry, 163,* 230–239.

Goenjian, A. K., Molina, L., Steinberg, A. M., Fairbanks, L. A, Alvarez, M. L, & Pynoos, R. S. (2001). Posttraumatic stress and depressive reactions among adolescents in Nicaragua after Hurricane Mitch. *American Journal of Psychiatry, 158,* 788–794.

Goenjian, A., Najarian L. M., Pynoos, R. S., Steinberg, A. M., Petrosian, P., Sterakyan, S., et al. (1994). Posttraumatic stress reactions after single and double trauma. *Acta Psychiatrica Scandanavica, 90,* 214–221.

Goenjian, A. K., Pynoos, R. S., Steinberg, A. M, Najarian, L. M., Asarnow, J. R., Karayan I., et al. (1995). Psychiatric co-morbidity in children after the 1988 earthquake in Armenia. *Journal of the American Academy of Child and Adolescent Psychiatry, 34,* 1174–1184.

Goenjian, A. K., Stilwell, B. M., Steinberg, A. M, Fairbanks, L. A, Galvin, M. R., Karayan, I., et al. (1999). Moral development and psychopathological interference with conscience functioning among adolescents after trauma. *Journal of the American Academy of Child and Adolescent Psychiatry, 38,* 376–384.

Kassam-Adams, N., & Newman, E. (2005). Child and parent reactions to participation in clinical research. *General Hospital Psychiatry, 27,* 29–35.

Layne, C. M., Pynoos, R. S., Saltzman, W. R., Arslanagic, B., Black, M., Savjak, N., et al. (2001). Trauma/grief-focused group psychotherapy: School-based postwar intervention with traumatized Bosnian adolescents. *Group Dynamics: Theory, Research and Practice, 5,* 277–290.

Norris, F. H., Friedman, M. J., Watson, P. J, Byrne, C. M., Diaz, E., & Kaniasty, K. (2002). 60,000 disaster victims speak. Part I: An empirical review of the empirical literature, 1981–2001. *Psychiatry, 65,* 2007–2039.

North, C., Pfefferbaum, B., & Tucker, P. (2002). Ethical and methodological issues in academic mental health research in populations affected by disaster: The Oklahoma City experience relevant to September 11, 2001. *CNS Spectrums, 7,* 580–584.

Pfefferbaum, B., Call, J. A., & Sconzo, G. M. (1999). Mental health services for children in the first two years after the 1995 Oklahoma City terrorist bombing. *Psychiatric Services, 50,* 956–958.

Pfefferbaum, B., Nixon, S. J., Tivis, R. D., Doughty, D. E., Pynoos, R. S., Gurwitch, R. H., et al. (2001). Television exposure in children after a terrorist incident. *Psychiatry, 64,* 202–211.

Pfefferbaum, B., Seale, T. W., McDonald, N. B., Brandt, E. N., Rainwater, S. M., Maynard, B. T., et al. (2000). Posttraumatic stress two years after the Oklahoma City bombing in youths geographically distant from the explosion. *Psychiatry, 63,* 358–370.

Pynoos, R. S., Ritzmann, R. F., Steinberg, A. M., Goenjian, A., & Prisecaru, I. (1996). A behavioral animal model of PTSD featuring repeated exposures to situational reminders. *Biological Psychiatry, 39,* 129–134.

Pynoos, R. S., Steinberg, A. M., & Piacentini, J. V. (1999). A developmental psychopathology model of childhood traumatic stress and intersection with anxiety disorders. *Biological Psychiatry, 46,* 1542–1554.

Pynoos, R. S., Steinberg, A. M., & Wraith, R. (1995) A developmental model of posttraumatic stress disorder in children and adolescents. In D. Cicchetti, & D. J. Cohen (Eds.), *Manual of developmental psychopathology* (pp. 72–93). New York: Wiley.

Roussos, A., Goenjian, A. K., Steinberg, A. M., Sotiropoulou, C., Kakaki, M., Kabakos, C., et al. (2005). Posttraumatic stress and depressive reactions after the 1999 Ano Liosia earthquake in Greece. *American Journal of Psychiatry, 162,* 530–537.

Saltzman, W. R., Steinberg, A. M., Layne, C. M., Aisenberg, E., & Pynoos R. S. (2002). A developmental approach to school-based treatment of adolescents exposed to trauma and traumatic loss. *Journal of Child and Adolescent Group Therapy, 11,* 43–56.

Stein, B. D., Jaycox, L. H., Kataoka, S. H., Wong, M., Tu, W., Elliott, M. N., et al. (2003). A mental health intervention for school children exposed to violence: A randomized controlled study. *Journal of the American Medical Association, 290,* 603–611.

Steinberg, A. M., Brymer, M. J., Decker, K., & Pynoos, R. S. (2004). The UCLA PTSD Reaction Index. *Current Psychiatry Reports, 6,* 96–100.

Steinberg, A. M., Pynoos, R. S., Goenjian, A. K., Sossanabadi, H., & Sherr, L. (1999). Are researchers bound by child abuse reporting laws? *Child Abuse and Neglect, 23,* 771–777.

Steinberg, A. M., & Ritzmann, R. F. (1990). A living systems approach to understanding the concept of stress. *Behavioral Science, 35*(2), 138–146.

U.S. Department of Education (2000). *Family educational rights and privacy: Final rule.* Fed. Reg. 41852 (34 CFR, Part 99).

CHAPTER 16

Conducting Research with Military and Uniformed Services Workers

CAROL S. FULLERTON, JAMES E. MCCARROLL,
and ROBERT J. URSANO

Conducting research within military and other uniformed organizations presents unique challenges. The study of emotional reactions to trauma and disasters began with observations of military units and soldiers during wartime. However, research on nonmilitary uniformed services workers, such as firefighters, public safety workers, and other disaster/rescue workers, lagged behind the study of soldiers and primary victims of trauma and disasters. Disasters and terrorist events of the past decade, such as the terrorist attacks of September 11, 2001, the terrorist attacks on the Murrah Federal Building in Oklahoma City in 1995, and others, have highlighted the importance of investigating psychological, behavioral, and psychosocial responses in disaster/rescue workers and first responders (e.g., Fullerton, Ursano, & Wang, 2004; McCarroll, Ursano, Fullerton, Liu, & Lundy, 2002; Marmar, Weiss, Metzler, Ronfeldt, & Foreman, 1996; North et al., 2002; Ursano, Fullerton, Vance, & Kao, 1999). This chapter addresses the challenges of conducting research in military and other uniformed services worker populations (e.g., firefighters, public safety workers, and other disaster/rescue workers). We draw primarily from lessons learned from the authors' own experience in conducting research in the military. In this chapter we examine gaining entrée to military and uniformed personnel as well as military and other uniformed cultures, developing the research plan, volunteerism and confidentiality for military research participants, military and uniformed comparison groups, the military spouse and family as research participants, the benefits of research participation for military and uniformed personnel, and providing feedback to military leaders and other uniformed organizations.

GAINING ENTRÉE

Gaining access to the field can be extremely difficult in disaster situations involving military and uniformed personnel. In any research situation, those in authority will be cautious about granting access. In disaster situations involving military and uniformed personnel, the level of concern of those in charge can be formidable. Most organizations have a formal "entry portal." In uniformed organizations permission to conduct research is usually required at several formal levels of authority. This may involve permission from governmental or other high-level institutions as well as from the leadership on site. In the military, the primary working contact for the researcher may be the mental health clinic or other health care facility commander, family services director, or chaplain. Typically one member of the research team will establish and maintain communication with the primary contact person in the organization. This contact should be established prior to arrival at the site and is critical to coordinating follow-up research (see Table 16.1 for guidelines for gaining entrée).

Frequently research with military and uniformed services workers is conducted at the request of the leadership. The expectation is that the results will have policy implications or generate recommendations for interventions to improve, for example, performance, unit cohesion, and retention. Such research is often requested to better understand and manage the consequences of traumatic events, for example: working in isolated or contaminated environments, exposure to the grotesque (e.g., body recovery and identification), multiple losses within a unit or squadron, and the effect of deployment on soldiers, spouses, and families. Leaders expect rapid— real-time—feedback to inform policy and recommendations for intervention programs. Research questions typical of military and unformed service workers are presented in Table 16.2.

When a disaster occurs, understanding who is in charge is critical and complex. Only with this knowledge and contacts within the organization can the researcher integrate into the disaster environment. Although each element within the military setting (whether officer, enlisted personnel, re-

TABLE 16.1. Guidelines for Gaining Entrée

- Establish points of contact within the organization at different levels within the hierarchy prior to arriving on site.
- Understand and follow appropriate organizational protocol at all times.
- Be aware of and respect jurisdictional boundaries when deployed to a disaster site.
- Define your research team's role and remain aware of your primary goal (avoid conflicting roles on site).
- Do not raise expectations for assistance; however, be prepared to respond to appropriate requests for consultation.
- Do not disrupt the environment or interfere with the mission of the organization.
- Time your arrival and respect the need for rest and respite of disaster/rescue workers.
- Do not make demands of people.
- Do not be judgmental.
- Be seen as someone who cares.
- Do not overstay your welcome.
- Plan a follow-up visit to establish closure and reinforce the research agenda.

servist, guard, or civilian) has a particular role, and these roles are generally well established in the organization, roles may change amid the chaos of disasters, and members of other organizations and jurisdictions may be deployed to the disaster site. Assistance is often requested from various sources and can cause confusion at the disaster site. Coordination of the disaster site presents complex leadership and management issues. When deployed to a disaster site, the research team must be aware of, and respect, jurisdictional boundaries. For example, members of our research team deployed following a civilian plane crash at an airport shared by civilian, military, and Air National Guard units (see McCarroll, Ursano, Fullerton, & Wright, 1992). When a crash occurs at an airport such as this, the jurisdiction may be taken by the federal government, the state government, or a city or county official. Jurisdiction may also change during the operation. Senior military personnel are often reluctant to give up jurisdiction, particularly when they have been in charge of initial phases of an operation. Regardless of the overall operational jurisdiction, the military commander usually remains in charge of the personnel and granting access to a research team.

With a formal invitation to enter a military or other uniformed environment and primary contacts in place, the research team may arrive and establish its role on site. It is critical for the team to remain aware of the primary goal, which is always to establish a research collaboration. In the chaos that surrounds a disaster site, there may be suspicions raised about

TABLE 16.2. Research Questions Typically Relevant to Military and Uniformed Services Workers

- How can leadership better prepare soldiers, uniformed workers, and families for all phases of deployment (e.g., anticipation and preparation predeployment, stressors during deployment, and readjustment postdeployment)?

- What should leaders, soldiers, or uniformed workers look for following deployment or other high-stress duty assignment in order to determine whether they should seek mental health consultation (e.g., what is the "recovery curve" following traumatic events)?

- How long after deployment should soldiers or uniformed workers be required to return to work (what are the indicators that a unit has returned to pre-event functioning)?

- What are the individual (e.g., age, gender, prior experience) and unit (e.g., unit cohesion, morale) risk factors for problems after duty in high-stress environments?

- What are the effects of volunteerism versus mandatory duty assignment in high-stress/traumatic environments?

- What interventions are effective for military and uniformed services workers working with the dead following war and other traumatic events (e.g., teach not to look at faces and hands which promotes identification with the dead)?

- In what the ways can leadership assist a military or uniformed services unit or military community in recovering from multiple losses (e.g., "grief leadership," replacement of unit members)?

the motivations of outsiders. The team's primary contacts become the critical link for gaining acceptance and lowering suspicions about motives. Introduction of team members and clarification of the research team's role and agenda by the primary contact person is important to this task. It is important not to raise expectations of assistance, for example, the research team is not at the disaster site to provide therapeutic interventions. However, the team leader must be prepared to respond to appropriate requests for consultation on unexpected topics, for example, therapeutic interventions or working with the media.

The research team must not disrupt the environment or interfere with the mission of the organization. The timing of arrival at the disaster site is critical. First and foremost, the research team must respect disaster workers' needs for rest and respite immediately following a disaster event. It is important not to make demands of people (e.g., do not ask people to complete a research survey when they have just come in from search and rescue and are exhausted). It is important for the researchers not to be judgmental and to be seen as people who care. Importantly, they must not overstay their welcome. Follow-up visits to establish closure and reinforce the research agenda are preferable to prolonged visits. Because the research team has an outside role in the disaster community, it is often best not to plan the follow-up visit during the first anniversary of the disaster. The anniversary is an important point that usually stirs feelings and can serve as a point of closure for many people.

MILITARY AND OTHER UNIFORMED CULTURES AND THE RESEARCH TEAM

The military as well as civilian uniformed services often have very specific cultural behaviors and structure. Military and other uniformed services represent organizations within the community with cultural similarities and differences. We will focus primarily on the military, in which the culture is more clearly defined and evident, but the issues are present in all uniformed responders. Military culture is deeply rooted in tradition and is defined by rank structure, language, dress, rituals, and ceremony. In order to conduct research within the military the researcher must become familiar with the culture, structure, and hierarchy. To facilitate this, the research team should have at least one uniformed individual and a primary contact person within the organization to help understand the unique cultural aspects of the organization. For example, it is important for the researcher to determine who can grant access to a site, to personnel, and to the logistical support necessary for conducting the research. In addition, knowledge of the military rituals and ceremony can help a researcher determine alternative ways of showing appreciation for research participation that are in keeping with military tradition.

Understanding the military culture is important to the way the research team presents itself in terms of dress, demeanor, language, and the observance of rituals and ceremony. The team must respect the culture, dignity, and pride of the organization. Team members must understand and follow appropriate protocol at all times. Knowing the correct name and rank structure of the organization is important. Understanding the traditions and social structure is not only respectful but provides opportunities for learning and adapting the research methodology. For example, after search and rescue following an airplane crash, joining firefighters around the firehouse table to share coffee and donuts provides an opportunity for the researcher to learn through listening and hearing stories told in an informal setting. In terms of dress, it is important to consider the type of people the team will be interacting with. The way people interact with the research team depends not only on how team members act but also what they are wearing. The research team should be inconspicuous in dress. Military personnel on the research team should wear the same uniform as the military at the disaster scene. Civilians on the research team should wear clothing similar to that worn by the military. For example, if the military personnel at the disaster site are dressed casually, as in the work uniform, the research team should also dress casually. Wearing bright or provocative clothing and jewelry would be conspicuous and elicit negative responses.

Similar to research in the general population, conducting research with military and uniformed service workers requires research teams that are diverse in composition, experience, knowledge, and areas of expertise. Ideally, the research team should include members of different ages, genders, and ethnic backgrounds. In working with the military, it is important to include people with prior military experience. The branch of service is not as important as the fact that the individual will understand military culture and operations. In addition to active duty military personnel, team members will need to interact with civilians working at military installations, reservists, guard personnel, and family members, including children.

DEVELOPING THE RESEARCH PLAN

As with any research investigation, a formal research protocol must be submitted to participating institutions, and institutional review board (IRB) approval must be granted prior to formal data collection. An official letter from the leadership requesting that your research team conduct research in their organization is usually required for research in military and other uniformed settings. The research team's primary contact can secure permission for access to "alpha rosters" (military personnel lists) for contacting potential research participants as well as providing motivation on-site for research participation. Such a roster can facilitate sampling and documentation of participation by rank and demographics. An explanation and discussion of the purpose of the research with key personnel, particularly noncommissioned officers, can help to increase participation in the research as well as facilitating longitudinal studies.

VOLUNTEERISM AND CONFIDENTIALITY

Recruitment and volunteerism among military and other uniformed service members raise unique issues for IRBs and human research committees. It is not uncommon for a military unit to be mobilized and ordered to perform duty following natural disasters, accidents, and other emergency situations. However, military and other uniformed personnel must volunteer in order to participate in a research study. Although military personnel can be ordered to show up to take a survey or participate in a research interview, they cannot be ordered to volunteer. Research protocols must document and verify that no coercion was applied and that participation was completely voluntary. Since the military community is highly structured, particular options for ensuring volunteerism are required. For example, to avoid feelings of obligation to participate in a research study by service members, survey distribution should not be done by leaders. Distribution can be accomplished through the chaplain or other people seen as neutral. Potential participants must be informed about their options to not participate or to drop out of the study at any time with no consequences to them either professionally or personally. It is important to make clear to potential participants that leaders will not be privy to information on who participated and who did not.

Confidentiality of research findings also raises important issues with military and other uniformed populations. Because of potential stigma and perceived job risk, military and uniformed personnel must be assured that they will not be identified in any research findings by name, organization, or other identifier such as a combination of age, sex, and rank. In addition, military and uniformed workers may have concerns about their security clearance and other career issues. Often military members express concern about mental difficulties revealed by research being reported to the leadership. For example, the revelation of emotional problems can put an Air Force flier's career in jeopardy. Forensic examiners may fear that contact with mental health could be seen as compromising their judgment and the ability to perform their duty or to testify in court. Military and other uniformed services workers especially in government operations are concerned about maintaining their security clearance, which may be the lynchpin upon which their career rests. The suspicion of a mental health problem may make an individual a pariah, one who others feel cannot be counted on in a "hot environment."

One solution to concerns about confidentiality is conducting research without identifiers. In longitudinal studies, however, the researcher needs unique identifiers in order to match surveys over time. A solution is to create a unique identifier that does not reveal the actual identity of the participant. Such an identifier might include: (1) the last letter of your last name (if married, use the last letter of your maiden name), (2) the first letter of the city you were born in, (3) the first letter of the month in which you were born, (4) the last digit of the day of the month on which you were born, or (5) last digit of the year you were born.

COMPARISON GROUPS

In disaster research, comparison groups are helpful, especially if there are no baseline data and randomized stratified sampling is not possible. As in research with civilians, it is important to make comparison groups similar on demographic variables. An advantage of conducting research in military samples is the availability and ease of recruitment of comparison groups in contrast to other disaster populations. Military samples need to be matched on rank (e.g., officers vs. enlisted personnel) as well as job, duty assignment, active duty versus reserve, service, and the location of the military installation. This can be difficult due to limitations in the availability of matched groups. The value of using a comparison group when no baseline data are available is illustrated by our study of disaster workers at Sioux City (see Fullerton et al., 2004). Exposed disaster workers had significantly higher levels of acute stress disorder, posttraumatic stress disorder (PTSD) at 13 months, and depression at 7 and 13 months than comparisons. Importantly, exposed disaster workers had significantly higher levels of health care utilization for emotional problems than comparisons, and more disaster workers indicated needing but not obtaining health care than comparisons during the 13 months postaccident.

SPOUSE AND FAMILY
AS RESEARCH PARTICIPANTS

During disaster operations, the concern of disaster workers for their families is extremely important to their functioning, as is the support provided by spouses and other family members. Military families, and spouses in particular, provide an important source of support before, during, and after disaster work and deployment operations. However, spouses experience their own stressors and may also experience support provision as stressful. The complexity of spousal support in the military is exemplified by the lack of support for the spouse due to distance from the family. Often the military spouse living on a military installation lacks the close availability of an extended family. If possible, research in military and disaster worker populations should include spouses and other family members. An advantage of research with military spouses is that recruitment can be facilitated through the use of military-sponsored groups and programs such as unit support groups and family support services. There are several good examples of studies involving military and disaster worker spouses (e.g., see Fullerton & Ursano, 1997; Fullerton, Wright, Ursano, & McCarroll, 1993; Pfefferbaum et al., 2002). Research findings have implications for further development of spouse and family support programs.

RESEARCH PARTICIPATION
BENEFITS, RECOGNITION, AND AWARDS

There are informal benefits to leaders as well as uniformed personnel participating in research. However, unless the research involves treatment trials, the researcher should make clear to potential research participants that there are no direct benefits of participation in the study. Research participation does provide a unique opportunity for those who have been through a stressful experience to help people in the future deal with similar experiences. A helpful question to ask participants is what advice they would give to others who might experience similar events. Such sharing is often felt as helping the next group that is exposed to a similar stressor. Some participants will simply want to get something "off their chest." Some may want to hear what others think and did (e.g., in a group setting). Others may feel that participating in research will provide access to a mental health professional. Although remembering a disaster experience can stir intense feelings, the vast majority of research participants feel that sharing their experience either via interviews or surveys provides an opportunity to reevaluate their experience and put closure on the event.

Awards, medals, decorations, and certificates of appreciation are traditional ways the military recognizes outstanding performance. Although decorations are rarely given for disaster work, in many cases, a simple "thank you" from officials in charge and higher-level officials is very meaningful. One important way for leaders and public officials to acknowledge disaster workers is simply to be visible to the workers. This shows their interest and support of the work. In operations such as body recovery and identification, leaders and officials may have a difficult time visiting the scene. However, their appearance and occasional presence are very meaningful to the workers.

Military and other uniformed personnel usually cannot accept monetary payment for research participation. However, certificates of appreciation are a good way to recognize participation in research. Certificates are in keeping with how the military recognizes achievement and can be produced and distributed at a reasonable cost. Token gifts such as mugs with logos, photographs, or caps are alternative ways to recognize research participation.

PROVIDING FEEDBACK

Rapid reporting of survey or interview data is a critical component of research requested by military leaders or other uniformed organizations. Univariate and bivariate frequency and qualitative data provide leadership with valuable insight into how soldiers are doing following participation in disaster operations and deployments. For example, leaders may want to know whether newsletters provided to spouses during soldier deployments help families cope with stressful separations. In order to address this type of question the researcher first needs to determine whether spouses know about the newsletter and then, of those who do know about the newsletter, whether the information is useful to them. Implications of these data can address whether the leadership needs to focus on making spouses aware of the newsletter and then whether the content is useful and, if not, what changes should be made. Reports of findings can be distributed rapidly as technical reports and later can be combined with other data for journal publications.

CONCLUSIONS

Disaster research with military and uniformed services workers done in a sensitive manner can set the tone for future research to be an integral part of the disaster site involving military personnel and disaster workers. Deployment to the disaster site by the research team helps to establish a trusting relationship and benefits the research. For example, the researcher can design surveys and interviews to address unique aspects of the disaster work, using the language of the operation. Learning about the environment and the functioning of the organization will enable the research team to gain entrée and facilitate research by providing important information unique to an event that can be used to design surveys or interviews. For example, visiting the runway where a plane crashed, viewing the naval ship gun turret where an explosion occurred, viewing the mortuary where bodies are being identified, being inside an army tank, going into a protective shelter designed for chemical and biological attacks, wearing protective gear and masks, and visiting with spouses of military and disaster/rescue workers. All such field work requires on-site visits—not only questionnaires, surveys, or interviews conducted from afar. In addition, being on-site allows the team to form primary contacts in order to facilitate the research, for example, obtaining alpha rosters for contacting potential participants.

Military and uniformed personnel represent other populations in addition to their service and therefore fulfill other roles that interact and affect their duties while wearing a uniform. For example, they are spouses, parents, and members of a community. Many hold civilian jobs. Research with military and uniformed personnel should include data on these roles because they may increase stress or serve as sources of support.

No two situations are identical with uniformed populations. The guidelines regarding research with military and uniformed service workers must be adapted to the situation being studied. The team must become familiar with the uniformed culture in order to gain entrée to the disaster site. The arrival of a researcher with a rigidly structured questionnaire in the immediate aftermath of a disaster will cause suspicion and concern and interfere with operations and the need for rest and respite. In the field, it is often necessary for the researcher to develop a chameleon-like adaptability— blending into unique uniformed cultures and contexts. Research with military and uniformed services workers has the potential for design and implementation of intervention programs as well as policy change.

REFERENCES

Fullerton, C. S., & Ursano, R. J. (1997). Posttraumatic responses in spouse/significant others of disaster workers. In C. S. Fullerton & R. J. Ursano (Eds.), *Posttraumatic stress disorder: Acute and long-term responses to trauma and disaster* (pp. 59–75). Washington, DC: American Psychiatric Press.

Fullerton, C. S., Ursano, R. J., & Wang, L. (2004). Acute stress disorder, posttraumatic stress disorder, and depression in disaster or rescue workers. *American Journal of Psychiatry, 161,* 1370–1376.

Fullerton, C. S., Wright, K., Ursano, R. J., & McCarroll, J. E. (1993). Social support of disaster workers: The role of significant others. *Nordic Journal of Psychiatry, 47,* 315–324.

Marmar, C. R., Weiss, D. S., Metzler, T. J., Ronfeldt, H. M., & Foreman, C. (1996). Stress responses of emergency services personnel to the Loma Prieta Earthquake Interstate 880 freeway collapse and control traumatic incidents. *Journal of Traumatic Stress, 9,* 63–85.

McCarroll, J. E., Ursano, R. J., Fullerton, C. S., & Wright, K. M. (1992). Community consultation following a major air disaster. *Journal of Community Psychology, 20,* 271–275.

McCarroll, J. E., Ursano, R. J., Fullerton, C. S., Liu, X., & Lundy, A. (2002). Somatic symptoms in Gulf War mortuary workers. *Psychosomatic Medicine, 64,* 29–33.

North, C. S., Tivis, L., McMillen, J. C., Pfefferbaum, B., Spitznagel, E. L., Cox, J., et al. (2002). Psychiatric disorders in rescue workers after the Oklahoma City bombing. *American Journal of Psychiatry, 159,* 857–859.

Pfefferbaum, B., North, C. S., Bunch, K., Wilson, T. G., Tucker, P., & Schorr, J. K. (2002). The impact of the 1995 Oklahoma City bombing on the partners of firefighters. *Journal of Urban Health, 79,* 364–372.

Ursano, R. J., Fullerton, C. S., Vance, K., & Kao, T. C. (1999). Posttraumatic stress disorder and identification in disaster workers. *American Journal of Psychiatry, 156,* 353–359.

CHAPTER 17

Conducting Research in Diverse, Minority, and Marginalized Communities

RUSSELL T. JONES, JAMES M. HADDER, FRANKLIN CARVAJAL, SARA CHAPMAN, and APRYL ALEXANDER

There are several reasons why disaster research among racial/ethnically diverse and marginalized communities is needed. First, and most fundamentally, few postdisaster samples have included sufficient numbers of members of ethnic and marginalized communities, and thus few studies have been able to examine disaster effects across and within these groups.

Second, there is reason to suspect that prevalence of exposure to predisaster trauma may be higher than average within economically disadvantaged urban environments (Breslau et al., 1998; Selner-O'Hagan, Kindlon, Buka, Raudenbush, & Earls, 1998), and, if so, these communities may have a greater prevalence of predisaster trauma-related psychopathology. Knowledge of the epidemiology of trauma and posttraumatic stress disorder (PTSD) within specific minority populations is limited by the shortcomings of most previous studies. For example, in the National Comorbidity Survey (Kessler, Sonnega, Bromet, Hughes, & Nelson, 1995), the Hispanic, Asian, and Native American samples were small in size, heterogeneous in terms of national origin, and limited to English-speaking persons (see Norris & Alegria, 2005).

Third, it can be hypothesized that minority and marginalized communities are at greater risk following disaster than other groups and therefore need greater research attention (Norris & Alegria, 2005). The relative impact of race, female gender, exposure levels, preexisting psychiatric disorders, family history, childhood trauma, exposure to violence, race-related stressors, lack of support, and underutilization of mental health services has yet to be systematically examined (Breslau, 2002; Vernberg, La Greca, Silverman, & Prinstein, 1996). A host of factors including racism and discrimination may render ethnic minority individuals more prone to negative outcomes resulting from disasters. The examination of race-related stressors that include social and economic effects of racial prejudice or stigmatization as well as bicultural identification (Jones, Brazel, Peskind, Morelli & Raskind, 2000; Loo, 2003) may be essential to the discovery of linkages between risk factors and symptom expression. In our program of research investigating the impact of fire, we have highlighted the need to study further the influence of gender, race, socioeconomic status, social support, parents' reactions, and coping on African Americans' functioning following trauma exposure (Jones & Ollendick, 2002).

Fourth, the question of whether the expression of certain psychiatric disorders is the same across ethnic/racial groups has yet to be adequately addressed (Breslau et al., 1998; Kessler et al., 1995). This question can be answered only through systematic investigations by trauma researchers targeting members of minority and marginalized communities. For example, in a study by Perilla, Norris, and Lavizzo (2002) following Hurricane Andrew, culture was found to have an effect on the types of symptoms minority groups displayed. African Americans tended to express distress in terms of arousal, while Spanish-speaking Latinos were more likely to express distress in terms of intrusive thoughts. Consistent with this, African Americans have higher levels of cardiovascular reactivity in response to a wide assortment of behavioral stressors (Anderson, McNeilly, & Myers, 1992; Parker & Jones, 1999). Lawson (2000) likewise suggested that PTSD symptom expression in African Americans might be different than in other racial groups and may result in misdiagnosis.

Fifth, treatment efficacy among these minority groups remains underresearched. The dearth of outcome studies, including clinical trials, psychotherapy, and cognitive behavior therapy, has been embarrassingly great (Zoellner, Feeny, Fitzgibbons, & Foa, 1999). Issues related to the retention of ethnic minorities in therapy have yet to be systematically examined (Rosenheck & Fontana, 1995).

Recognizing the importance of conducting research in these populations, we aimed in this chapter to identify (1) barriers to research among minority/marginalized communities and (2) solutions to facilitate the conduct of research with these populations following disasters.

BARRIERS TO RESEARCH IN MINORITY/MARGINALIZED COMMUNITIES

Mistrust

Perhaps one of the greatest barriers for researchers is the lack of trust. When asking a group of minorities why they did not participate in research, Roberson (1994) documented the three most frequent responses: fear, mistrust, and a lack of knowledge about scientific research. African Americans' fear and mistrust of researchers has been well documented. Gamble (1993) noted that, as early as the 1920s, African Americans avoided entering hospitals for fear of being used as test subjects. It is not unreasonable to suggest that African Americans' reluctance to participate in the white medical/ scientific community's research programs may be a product of the historical relationship between them and whites in the United States (in particular, the social and medical abuse that has been visited upon African American populations; Shavers-Hornaday, Lynch, Burmeister, & Torner, 1997). The horrific impact of the Tuskegee Study, where infected African Americans were neither informed of their disease status nor treated (King, 1992), remains a constant reminder to this community of potential abuses of science. In a survey of 220 African Americans, Million-Underwood, Sanders, and Davis (1993) found that 57% of respondents were either (1) of the opinion that scientific research was unethical in the United States or (2) wary of scientific research although they required more information to make a definitive judgment.

Bonham (2002) also documented forms of distrust with other minority and marginalized populations. For instance, undocumented Latino immigrants reported fear of deportation and, therefore, were naturally wary of strangers who approached them to provide information on a given issue (Marín & Marín, 1991). A related reason Latinos may be wary of research is the fact that they are frequently targeted by unscrupulous business organizations (Marín & Marín, 1991).

Mistrust is also evident in the domain of treatment and impedes successful recruitment of minorities for research. For example, Corbie-Smith, Thomas, and St. George (2002) found that African Americans had a greater distrust of research than whites even when controlling for social class. Mistrust of physicians, cultural misunderstandings, misdiagnoses of illnesses, and financial constraints collectively contribute to mistrust on the part of the minority groups (Boulware, Cooper, Ratner, LaVeist, & Powe, 2003; Johnson, Saha, Arbelaez, Beach, & Cooper, 2004).

Access

There are several barriers to access for researchers interested in working with minority or marginalized populations. These populations may not be familiar with the research process and may have limited time to talk to researchers. Additionally, the array of social, demographic, and geographic barriers also prohibit racial and ethnic minorities from receiving needed attention following disasters.

Culture and Linguistics

The third major barrier relates to culture and linguistics. Disaster researchers' lack of attention to issues related to these constructs has left huge gaps in their knowledge base and ability to work effectively with marginalized populations. Researchers' inability to address issues related to culture is a major hindrance to progress in this area. For example, their lack of understanding and appreciation of constructs of thoughts, communications, actions, customs, beliefs, values, and institutions of those represented in marginalized, minority, and underserved groups seriously jeopardizes their access to these groups. Without careful consideration to culture, our research paradigms, data collection methods, and interpretation of findings will continue to be significantly flawed. The interpretation of variables including gender, social support, coping, family environment, and family composition must all be examined through "cultural lenses" if valid conclusions are to be drawn.

Language has also proven to be a major barrier for non-English-speaking individuals to participate in mental health research and care. Language refers to words, syntax, and local idiomatic expressions as well as symbols and concepts shared by the cultural group (Jones et al., 2001). For example, a major obstacle for Hispanic and Asian Americans is the absence of bilingual mental health workers. Nearly one out of every two Asian Americans has difficulty accessing mental health treatment because he or she does not speak English or cannot find services that meet his or her language needs (U.S. Department of Health and Human Services, 2001a). This shortcoming is certainly mirrored in many disaster research efforts.

The consequences of linguistic problems have resulted in frequent misdiagnosis and in poor quality of treatment (Norris & Alegria, 2005). Frequently, immigrants who have trouble communicating in English are more likely not to receive care (Norris & Alegria, 2005). Additionally, many instruments used in assessment rely on an understanding of the English language, which makes it impossible for a non-English-speaking individual to participate in research activities. Consequently, there is a strong need to devise appropriate instruments for Latinos and others (Perilla et al.,

2002). Furthermore, understanding the meaning of body language, gestures, postures, and inflections within a minority group may increase rapport.

Summary of Barriers

These challenges present major obstacles to research among minority and marginalized communities, including recruitment of study participants and enrollment of participants into treatment research. Solutions to overcome these obstacles are becoming of even greater importance in light of the fact that the United States is becoming more ethnically and racially diverse than ever before (Betancourt, Green, & Carrillo, 2002). However, there are potential solutions that can help researchers overcome these barriers, as discussed in the following section.

SOLUTIONS

In light of the fact that there exists no empirically validated model that spells out guidelines for addressing issues related to mistrust, access, and culture/language in disaster research, we are proposing such a model: the "cultural competence model for accessing minority and marginalized communities affected by disaster" (Figure 17.1). This working model is based on the "dose–response" notion whereby it is assumed that the greater the impact of the disaster, the greater the likelihood of more negative outcomes. This model is similar to the model used in our exploration of child and adult survivors of residential fire (see Jones & Ollendick, 2002). In this model, the relationships between the "event" and the "outcomes" are influenced (mediated or moderated) by the availability of resources (i.e., trust, access, and cultural/linguistic capabilities) to address challenges that have long plagued minority communities. With reference to the third step in the model, "resources," we hypothesize that, to the extent that such resources are provided by a culturally competent approach, there is a greater likelihood that challenges will be lessened and that "outcomes" in the acute, data analytic, and recovery phases will be more desirable.

A major predictor of success within this model is a culturally competent perspective. Betancourt et al. (2002, p. v) defined cultural competence as "the ability of systems to provide care to patients with diverse values, beliefs, and behaviors, including tailoring delivery to meet patients' social, cultural, and linguistic needs." We strongly suggest that a cultural competence perspective serve as the lens through which disaster-related initiatives are conceptualized and implemented. If disaster researchers are serious about learning more about the nature and course of the impact of disaster on minorities and marginalized communities, it is essential that such a

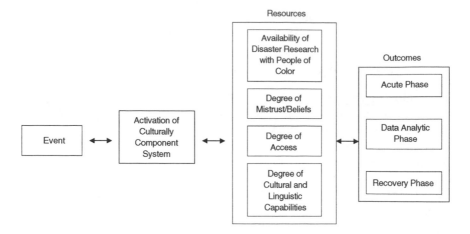

FIGURE 17.1. Cultural competence model for accessing minority and marginalized communities affected by disaster.

framework be adopted. We feel that its adoption and implementation will lessen the negative impact of the obstacles of mistrust, barriers to access, and cultural and linguistic challenges. Solutions for each challenge will be presented in turn.

Mistrust

From the perspective of our model, the following three suggestions are presented that may assist in remedying issues resulting from mistrust. First of all, the reader is directed to the recommendations in Table 17.1 for a list of very practical suggestions including assessing and discussing levels of distrust, involving community gate keepers, and articulating the research project's benefit to community members. Second, it is important to recognize the fact that there is a problem. As researchers and mental health professionals, we can ill afford to continue to deny the fact that negative practices with reference to minorities exist. While there is indeed a role to play on the part of minorities (e.g., voicing problems resulting from disaster and seeking help), the bulk of the responsibility is on the part of the mental health professional. After all, our mission is to assist those who fall prey to the vicissitudes of disasters.

Third, it is paramount that the reader recognize that maximal participation of minority and marginalized groups in research efforts will be forthcoming in instances where meaningful relationships have been

TABLE 17.1. Recommendations for Overcoming Barriers in the Conduct of Research with Minority and Marginalized Communities

Mistrust/beliefs

- Assess and discuss levels of mistrust.
- Find community gatekeepers and request their involvement.
- Interact with leaders and members of the target community.
- Build rapport by establishing bonds with members of the community.
- Include representatives from the target groups as part of the research team.
- Use people of color and individuals from marginalized communities as role models.
- Understand current needs and realities of the target group.
- Recognize and respect differing cultural beliefs and practices.
- Recognize the importance of churches and other community organizations as legitimate support systems.
- Contact people personally when possible.
- Articulate the fact that the program will benefit the target group.
- Demonstrate how the benefits will outweigh risks.
- Ensure research will be conducted ethically.
- Assure all data are confidential and will be used for research only.
- Use culturally sensitive instruments.

Barriers to access

- Find study sites proximate to communities/convenient location.
- Use publicity campaigns directed at minorities.
- Use door-to-door subject recruitment.
- Develop convenient hours of operation.
- Provide/find transportation services to research/treatment sites or reimbursement for transportation costs.
- Provide financial assistance, fee waivers, and incentives.

Culture/linguistics

- Develop, implement, and assess specific plans that outline goals, policies, and systems of accountability when engaging in culturally and linguistically appropriate services.
- Train all research team members in culturally and linguistically appropriate service delivery and research methods.
- Appropriately translate and interpret research materials and measures when research participants are not comfortable with the English language.

forged and are operative prior to the event. No matter how rudimentary or tenuously established these relationships might be, their presence is essential to ensure success in times of crisis. During and after disasters, individuals are most likely to turn to trusted and enduring support systems where previous successes have been demonstrated. The prerequisite for any type of meaningful entry into communities is the development of relationships.

For this purpose, it is useful to consider the conceptual framework for the National Academic Centers of Excellence for Youth Violence Prevention (ACE), which offers the following suggestions. First, the establishment of a participatory process consisting of diverse local, state, and national stakeholders was recommended. Having key representatives of minority and disadvantaged populations at the table during the early planning phases of projects is imperative and is also an important element of the cultural competence model. Second, the requirements of relationship building and careful planning are also key components of this model and are essential prerequisites for successful ventures with minority communities.

Another essential component of this model is building capacity. Requiring researchers to work hand in hand with a variety of individuals within a given community, ranging from laypersons to professionals, is a major component for relationship building. For example, from the initial stages of forming consensus on "the plan of action" to the actual obtaining of data following disaster, researchers should openly and consistently solicit input from community partners. The openness of the researcher to receive input from the targeted group at any point in the process should have an important impact on communities' acceptance of various aspects of the project. A culturally competent team, sensitive to the unique needs of a given community, should play a major role in the training, mentoring, and provision of technical assistance to community participants. Once the data are collected and analyzed, input from these community partners in the interpretation of findings as well as their translation into practice and policy should be obtained.

Given that cultural sensitivity is a *sine qua non* of these types of efforts, a second example is in order. Israel, Schulz, Parker, and Becker (1998) described a collaborative approach to community-based research in which studies are conducted in community settings utilizing input and active participation of actual community members in the research process. Israel et al. (1998) cited multiple features and benefits to community-based research approaches. These research designs build on the strengths and preestablished networks already in place within the community. Additionally, a collaborative partnership is facilitated between researchers and community members, thereby increasing ownership and control of the studies being conducted. Another benefit of community-based research designs is that they involve partnerships of individuals with a diverse array of skills. This wide selection of different skills is often quite valuable in solving the complex problems addressed by community-based research designs. When formed and implemented correctly, collaborative community-based research designs can be an effective way to work with individuals in minority and marginalized communities.

Access

A number of very practical suggestions are provided in Table 17.1. Readily adaptable strategies targeting a variety of practical issues include using publicity campaigns to recruit participants, use of door-to-door recruitment, and providing transportation to research sites as well as incentives for participation. An additional course of action is the use of educational efforts to enhance potential participants' involvement in the research study. Information regarding the research process, as well as the relative benefits of data collection to community members, is a vital step in gaining access to these communities. The need for individuals to become aware of the relative merits of sharing their experiences during the disaster as well as their resulting fears and needs (both psychological and physical) is of vital importance. Both recovery on the part of survivors and knowledge to be gained by the research can be facilitated.

A fairly successful strategy was implemented in our National Institutes of Mental Health (NIMH) funded project designed to assess the impact of residential fire. In light of the fact that African Americans are among those most at risk to experience injury and death resulting from fires, access to this was group was essential. Therefore, to gain the acceptance of churches and/or church members we incorporated a religious component within our protocol to capture "culturally sanctioned ways of coping." More specifically, a measure of religious coping was administered where questions pertaining to the role of prayer, attending church, and looking to religious leaders in times of crises were examined. When approaching various religious organizations, we were able to inform them of the inclusion of these questions, with the goal of determining the relative role of such religious practices in their recovery. Given that we found this practice to be particularly helpful, we strongly advocate for the inclusion of instruments that tap culturally specific modes of dealing with disasters.

The extent to which the researcher's goals overlap with those of community members may do much to enhance participation. Addressing the age-old questions of "what's in it for me?" up front and in a straightforward manner is likely to enhance participation even in the face of historical challenges. For instance, if parents are informed that disasters have been found to interfere with academic performances of some children, they may be open to finding out how their child's academic performance might have been affected. Consequently, their willingness to participate might be greatly enhanced. If intervention strategies are promised following assessment, this may be an even greater reinforcer for those whose children might benefit.

In communities where such elaborate cultural competent systems are yet to be established, a similar approach can be taken whereby disaster studies may be endorsed by, and carried out in, culturally sanctioned entities. For example, in several investigations designed to assess the impact of fire-related trauma on children and their families, we found a great resource within the culture of the Red Cross. That is, after informing Red Cross officials of our work and its potential for developing a knowledge base regarding the psychosocial impact of disaster on families, they not only embraced several of our projects but also provided actual sites where we were able to recruit and interview participants. The essential point here is that conceptualizing existing cultures as resources can provide another means of gaining access to minority communities. We should add that this strategy is particularly applicable to situations where relationships were not previously established. The leveraging of existing entities within communities may be the most effective route to pursue.

Culture and Linguistics

Table 17.1 provides several suggestions to address issues related to cultural/ linguistic challenges in research. These challenges are similar to those faced by practitioners. The U.S. Department of Health and Human Services' Office of Minority Health established a set of 14 standards to ensure that all people receive equitable and effective health care (U.S. Department of Health and Human Services, 2001b, 2001c). Perusing the standards proposed, we feel that the following recommendations would aid research teams interfacing with minority communities:

1. Ensure that all participants are treated respectfully in a manner compatible with their culture, health beliefs and practices, and preferred language.
2. Include, retain, and promote individual representatives of the traumatized community on the research team.
3. Ensure that all members of the research team receive ongoing education and training in culturally and linguistically appropriate service delivery or research.

4. Offer and provide language assistance capabilities, including bilingual members and interpreter services to all participants with limited English proficiency, at no cost.
5. Develop, implement, and routinely assess a written strategic plan outlining goals, policies, and systems of accountability to engage culturally and linguistically appropriate research.
6. Use culturally and linguistically appropriate measures and assess participants' satisfaction with such measures.
7. Establish collaborative partnerships with traumatized communities where individuals representative of these communities are involved in the designing and implementing of research initiatives.

In summary, if research participants of color are to be ensured culturally and linguistically appropriate inclusion, it is incumbent upon the research team to systematically implement the above recommendations. Furthermore, interviewers need to understand the meaning of body language, gestures, postures, and inflections within minority groups so as to enhance the overall effectiveness of the interview process.

SUMMARY

Challenges of conducting research in minority and marginalized communities include mistrust on the part of minorities toward researchers as well as the mental health system, lack of access, and cultural and linguistic issues. These barriers are best addressed through the adoption of attitudes, behaviors, and processes embedded within culturally competent approaches. The benefits of a culturally competent framework to the trauma researcher are enormous. The wealth of resources resulting from relationship building, engagement of indigenous professionals, paraprofessionals, and community leaders, sensitivity in the training, mentoring, and provision of technical assistance to participants and "openness" of the researcher to receive input from the community are certain to enhance the quantity and quality of interaction between the traumatized communities and researchers. It is hoped that this union will do much both to enhance our knowledge of the impact of disasters on these groups and to enable mental health professionals to better assist them during the recovery process.

ACKNOWLEDGMENT

Preparation of this chapter was supported in part by Grant No. 546770 from the UCLA/National Center for Child Traumatic Stress to Russell T. Jones.

REFERENCES

Anderson, N. B., McNeilly, M., & Myers, H. (1992). Toward understanding race difference in autonomic reactivity: A proposed contextual model. In J. Turner, A. Sherwood, and A. Light (Eds.), *Individual differences in cardiovascular response to stress* (pp. 125–145). New York: Plenum Press.

Betancourt, J. R., Green, A. R., & Carrillo, J. E. (2002). *Cultural competence in health care: Emerging frameworks and practical approaches* (field report). Boston and Syracuse: Commonwealth Fund.

Bonham, V. L. (2002, June). *Ethical, legal, and social implications: A community view.* Paper presented at the Symposium on Genomic Medicine, National Medical Association, National Human Genome Institute, Bethesda, MD.

Boulware, L. E., Cooper, L. A., Ratner, L. E., LaVeist, T. A., & Powe, N. R. (2003). Race and trust in the health care system. *Public Health Reports, 118*(4), 366–367.

Breslau, N. (2002). Epidemiologic studies of trauma, posttraumatic stress disorder, and other psychiatric disorders, *Canadian Journal of Psychiatry, 47,* 923–929.

Breslau, N., Kessler, R. C., Chilcoat, H. D., Schultz, L. R., Davis, G. C., & Andreski, P. (1998). Trauma and posttraumatic stress disorder in the community: The 1996 Detroit area survey of trauma. *Archives of General Psychiatry, 55*(7), 626–632.

Corbie-Smith, G., Thomas, S. B., & St. George, D. M. M. (2002). Distrust, race, and research. *Archives of Internal Medicine, 162,* 2548–2463.

Gamble, V. N. (1993). A legacy of distrust: African Americans and medical research. *American Journal of Preventative Medicine, 9*(Suppl. 6), 35–38.

Israel, B. A., Schulz, A. J., Parker, E. A., & Becker, A. B. (1998). Review of community-based research: Assessing partnership approaches to improve public health. *Annual Review of Public Health, 19,* 173–202.

Johnson, R. L., Saha, S., Arbelaez, J. J., Beach, M. C., & Cooper, L. A. (2004). Racial and ethnic differences in patient perceptions of bias and cultural competence in health care. *Journal of General Internal Medicine, 19*(2), 101–110.

Jones, L., Brazel, D., Peskind, E. R., Morelli, T., & Raskind, M. A. (2000). Group therapy program for African-American veterans with posttraumatic stress disorder. *Psychiatric Services, 51,* 1177–1179.

Jones, R. T., Kephart, C., Langley, A. K., Parker, M. N., Shenoy, U., & Weeks, C. (2001). Cultural and Ethnic Diversity Issues in Clinical Psychology. In C. E. Walker & M. C. Roberts (Eds.), *Handbook of Clinical Child Psychology* (pp. 955–973). New York: Wiley.

Jones, R. T., & Ollendick, T. H. (2002). The impact of residential fire on children and their families. In A. La Greca, W. Sliverman, E. Vernberg, & M. Roberts (Eds.). *Helping children cope with disasters: Integrating research and practice* (pp. 175–202). Washington, DC: American Psychological Association.

Kessler, R. C., Sonnega, A., Bromet, E., Hughes, M., & Nelson, C. B. (1995). Posttraumatic stress disorder in the National Comorbidity Survey, *Archives of General Psychiatry, 52,* 1048–1060.

King, P. A. (1992). Twenty years after. The legacy of the Tuskegee syphilis study. The dangers of difference. *Hastings Center Report, 22,* 35–38.

Lawson, W. B. (2000). Issues in pharmacotherapy for African Americans. In P. Ruiz, J. M. Oldham, & M. B. Riba (Eds.), *Ethnicity and Psychopharmacology: Vol. 19. Review of Psychiatry. (pp. 37–52).* Washington, DC: American Psychiatric Publishing, Inc.

Loo, C. M. (2003). PTSD among ethnic minority veterans: A National Center for PTSD fact sheet. Retrieved September 24, 2003, from www.ncptsd.org/facts/veterans/fs_ethnic_vet.html.

Mar'n, G., & Marín, B. (1991). *Research with Hispanic populations.* Newbury Park, CA: Sage.

Million-Underwood, S., Sanders, E., & Davis, M. (1993). Determinants of participation in state-of-the-art cancer prevention, early detection/screening, and treatment trials among African-Americans. *Cancer Nursing, 161,* 25–33.

Norris, F. H., & Alegria, M. (2005). Mental health care for ethnic minority individuals and communities in the aftermath of disasters and mass violence. *CNS Spectrums, 10*(2), 1–9.

Parker, M. N., & Jones, R. T. (1999). Minority status stress: Effect on the psychological and academic functioning of African American atudents. *Journal of Gender, Culture, and Health, 4*(1), 61–82.

Perilla, J. L., Norris, F. H., & Lavizzo, E. A. (2002). Ethnicity, culture, and disaster response: Identifying and explaining ethnic differences in PTSD six months after Hurricane Andrew. *Journal of Social and Clinical Psychology, 21*(1), 20–45.

Roberson, N. L. (1994). Clinical trial participation. Viewpoints from racial/ethnic groups. *Cancer, 74,* 2687–2691.

Rosenheck, R. A., & Fontana, A. F. (1995). The effect of clinician–veteran racial pairing in the treatment of posttraumatic stress disorder. *American Journal of Psychiatry, 152,* 555–563.

Selner-O'Hagan, M. B., Kindlon, D. J., Buka, S. L., Raudenbush, S. W., & Earls, F. J. (1998). Assessing exposure to violence in urban youth. *Journal of Child Psychology, 39*(2), 215–224.

Shavers-Hornaday, V. L., Lynch, C. F., Burmeister, L. F., & Torner, J. C. (1997). Why are African Americans under-represented in medical research studies? Impediments to participation. *Ethnicity and Health, 2,* 31–45.

Vernberg, E. M., La Greca, A. M., Silverman, W. K., & Prinstein, M. J. (1996). Prediction of posttraumatic stress symptoms in children after Hurricane Andrew. *Journal of Abnormal Psychology, 105*(2), 237–248.

U.S. Department of Health and Human Services (2001a). *Mental health: Culture, race, and ethnicity—a supplement to mental health: A report of the Surgeon General.* Rockville, MD: U.S. Department of Health and Human Services, Substance Abuse and Mental Health Services Administration, Center for Mental Health Services.

U.S. Department of Health and Human Services (2001b). *National standards for culturally and linguistically appropriate services in health care* (final report). Rockville, MD: Office of Minority Health.

U.S. Department of Health and Human Services (2001c). *Cultural competence works: Using cultural competence to improve the quality of health care for diverse populations and add value to managed care arrangements.* Rockville, MD: U.S. Department of Health and Human Services, Health Resources and Services Administration.

Zoellner, L. A., Feeny, N. C., Fitzgibbons, L. A., & Foa, E. B. (1999). Response of African American and Caucasian women to behavioral therapy for PTSD. *Behavior Therapy, 30,* 581–595.

CHAPTER 18

Conducting Research in Other Countries

ARTHUR D. MURPHY,
JULIA L. PERILLA, and ERIC C. JONES

Over the years, we have participated in interdisciplinary collaborations with colleagues from various countries and disciplines as wide ranging as engineering, urban planning, architecture, medicine, and theology. As a result, we have learned a great deal about crossing not only disciplinary boundaries but also about the negotiations involved in the international research process. Along the way, we have found that collaborating with colleagues from other nations is one of the most rewarding parts of our academic careers. It takes a great deal of personal and administrative energy, but when it works the process has enriched us in ways that are difficult to enumerate. In this chapter we hope to provide the reader with a summary of some of what we have learned in the process of conducting international collaborative research. In every project we have undertaken, we have learned as much from our mistakes as from our successes. Some of the experiences were painful, others humbling, and some humorous, while yet others provided us with unexpected insights into our profession and ourselves. The sections below are a compilation of the collective wisdom we have gathered in that process. We note that we bring to this chapter our

North American perspective and primarily rely on our experience working with colleagues in less wealthy countries. There are of course challenges inherent in work with colleagues in other wealthy countries, some of which are similar and some of which are different from the challenges discussed here.

BRINGING COLLEAGUES FROM FOREIGN COUNTRIES INTO RESEARCH PROJECTS: TRUE COLLABORATION ACROSS BORDERS

There are several concerns we keep in mind when undertaking a project across cultural and national boundaries: collaboration, financial issues, language, validity, protection for human participants, engaging the study community, and being a guest researcher.

The Colleague Facilitator

Our first step in carrying out international collaborative work is putting together a research team that can truly help us get the project completed. In doing so, it is important to find someone who has experience working with government and research personnel in the place where we will carry out our project. This might not be a person in our discipline. What is important is that local colleagues have experience working through the bureaucratic, political, and cultural issues that are involved with research in the target area. We look for a colleague who is able to spend the time guiding our project through the local system. An individual who has spent time on the faculty at a local university is ideal. We often find that our collaborator is able to give our conclusions and analysis a "reality check," placing our analysis in a context with which we may not be experienced. For further reading about collaborative research, we recommend Stull and Schensul (1987) and LeCompte, Schensul, Weeks, and Merrill (1999).

Reward Mechanisms

One of the first issues we often confront, and admit it is still a difficult one for us to overcome, involves differences in avenues for professional advancement between us and foreign colleagues. In many non-Western nations, advancement is not based on the number of publications or research grants but rather on seniority and the contract negotiated between the union and the administration. Academics in many countries do not earn enough to maintain their family and are working secondary jobs in order to make ends meet. Academics often consider such grants as an opportunity for supplemental pay. In many institutions in Africa, Asia, the Middle East, Latin America, and eastern Europe, there is no mechanism comparable to augment fixed salaries with external grant funding, as is the norm in North American academic institutions. This often means that not only must we find creative ways to compensate local collaborators, but that we must also work with the financial disbursement structure of the institution managing the relevant compensation portion of the grant so that the financial relationship is acceptable to local colleagues.

Differences in Training, Research, and Professional Expectations

The implicit hierarchical structure within the Western academic tradition has at times made it difficult to bring foreign colleagues into every stage of the research process. First, the power differential between the principal investigator and all other participants in a project is exacerbated when the study is funded in a wealthy country but carried out in a foreign locale, particularly if we are working with colleagues in one of the secondary institutions in a nation where academic research funds tend to be focused at a single leading national university. It is helpful to remember that our location in a Western institution has allowed us a privileged position. However, this does not necessarily afford us access to the research site. Also, we try to remember that our colleagues are the persons who give us access to participants in *their* country and, as such, also have a more nuanced understanding of how research is conducted in their country.

One point worth reinforcing is that one should try not to become too focused on formal faculty degrees. In many places in the world, individuals with what in the United States would be considered an honors BA degree are teaching and doing research at major universities. In our experience, this is one of the hardest obstacles for Western-trained academics to overcome. We are bound to our notion that a PhD or other advanced degree confers authority over others who have not achieved that status. Investigators working with colleagues in other environments need to remember that there are different norms in other settings that may determine academic tenure, rank, and the criteria for promotion. In many countries promotion and/or salary increases are not based on one's academic track record. Instead, they are commonly based on longevity and service to the institution. Publications are secondary, as is research. Service, on the other hand, is primary. We try to keep in mind that only wealthy nations can afford the luxury of what we call "basic" science, and we try to be prepared to respond to foreign colleagues' questions about the project's benefit.

CHALLENGES IN STUDY DESIGN
AND IMPLEMENTATION

Institutional Review Board Clearance and
Informed Consent

In a foreign context, this can be a challenging and culturally loaded issue. We are not surprised if the local institutional review board (IRB) is more concerned with issues of relevance than with confidentiality and compensation to the participants. It may be concerned with the origin of the funding and who in the United States will be the ultimate recipient of the data. That is to say, the local IRB may be concerned with the possible harmful use of data not only against an individual, but also its institution or the nation. We try to answer such questions directly and honestly. In most of the places we work, there is much stronger awareness of the link between research and political and economic ideology than that to which we are normally willing to admit in Western science.

Privacy and associated stress and harm are cultural constructs. For example, in the United States we see domestic violence as a private matter, something to be dealt with between husband, wife, and the authorities— not as a public issue. In many places, domestic violence is a public issue. Men and women know when it is happening; they talk about it, and often it is because of this social collective pressure that change occurs, not because the spouse had to spend time in the local jail. In such situations it is much more stressful to "keep a secret" than to discuss it publicly. In many contexts the very act of placing the individual in a secluded environment will raise the level of anxiety and stress. Our participant may be concerned about what others are thinking about him or her, the community, or other family members behind those closed doors. These are real concerns. We cannot expect assurances of confidentiality either to the subject or to his or her family and community to alleviate these concerns. They will not. However, this is an opportunity to develop creative and sensitive ways to meet our IRB obligations. For further reading about issues of informed consent, see Fleischman, Collogan, and Tuma (Chapter 5, this volume) and Dunn and Chadwick (2002).

Informed consent and permission is another issue to be addressed. In many parts of the world, people are reluctant to sign anything because, more often than not, their signature on a piece of paper has resulted in harm rather than protection. What would a Mayan during the dirty war in Central America have thought if a stranger had come up and had asked him or her to read a document and to sign the line at the bottom, indicating that he or she understood the form and was in agreement? In all probability, the Mayan would either have refused to sign simply because he or she did not trust us or perhaps believed the researcher to be a collaborator with the military or government.

Clearly, we are not suggesting that one should not secure informed consent; we simply ensure that we do so in a manner that is consistent with the cultural constructs of the community with which we are working while at the same time meeting the needs of our own IRB. This is often a multitiered, time-consuming process, but the last thing we want is to have a community leader stop us and question our activities. Our explanation that the mayor gave his blessing to our study will not be sufficient. He will want to know why we did not stop by and see him before starting our work. Our recommendation is to ask for advice from local contacts about the appropriate way to obtain these forms. Our experience is that if a participant asks about authorization to do research, what he or she wants to know is not if the Ministry of Health has approved the study but whether we have talked with the president of the local community organization or the village elder and whether they have approved it. It saves a great deal of difficulty when we take the time to learn how local processes of authority and community structures serve to protect their citizenry.

Participant Compensation

Compensation for participants in research projects in host countries can be a complex issue. Undoubtedly, people's time and effort should be acknowledged and recognized. We are constantly reminded by our IRB guidelines to specifically spell out the amount and type of compensation that we will provide for participants. At the same time, we are admonished to make sure that we are not coercing people into participating in our studies. When we conduct research with low-income or vulnerable populations, we are also aware of the potential coercive nature of any incentives or the level of compensation offered. If we are offering $10 for 2 hours of work to a person in a country in which the daily wage is $5, it will be difficult for a person to turn down the opportunity, even if he or she would prefer not to participate. Incentives and compensation for study participants should definitely be decided after consultation with colleagues in each host country, and deference should always be give to local customs.

Use of Appropriate and Comprehensible Language

Language is critical. We assume that language is relatively constant and universal—English is English, Spanish is Spanish, French is French, or Hindi is Hindi. Nothing could be further from the truth. The internal variation within a language is extraordinary. In some places, one version of the language is spoken by the elite, and another is spoken by the common people.

In other cases, a particular word may be different from one location to another. An instrument devised in the United States is generally not appropriate for work in Australia. Whether using romance languages spoken over large areas of the globe (e.g., Spanish, French, and English) or native languages spoken in several localities or regions of a continent (e.g., Swahili, Hindi, and Maya), all languages deserve equal respect. Each will have regional variations that will affet results and the ways in which we are perceived by our colleagues. When working in a foreign language, it is important to be conscious both of variations in language and of the particular variations in language used by specific audiences. This issue is probably most important when considering the validity of the instrument or interview guide that will be used in the field, and for interpreting participant responses.

Validity and Reliability

Validity is something we try to consider before going to the field. We will already have spent time and resources to get a research team ready and into the field, and we want to avoid, at a later stage in the process, retranslation, retesting, or even doing further ethnographic research to get a handle on the effectiveness of our protocol.

What is the validity of the translated version of our instrument? In other words, can an instrument translated in France be used all over Francophone Africa? Or, can a Dehli version of an instrument be used in other large cities in India or even in rural areas of India? Of course, this depends in part on the issues being addressed. Answering these questions requires some initial fieldwork. We take the instrument to the field and ask people what they understand by each question. Local translators are key to this process. It may take many hours to explain conditions and symptoms to a translator, but this is necessary to attain the appropriate local wording.

In cross-cultural settings, internal validity is challenged by the same issues as in the country where the instrument originated: changes over time due to factors other than the independent variable, contamination through repeated measures due to familiarity with the instrument, changes in the way the instrument is administered, and participant dropout. None of these propose significantly greater problems for cross-cultural settings. However, a local understanding of history and of potential developmental factors helps us provide alternative hypotheses rather than assuming that the change in the dependent variable necessarily results from changes in the independent variable.

While language is the single most important factor influencing cross-cultural or external validity, there are other concerns. One is the willingness of people in different places to answer questions that may be considered taboo or shameful. Given a particular social or political context, the study participant might even give us an untruthful answer because he or she is not comfortable giving us a truthful answer. Working with someone who knows the general belief system of the study population is helpful for addressing these kinds of challenges to generalizability.

Another challenge to external validity is that the household composition and the geographic distribution and density may be quite different from that which we have encountered before. Thus, knowledge of the residence pattern and household systems will help direct appropriate sampling techniques. Of course, choosing control study sites or multiple research sites for study may improve generalizability. However, additional sites should be chosen for theoretical reasons and not just for external validity.

Engaging the Local Community

Not unlike the reaction we would have if a stranger came into our neighborhood and began asking probing questions regarding our health, our habits, our family, or our house, the communities in which we conduct research usually have many questions and opinions about the relevance, feasibility, and need for our project. We have found that we have been most successful when we have taken the time to dialogue with members of the community and hear their ideas, concerns, and questions regarding our study before we finalize our design and data collection procedures. The issues that are raised and the questions that are asked help us to think through our assumptions and strategies and, undoubtedly, result in tremendous savings of time, and money. Our greatest challenges have come from the times when we were developed our questionnaires, strategies, procedures, and timelines without consulting colleagues in the host country: questions they perceive to be disrespectful or dangerous to participants; procedures that that seemed reasonable and ethical but were impossible or potentially harmful for interviewers; and compensation schemes that might be hard for local investigators to meet in future studies.

One of the advantages of a presence in the community is the added potential to invite people to become part of the research process. Community consultants help us understand the possible pitfalls of our procedures, give us guidance regarding community dynamics and politics that can affect the feasibility of our study, and aid us in addressing the problems that arise during the project. Their voices are also essential in creating a more in-depth understanding of the findings of our studies and the latent cultural misinterpretations that, as outsiders, we might not fully appreciate. The insight that community members have given our research teams has been extremely beneficial to our writing and dissemination strategies once the project is finished. At the same time, the involvement of community members as recipients of the knowledge and information we gained from our study is a symbolic and practical way to give useful information back to the people from whom we obtained the original data.

LOGISTICAL CHALLENGES

Hidden Costs

International research contains hidden costs that affect all research budgets. First, are there currency transfer laws between the United States and the host nation? Many countries set limits to the amounts that may be transferred, or otherwise define the mechanisms for carrying out these transactions. The advent of ATMs has made it easier to access funds around the world, but there are limits to the amount that can be withdrawn at any one time. We have found ourselves making several trips to the ATM to withdraw our weekly payroll. In addition foreign banks often charge a significant fee for use of the ATM in addition to any charge our home bank may levy.

An option is electronic transfer from the United States to a local bank. This has the advantage of being able to move larger amounts of money in a single transaction. However, it has some drawbacks. First, there are often hefty transaction fees levied by both the sending bank and receiving bank. It is important to calculate these fees into your budget. Second, such transactions require a bank account in an appropriate banking institution in the host country. In each country, a different culture of banking exists, and different laws and regulations govern the system. It is not unusual for banks in some places to hold funds transferred from our country for several days or weeks before releasing them. Also, once the funds are in the local account, we might have only limited access to them, potentially not being able to withdraw more than a fixed amount at any one time, or we may be required to keep the funds in a local currency that is constantly fluctuating against the dollar.

We are always prepared to carry out all local transactions in cash. In many countries, even middle-class households do not have bank accounts. Thus, we have to be prepared to pay our workers or participants with cash and to adapt to the accepted pay period. In some places it is customary to liquidate all payroll debts on Friday or Saturday. We recommend that researchers never let the pay period go for longer than 2 weeks so that any issues are resolved quickly. This leads to the question of accounting.

Accounting and payroll practices vary across the globe. Most agencies and foundations that fund international research expect the local institution to adhere to "accepted" procedures or standards. We have had to work closely to establish a clear procedure for disbursement of funds that meets the requirements of our home institution, as well as what is expected at the local level. In many cases, this has required that we or one of our colleagues take on the role of "accountant"—that is, be responsible for the disbursement of funds, the justification of those payments, and the collection of proper documentation. We are careful to make certain that payments are made in accordance with local laws and customs. We do not want to assume, for example, that local consultants will be responsible for health insurance, taxes, and the like, only to discover that local law requires that we pay such costs.

It is usually far more costly to carry out a project across national borders than within a single country. Our experience is that, once we have a budget, we anticipate an additional 10–25% in each of our categories—the lower figure if we have previously carried out research in the location with the same researchers and institutions, the higher if this is our first attempt at such a project.

Hiring of Local Staff

This is a highly complex process, and how one goes about it depends on what tasks need to be performed. If we are looking for a specific set of skills—for example, laboratory technician or statistician—we use local colleagues to help us find these individuals. Our local colleagues know who in their institutions has the skills and how best to approach them. Hiring field staff is an even more complicated process.

Our experiences, and those of colleagues with whom we have worked, have taught us not to try to predict who will be the best interviewer or field data person. We are particularly cautious when the field research involves individuals of varying class backgrounds. The best solution for these problems is ensuring uniform and consistent training for all research assistants and interviewers and constant review of field work by local colleagues who are aware of the pitfalls that class and education bring to the process. If inadvertent bias on the part of a staff person is found, it can often be remedied by additional training and through role playing. This is one of those areas that requires constant vigilance by us and our local colleagues.

CONCLUSION: THE RESEARCHER
AS A GUEST OF THE HOST COUNTRY

Along with the advantages and privileges that come with being funded investigators from North America, there is always the risk of forgetting that we are—and always will be—guests of the host country. Those of us who have spent long years working in another country are particularly susceptible to this error. We cannot think of a more harmful approach to the research project, the quality of the data we will be collecting, or the potential for future collaborations than the belief or attitude that our ability to provide most or all of the economic support for a project accords us special privileges. At times, the graciousness with which our invitation to collaborate is met lets us forget that it is a unique opportunity to be allowed to advance our fields and our personal careers and that we must reciprocate by making sure that we follow the unwritten rules of etiquette governing such cooperative efforts.

Although the expectations and understandings may differ from country to country, it is always best to err on the side of formality, as an informal approach to interactions may be taken as lack of respect. Negotiations and discussions are a given and must be carried out in such a way that they are not perceived as assumptions of entitlement. What we have learned is that flexibility is not only necessary but can actually increase the quality of our study and the potential to uncover information that, while not part of the original design strategy, can enhance our understanding of the issue we are studying. It goes without saying that criticism of host country institutions, people, society, etc., will not assist our research efforts.

Sense of Humor

As researchers we tend to take ourselves very seriously. As a result, our work may take on a critical and urgent attitude that often may not be shared by our colleagues and researched communities. This difference in priorities calls for a strong sense of humor to manage the anxiety that is provoked by delays, no-shows, changes in administrative staff, government office shutdowns, long holidays during which the entire country is off work, the intermittent availability of electricity and other utilities, and equipment malfunction, just to name a few of the circumstances we have encountered. Our experience has taught us to laugh at the unexpected and to rethink, within the context of our entire lives, the meaning of our work and the knowledge derived from our studies.

Respect

Quite possibly, the quality that is most universally considered central to any cross-cultural collaboration is respect. Respect is a reciprocal association in which both parties expect to give and receive respect while being aware of the inherent differences conferred by social status. All of us are aware that people in positions of power in our host country have the ability to accept our offer of collaboration or refuse permission to conduct a study in their territory. Somewhat further down the hierarchical scale are our colleagues. Even further from the hierarchical top are the people who will be conducting the interviews or surveys and the community members from whom we will collect the data. We strongly believe that the quality of our data is closely tied to the degree to which the research team members from our host country and the participants of our study feel respected by and in turn respect the investigators.

Having Fun

Not everything about conducting research in other countries is about hard work and serious issues. There are naturally occurring opportunities for the research team to get together and jointly celebrate the work that is being accomplished. Maintaining morale in the field is of paramount importance. If researchers do not plan to be on site for the duration of the project, they would be well advised to take every opportunity to visit. The daily challenges, frustrations, and successes that occur as a natural part of any study of this type should be shared by both field workers and investigators. The researchers will undoubtedly obtain a better sense of the possibilities and limitations of the project and thus be able to make more informed decisions if there is ongoing dialogue with people in the field. These visits are excellent times for having fun together and enjoying the unique opportunities available to enhance the personal and collective understanding of the host culture. We hope that our experiences may prove useful to North American investigators thinking of conducting work that involves data collection in other countries.

REFERENCES

Dunn, C. M., & Chadwick, G. (2002). *Protecting study volunteers in research: A manual for investigative sites* (2nd ed.). Boston: CenterWatch.

LeCompte, M. D., Schensul, J., Weeks, R., & Singer, M. (Eds.). (1999). *Research roles and research partnerships.* Walnut Creek, CA: Altamira Press.

Stull, D., & Schensul, J. (Eds.). (1987). *Collaborative research and social change: Applied anthropology in action.* Boulder, CO: Westview.

CHAPTER 19

Disaster Mental Health Research

Challenges for the Future

MATTHEW J. FRIEDMAN

The purpose of this volume was to promote the best methodological approaches to disaster mental health research. The preceding chapters have provided a comprehensive review of the current state of knowledge and have identified important gaps in our current scientific understanding. Several authors suggested that the field of disaster mental health research has matured considerably since its inception but that disaster research methods need to improve in several ways. These chapters then are important calls to action that bear serious consideration. The aims of this volume were both to help the interested reader design methodologically sound research projects and to utilize such methodology for the best purposes. In this concluding chapter I present a synthesis of the areas of research that the other editors and I feel are key challenges for the future. Although we build on the preceding chapters, ultimately the areas we highlight here are based on our judgment and experience in the field. In the sections that follow I discuss what research areas need the greatest attention in the future and then consider important implementation challenges that must be addressed to achieve this end. I conclude by discussing public and research policy considerations toward achieving these goals.

THE TEMPORAL DIMENSION

The temporal dimension of postdisaster reactions is particularly important. At this time we don't have a good idea about the full range of postimpact reactions, from the acute aftermath through intermediate phases to the long term. As a field, we have become much better at implementing protocols that tap acute-phase reactions, especially utilizing telephone and Web-based approaches. Progress has been much less evident with regard to long-term follow-up. As noted by Norris and Elrod (Chapter 2, this volume), few studies have assessed survivors for more than 2 years after the event.

In addition to the obvious deficits in scientific understanding of the longitudinal psychological experience of individuals and communities impacted by disasters, this lack of information has major consequences for public policy and the funding of disaster relief programs. In the United States, postdisaster crisis counseling services are funded by the Stafford Act for only 1 year, although services sometimes continue through no-cost extensions. There are some data indicating that postdisaster psychological consequences extend far beyond this 1-year window (Norris, Friedman, Watson, Byrne, et al., 2002; Norris, Friedman, & Watson, 2002). Longitudinal research is clearly needed to decide this issue one way or the other or to show when, where, or for whom the effects are long-lasting. Should it be shown, conclusively, that a year's worth of federal support for disaster relief (at least under certain circumstances such as a terrorist attack) is inadequate to meet the needs of a significant percentage of survivors, it would be necessary to modify public policy and public funding in this regard.

ASSESSING DISASTER EXPOSURE

It is by no means obvious how best to measure exposure to disasters. There are three types of exposure that have been cited in the trauma literature. Many years ago, Terr (1991) differentiated Type I trauma, an instantaneous moment of terror resulting from a discrete event (such as a hurricane, rape, or motor vehicle accident) from Type II trauma, protracted, repetitive exposure (as in childhood sexual/physical trauma, domestic violence, war zone exposure, or living in a locale frequently subjected to natural disasters). She proposed that important differences between the event characteristics (e.g., acute vs. chronic) and differences in event-related expectations, appraisals, and coping strategies predicted different clinical phenotypes; Type I trauma tended to produce intrusive recollections, while Type II trauma was more likely to produce numbing and dissociation. Any possible qualitative differences between Types I and II trauma exposure are probably less important than dosage differences. For measurement purposes, it seems reasonable to suggest that, when estimating the severity of chronic trauma exposure, we should utilize some area-under-the-curve metric that integrates both intensity and duration of trauma exposure into the estimate.

To complicate matters even more, fear of ongoing threat is a third type of potentially traumatic experience that is quite relevant within the current context of global fear of terrorism. Since terrorism is primarily psychological warfare in which widespread fear is created through production of a credible threat, people may exhibit extreme emotional distress even though they have never been in any physical danger themselves. Galea et al. (2002) have addressed this issue in their research by distinguishing between New Yorkers who had direct exposure to the World Trade Center attacks and New Yorkers who were affected indirectly. Distress due to ongoing threat also applies to scenarios other than terrorism such as invisible toxic environmental contamination or living in an area that is frequently bombarded by hurricanes, earthquakes, and the like. The conceptual challenge is to determine whether fear of ongoing threat can be considered "traumatic" within the DSM-IV definition. The measurement challenge is how best to assess fear of ongoing threat and what instrumentation to use for this purpose.

Assessments of traumatic exposure are generally obtained after the fact, occasionally many years after the disaster has occurred. Such retrospective recollections are affected by recall bias and the emotional state at the time of assessment rather than at the time of the traumatic experience. This problem is endemic to all research of this sort. A question is: How important is the distinction between assessments that are "factual" (what actually happened) and "perceived" (what is believed to have happened at the time of assessment)? Whereas this distinction is crucial in legal proceedings, where a verdict may hinge on the veracity of a recollection, it may be of less consequence in psychological research. It has been demonstrated in research with geriatric and cancer patients that "perceived" health status is a better predictor of psychological and functional outcomes than "objective" health status as determined by a medical examination (Hong, Zarit, & Malmberg, 2004; Smith, Young, & Lee, 2004; Stewart, Hays, & Ware, 1992). Perhaps this also applies to disaster research. Within reasonable limits, we too should be more concerned about such perceptions than about the historical accuracy of trauma severity estimates by research participants.

WHAT OUTCOMES TO MEASURE

Another continuing challenge for the field is to identify and monitor the full range of acute/chronic postdisaster reactions. This can be accomplished with assessment strategies that focus on psychological and biolog-ical *mechanisms of change* hypothesized to mediate or moderate post-disaster outcomes. Longitudinal research, in which such psychological and biological mechanisms are monitored prospectively and sequentially, is particularly suited to the study of which reactions are adaptive, which are not, how to distinguish one from the other, and how to predict resil-ience and vulnerability. Therefore, in addition to measuring "the usual suspects" (symptom severity, diagnostic category, etc.), it is essential to utilize instruments that assess constructs such as social support, self-efficacy, locus of control, personality traits, cognitive strategies, genetic factors, stress tolerance, neurobiological reactivity, aspects of the recovery envi-ronment, and the psychological resources of survivors. Operationalizing and monitoring such constructs is an important challenge. Other relevant domains are physical health (e.g., medical diagnosis, physical symptoms, somatization, or medically unexplained pathology), concurrent stress, past history, attitudes such as trust in authorities, appraisals of personal safety, and coping strategies.

Most lists of this sort include "functional capacity." Although the im-portance of this construct is universally accepted, there is no agreement about how to standardize and operationalize such an important measure. A recent attempt to identify key components of functional status among chil-dren and adolescents cites the following factors (with the understanding that norms for such factors will vary depending on developmental level): school achievement and failure, quality of peer relationships, quality of family relationships, achievement of developmental milestones, empathic and prosocial behavior/citizenship, quality of work performance, romantic relationships, teenage sexual activity, alcohol and drug use, and delin-quency and antisocial behavior (Balaban et al., 2005). We are not suggesting this list as a template for assessment of functional status in future research but as an example of the scope and complexity of this key construct. Indeed, some investigators have suggested that functional status is a more impor-tant prognostic indicator of well-being than symptom severity or even than the presence or absence of a formal psychiatric diagnosis (Norris, Murphy, Baker, & Perilla, 2003; North & Westerhaus, 2003).

INDIVIDUAL VERSUS SOCIAL VARIABLES

Traditionally, disaster mental health research has focused on the impact of disasters on individual distress, psychopathology, and functional capacity (e.g., posttraumatic stress disorder [PTSD], depression, and substance abuse). Such an individual psychopathological orientation has also ad-dressed variables hypothesized to mediate or moderate adverse postdisaster outcomes such as vulnerability/resilience, ways of coping, peridisaster appraisals, cognitive processing, and genetic or psychobiological factors.

More recently, a greater emphasis on public mental health has emerged that is concerned with social and community factors that may influence both the onset of, and recovery from, mental illness after disasters. Although features of the social environment may plausibly influence wellness, illness, recovery, and chronicity, there are relatively few empirical studies that have explored the role of social context after disasters. If we define *disaster* as an acute, collectively experienced event with sudden onset (McFarlane & Norris, Chapter 1, this volume), we need to improve our capacity to both conceptualize and measure collective experience. This collective context lends itself to a social cognitive theoretical approach that postulates constructs such as agentic perspectives on social support, collective efficacy, and conservation of resources (see Benight, McFarlane, & Norris, Chapter 4, this volume).

For example, the agentic theoretical framework understands human adaptation as a dynamic interplay between environmental, intraindividual, and behavioral factors where outcomes depend on how each factor influences the other (Benight & Bandura, 2004). A good example of this is in military research that emphasizes the salutary impact of unit cohesion on individual psychological well-being (Bliese & Halverson, 1996; Oliver, Harman, Hoover, Hayes, & Pandhi, 1999). Likewise, international mental health relief workers who seek to promote the psychological well-being of children during the postwar reconstruction period (which has many similarities to postdisaster scenarios) are convinced that social or community-level interventions constitute the best way to promote individual recovery (Friedman & Mikus-Kos, 2005).

The methodological challenges are enormous. We must develop instruments that assess the full spectrum of individual postdisaster reactions, identify and operationalize collective outcomes and processes that are important in and of themselves, and also generate and test models that predict how individual and collective factors influence and change one another. Furthermore, since disasters precipitate a time-sensitive sequence of events consisting of a wide spectrum of individual and collective processes, we must conduct longitudinal studies that will enable us to monitor the key phases and trajectories that have been set in motion. Finally, constructing an assessment battery that can usefully map such individual and collective processes, outcomes, phases, and trajectories is a prerequisite to meaningful intervention research.

A good example of this challenge concerns the construct of social support. At the individual level there is an important distinction between received, in contrast to perceived, social support. At the collective level, social embeddedness encompasses the structural component of social support, describing the size, activeness, and closeness of the network. But there is also an interaction term, an agentic construct that has received less attention—the capacity of an individual to accept or utilize social support when it is made available (e.g., Benight & Bandura, 2004; Dougall, Hyman, Hayward, McFeeley, & Baum, 2001). This capacity will depend both on individual factors (such as past experience, personality traits, coping style, etc.) and social factors (such the structure of social support network, access to information, availability of resources, etc.). Furthermore, individual, collective, and interactional factors may vary longitudinally throughout the acute and long-term postdisaster period. This is clearly grist for the mill and an area deserving attention in future research.

EVIDENCE-BASED INTERVENTIONS

Although there is strong evidence for the efficacy of cognitive-behavioral therapy and pharmacotherapy for chronic PTSD, few randomized clinical trials (RCTs) have been conducted testing interventions during the first days or weeks following a disaster. Indeed, RCTs on early intervention following any traumatic episode are very rare. As summarized by Gibson, Hamblen, Zvolensky, and Vujanovic (Chapter 13, this volume), two findings have emerged so far. First, cognitive-behavioral therapy administered for acute stress disorder 10–14 days after traumatic exposure have been very effective. (Participants in these studies, however, have generally been exposed to motor vehicle accidents, industrial accidents, or nonsexual assault rather than disasters.) Second, psychological debriefing has failed to prevent long-term psychological sequelae and may even be harmful. There have also been a few small RCTs with medication that need to be replicated with larger cohorts. There are also some interesting Web-based trials in progress, and a Psychological First Aid manual is under development, as of this writing, for field testing. In short, research on evidence-based treatments for acutely traumatized disaster survivors is in its infancy.

A practical design issue is the problem of random assignment during the acute aftermath of a disaster. Given a strong disinclination among many clinicians to withhold treatment from a symptomatic disaster survivor, even when such treatment has not been proven to be effective, there is a growing belief in some circles that matched sample comparisons are more feasible. Such an approach would provide Treatment A to all potential participants in one locale who met entrance criteria (e.g., for PTSD, depression, etc.) whereas all potential participants in another locale would receive Treatment B, or treatment-as-usual. Such a design would probably be more acceptable to an institutional review board (IRB) as well as to clinicians assigned to one locale or the other.

There is a great need to rigorously investigate a wide spectrum of individual and community-level interventions. Research interventions for individuals should consider efficacy, effectiveness, timing, treatment setting, dosage, target population, cultural factors, and developmental level. Research on societal and community-level interventions should systematically evaluate predisaster preparation as well as the postdisaster community/societal interventions themselves. (Friedman, Foa, & Charney, 2003).

DISSEMINATION OF EVIDENCED-BASED TREATMENT

Marshall, Ansel, Neria, and Suh (Chapter 14, this-volume) addressed two predictable problems following a disaster. First, there will be a sudden increase in the prevalence of symptomatic survivors, many of whom would benefit from treatment. Second, there will be an insufficient number of clinicians who practice evidence-based treatments for PTSD. The challenge is to rapidly increase the pool of clinicians trained in evidence-based treatments in order to meet the surging demand for services. Marshall and associates provided a thoughtful description of their attempt to meet this challenge following the attacks of September 11, 2001, by offering a training program in cognitive behavior therapy to New York-based therapists.

Inclusion of this modest report in this volume is instructive because it underscores a generic problem that does not apply merely to knowledge deficits concerning early intervention. The larger issue is dissemination of evidence-based best practices to clinicians in any medical discipline. There is abundant evidence (Addis, 2002; Guptill, 2005; Shojania & Grimshaw, 2005) that development of evidence-based treatment guidelines does not, in and of itself, alter clinician behavior. The next step is to disseminate this information in such a way that it will be adopted in clinical practice settings. This process, which originated in the business community and is now finding its way into clinical care, is called "knowledge management." A discussion of the applicability of knowledge management techniques to change PTSD treatment is beyond the scope of this chapter but can be found elsewhere (Ruzek, Friedman, & Murray, 2005). In short, knowledge management approaches have much in common with in-person epidemiological research in community, school, military, and other settings. It requires sensitivity to the clinical culture, overcoming mistrust, obtaining buy-in from the community, engaging gatekeepers, creating incentives, and fostering communication. The goals are different, of course. Rather than data acquisition, the goal is to promote a change in the clinical culture. Ongoing program evaluation is essential to monitor two different results: clinician behavior and patient outcomes.

Knowledge management initiatives can, and should, be tested scientifically. Randomized trials can be designed to compare practical settings that continue to provide treatment-as-usual with settings targeted to adopt evidence-based treatments through a knowledge management intervention.

The bottom line is that we must begin to address postdisaster clinician behavior with the same methodological rigor as has been proposed for research with survivors of major disasters.

PREPARATION AND COORDINATION

Because events change quickly after a disaster and data are perishable, research must be launched with minimal delay and with focused attention to the way the event unfolds over time (McFarlane & Norris, Chapter 1, this volume). Well-designed research protocols must be ready for implementation as soon as first responders have been dispatched to the disaster area. This goal can only be achieved if a process is set in place whereby research protocols are written in advance, have already received IRB approval, have received extramural support (conditional on the occurrence of a disaster), and have already obtained entr e to the community or endorsement from gatekeepers.

There are two crucial components to preparation and coordination, top-down and bottom-up. Top-down issues concern funding mechanisms and IRB review procedures. The American experience after the September 11th terrorist attacks showed that the scientific and IRB review processes delayed the implementation of research projects well beyond the acute postdisaster phase. There were also administrative problems that constrained rapid funding of new projects. This matter can only be addressed at the policy level (see below).

Bottom-up issues are equally important. Ideally, cooperative agreements for critical research with potential target communities would be negotiated before a disaster occurs (Benight et al., Chapter 4, this volume; Marshall et al., Chapter 14, this volume). Although this might be feasible in communities that are frequently subjected to hurricanes, earthquakes, monsoons, etc., it is more often the case that disasters strike suddenly in unexpected locales.

Whether negotiations for such cooperative agreements take place before or after a disaster, the key to their success is obtaining buy-in from gatekeepers who are empowered to guard access to any potential pool of research participants. Community gatekeepers not only are highly protective of disaster survivors and suspicious of outside investigators, but also they often fear that research is potentially harmful or frivolous. Their support may be difficult to obtain unless they feel that the proposed research will benefit the community. When gatekeepers are on board, however, they are key allies whose endorsement can often ensure the success of a project. Enlisting gatekeeper support and promoting community ownership of the project is a major preliminary step that must be carried out with sensitivity to the leadership hierarchy, jurisdictional boundaries, social structure, and cultural issues.

Coordination of first responder and scientific activities is both a top-down and bottom-up challenge. At the national level, such coordination will require cooperation, legislative mandates, and joint participation of different governmental departments and agencies (see below). If such coordination and cooperation can be achieved nationally, it can only succeed through implementation of joint periodic regional preparation and training that involves both first responders and the local academic community.

One of the best ways to prepare for postdisaster research is through establishment of an ongoing mental health surveillance system that provides normative (predisaster or baseline) data on a local, regional, or national level (Galea & Norris, Chapter 11, this volume). Likewise, preparation and coordination of ongoing mental health services databases could also serve this purpose (Rosen & Young, Chapter 12, this volume).

ETHICAL ISSUES

Many of the authors of this volume cautioned readers on the ethical dilemmas that arise in disaster research; for example, the use of incentives in disaster research must be approached with care. Bromet and Havenaar (Chapter 6, this volume), in discussing the implementation of epidemiological surveys, mentioned the provision of physical exams, financial remuneration, "meaningful gifts," or medical referral for individuals at risk as useful techniques for recruiting subjects, boosting response rates, or obtaining permission to conduct research from community gatekeepers. Similar suggestions were provided with regard to research with children in school settings (La Greca, Chapter 9, this volume; Steinberg, Brymer, Steinberg, & Pfefferbaum, Chapter 15, this volume), with military cohorts (Fullerton, McCarroll, & Ursano, Chapter 16, this volume), with residents from minority and marginalized communities (Jones, Hadder, Carvajal, Chapman, & Alexander, Chapter 17, this volume), and in foreign countries (Murphy, Perilla, & Jones, Chapter 18, this volume). In all cases, authors were sensitive to the importance of maintaining an appropriate balance that will provide inducements to promote successful implementation of research protocols without crossing a line that will compromise informed consent. It can be a tricky balance. For example, the amount of financial compensation offered to impoverished residents of a marginalized community or poor country must not be potentially coercive if the research project seeks to conform to ethical guidelines.

Another ethical concern is the "therapeutic misconception," which refers to misperceiving participation in a research protocol as receiving direct clinical care for postdisaster problems (Fleischman, Collogan, & Tuma, Chapter 5, this volume). Although treatment may be provided in studies testing the effectiveness of a specific intervention, most disaster research has no therapeutic purpose. This must be spelled out clearly during the informed consent process. However, the line may be a fuzzy one, as discussed previously with respect to incentives. For example, in the Kyiv children's study of the Chornobyl disaster, physical examination and blood tests were provided not just to the 600 children who were preselected for the study but to any family member or neighbors who requested it (Bromet & Havenaar, Chapter 6, this volume). It is a complicated issue on which investigators may disagree with respect to the appropriate balance between misleading potential participants regarding the therapeutic misconception and providing humanitarian assistance, as in the Chornobyl study, in order to obtain buy-in from gatekeepers and the community (see below).

PUBLIC AND RESEARCH POLICY ISSUES

Recent high-profile disasters, including the terrorist attacks on New York, Bali, Madrid, and London, exposed major gaps in our current knowledge about the impact of disasters and other large-scale catastrophes. Such gaps included "limited understanding of the natural longitudinal postdisaster course of psychological consequences . . . inadequate scientific understanding of the psychological and psychobiological mechanisms that mediate and moderate underlying acute and long-term reactions to traumatic events . . . and best (evidence-based) practices for early and later interventions" (Friedman, 2005, p. 20). As a result, national research priorities have shifted in favor of support for initiatives that would address these important deficits.

By chance, a previously planned consensus conference, "Mental Health and Mass Violence," was convened several weeks after the attacks of September 11, 2001. Participants included national and international experts in disaster mental health, and the proceedings were published by the National Institute of Mental Health (NIMH, 2002) and made available on the Internet (www.nimh.nih.gove/research/massviolence.pdf). Research and evaluation was one of the major areas addressed. Key recommendations pertinent to the present volume are as follows (NIMH, 2002):

1. Research and program evaluation are critically important components of a national mental health disaster response.
2. The scientific community has an obligation to examine the relative

effectiveness of each intervention that seeks to reduce adverse outcomes and foster positive adaptations following mass violence and disasters.

3. A national strategy should be developed to ensure that adequate resources are available for systematic data collection, evaluation, and research to be carried out before, during, and after mass violence and disasters.
4. When the optimal forms of intervention are unknown, there is an ethical duty to conduct scientifically valid research to improve prevention, assessment, intervention, and treatment.
5. Systematic evaluation activities should be planned and carried out in conjunction with identified bodies that are responsible for organizing and delivering early intervention.
6. A standard taxonomy (categorization) and terminology need to be developed for program evaluation and research protocols.
7. A strategy should be developed for informing the broader research community, including IRBs, of the necessity of conducting research on sensitive topics.
8. Early intervention policies should be based on empirically defensible and evidence-based practices. An ethical duty exists to discourage the use of ineffective or unsafe techniques.

Efforts to implement many of these recommendations have begun, but there is a long way to go. Cooperation and coordination between a number of federal agencies (e.g., NIMH, the Substance Abuse and Mental Health Services Administration, the Centers for Disease Control and Prevention, the Department of Defense, and the Department of Veterans Affairs) is at an all-time high. Such joint efforts have accelerated efforts to improve assessment strategies to develop a national mental health surveillance system, to develop evidence-based early interventions, to place greater emphasis on research concerning children, and to disseminate evidence-based practices to first responders and clinicians providing acute or longer-term follow-up care. As we see it, the major challenges for the future are:

1. Launching longitudinal studies that begin measurement during the acute postimpact phase and provide prospective sequential assessment through the long-term follow-up phase.
2. Improving current methods for assessing disaster exposure.
3. Focusing on psychological and biological mechanisms of change hypothesized to mediate or moderate postdisaster outcomes.
4. Utilizing assessment strategies that monitor both individual and collective postdisaster outcomes as well as how they influence one another.

5. Testing early psychosocial and pharmacological interventions.
6. Developing and implementing methods to disseminate evidence-based treatments as widely as possible.

In summary, we suggest that improvements in current approaches are needed to move the field toward a more theoretical and longitudinal perspective. Looking ahead, we expect the field to gain a better understanding of the complex mechanisms underlying acute and long-term psychological reactions to disasters. Such progress is achievable and essential if we hope to provide timely and effective interventions for individuals exposed to such catastrophic events.

REFERENCES

Addis, M. E. (2002). Methods for disseminating research products and increasing evidence-based practice: Promises, obstacles, and future directions. *Clinical Psychology: Science and Practice, 9,* 367–378.

Balaban, V. F., Steinberg, A. M., Brymer, M. J., Layne, C. M, Jones, R. T., & Fairbank, J. A. (2005). Screening and assessment for children's psychological needs following war and terrorism. In M. J. Friedman & Mikus Kos, A. (Eds.). *Promoting the psychosocial well-being of children following war and terrorism* (pp. 121–161). Amsterdam: IOS Press.

Benight, C., & Bandura, A. (2004). Social cognitive theory of posttraumatic recovery: The role of perceived self-efficacy. *Behavior Research and Therapy, 42,* 1129–1148.

Bliese, P. D., & Halverson, R. R. (1996). Individual and nomothetic models of job stress: An examination of work hours, cohesion, and well-being. *Journal of Applied Social Psychology, 26,* 1171–1189.

Dougall, A. Hyman, K., Hayward, M., McFeeley, S., & Baum, A. (2001). Optimism and traumatic stress: The importance of social support and coping. *Journal of Applied Social Psychology, 31,* 223–245.

Friedman, M. J. (2005). Every crisis is an opportunity. *CNS Spectrums, 10,* 20–22.

Friedman, M. J., Foa, E. B., & Charney, D. S. (2003). Toward evidence-based early interventions for acutely traumatized adults and children. *Biological Psychiatry, 53,* 765–768.

Friedman, M. J., & Mikus-Kos, A. (Eds.) (2005). *Promoting the psychosocial well-being of children following war and terrorism.* Amsterdam: IOS Press.

Galea, S., Ahern, J., Resnick, H. S., Kilpatrick, D. G., Bucuvalas, M. J., Gold, J., & Vlahov, D. (2002). Psychological sequelae of the September 11 terrorist attacks in New York City. *New England Journal of Medicine, 346,* 982–987.

Guptill, J. (2005). Knowledge management in health care. *Journal of Health Care Finance, 31,* 10.

Hong, T. B., Zarit, S. H., & Malmberg, B. (2004). The role of health congruence in functional status and depression. *Journals of Gerontology: Series B: Psychological Science & Social Sciences, 59B,* P151–P157.

National Institute of Mental Health. (2002). *Mental health and mass violence: Evidence-based early psychological intervention for victims/survivors of mass violence: A workshop to reach consensus on best practices* (NIH Pub. No. 02-5138). Washington, DC: U.S. Government Printing Office.

Norris, F. H., Friedman, M. J., Watson, P. J., Byrne, C., Diaz, E., & Kaniasty, K. (2002). 60,000 disaster victims speak, Part 1: An empirical review of the empirical literature, 1981–2001. *Psychiatry, 65,* 207–239.

Norris, F. H. Friedman, M. J., & Watson, P. J. (2002). 60,000 disaster victims speak, Part II: Summary and implications of the disaster mental health research. *Psychiatry, 65,* 240–260.

Norris, F. H., Murphy, A. D., Baker, C. K., & Perilla, J. L. (2003). Severity, timing, and duration of reactions to trauma in the population: An example from Mexico. *Biological Psychiatry, 53,* 769–778.

North, C. S., Pfefferbaum, B., Tivis, L., Kawasaki, A., Reddy, C., & Spitznagel, E. L. (2004). The course of posttraumatic stress disorder in a follow-up study of survivors of the Oklahoma City bombing. *Annals of Clinical Psychiatry, 16,* 209–215.

North, C. S., & Westerhaus, E. T. (2003). Applications from previous disaster research to guide mental health interventions after the September 11 attacks. In R. J. Ursano, C. S. Fullerton, & A. E. Norwood (Eds.), *Terrorism and disaster: Individual and community mental health interventions* (pp. 93–106). Cambridge: Cambridge University Press.

Oliver, L. W., Harman, J. Hoover, E., Hayes, S. M., & Pandhi, N. A. (1999). A quantitative integration of the military cohesion literature. *Military Psychology, 1,* 57–83.

Ruzek, J. I., Friedman, M. J., & Murray, S. (2005). Towards a PTSD Knowledge Management System in Veterans Health Care. *Psychiatric Annals, 35,* 911–920.

Shojania, K. G., & Grimshaw, J. M. (2005). Evidence-based quality improvement: The state of the science. *Health Affairs, 24,* 138–150.

Smith, N., Young, A., & Lee, C. (2004). Optimism, health-related hardiness and well-being among older Australian women. *Journal of Health Psychology, 9,* 741–752.

Stewart, A. L., Hays, R. D., & Ware, J. E. (1992). Health perceptions, energy/fatigue, and health distress measures. In A. L. Stewart & J. E. Ware (Eds.), *Measuring functioning and well-being: The medical outcomes study approach.* Durham, NC: Duke University Press.

Terr, L. C. (1991). Childhood traumas: An outline and overview. *American Journal of Psychiatry, 148,* 10–20.

APPENDIX 1

Disasters Mentioned in the Text

SANDRO GALEA

Anthrax attacks. Beginning on September 18, 2001, a week after the September 11, 2001, terrorist attacks, letters containing anthrax bacteria were mailed to several news media offices in Florida and New York City and to two U.S. Senators at their Washington, DC, Senate offices. Five people died in the anthrax attacks, and, as of this writing, the crimes remain unsolved.

Ash Wednesday bushfires. The Ash Wednesday bushfires swept through South Australia in February 1983. Caused by the 1982 El Niño drought and an ongoing fire in eastern Victoria that went uncontrolled for almost a month, the bushfires affected much of Victoria and South Australia. Ninety-two people died in the fires, including 17 firefighters on account of the rapidly changing direction of the fires. More than 2,000 families lost their homes, and nearly 400,000 square kilometers of territory were destroyed.

Bali bombing. On October 12, 2002, in the town of Kuta on the Indonesian island of Bali, 202 people were killed and 209 were injured in a coordinated terrorist attack. A suicide bomb in a crowded tourist restaurant was followed by a powerful car bomb, killing many as they ran out of the restaurant. This was the deadliest terrorist attack on Indonesia. The majority of the dead were Australian or British tourists.

Beverly Hills Supper Club fire. On May 28, 1977, faulty wiring caused a fire at the popular Beverly Hills Supper Club in Southgate, Kentucky. The fire spread quickly through the overcrowded club, killing 165 people.

Bhopal gas leak. On December 3, 1984, methyl isocyanate gas leaked from a tank at the Union Carbide plant in Bhopal, India. Approximately 3,800 people died as a direct result of the gas exposure. Although the full extent of the injuries and the economic consequences related to the gas leak have not been definitively determined, the government of Madhya Pradesh Province has thus far provided economic compensation to close to 80,000 families in the area through a special relief fund.

Buffalo Creek dam collapse. On February 26, 1972, a dam constructed of coal waste collapsed near the town of Buffalo Creek, West Virginia. The poorly constructed dam was holding back a lake of water used for cleaning coal. Several small towns were washed away. Over the course of a few hours, 125 people died in the ensuing flood, approximately 1,000 persons were injured, and 4,000 were left homeless.

Chornobyl nuclear accident. The Chornobyl accident took place on April 26, 1986, at the Chornobyl power plant in the Ukraine (then part of the Soviet Union). The accident followed a test of the reactor's turbine generator gone awry. The accident produced a plume of radioactive debris that drifted over parts of the western Soviet Union, eastern Europe, Scandinavia, the United Kingdom, and the eastern United States. Large areas of the Ukraine, Belarus, and Russia were badly contaminated, resulting in the evacuation and resettlement of approximately 200,000 people. Accurate tallies of the number of deaths caused by the events at Chornobyl are not availble, with estimates ranging from hundreds to hundreds of thousands. The long-term effects of the accident are not yet completely understood.

Chi Chi earthquake. An earthquake measuring 7.6 on the Richter scale struck central Taiwan (Chi Chi township in Nantou County) on September 20, 1999, and was followed by a series of more than 9,000 aftershocks. More than 2,400 people died in the earthquakes, and approximately 9,000 people were injured.

El Al Boeing 747 crash. On October 4, 1992, an El Al 747 freighter crashed soon after takeoff from Schiphol Airport, Amsterdam. The plane plowed into a low-rise apartment building complex, killing all 4 people on board and approximately 50 people on the ground. Mechanical failure is believed to have caused the crash. It is possible that many more people died on the ground, since the apartment complex housed a large number of undocumented immigrants.

Exxon Valdez *oil spill.* On March 24, 1989, at about 12:04 A.M., the oil tanker *Exxon Valdez,* carrying a full load of oil, hit the Bligh Reef in Prince William

Sound, Alaska. Between 11 million and 35 million U.S. gallons of crude oil were spilled in the accident, affecting 1,900 kilometers of coastline. This was the most environmentally devastating domestic oil spill in the United States. The remote location of the accident made government and industry response efforts difficult and delayed efforts to remediate the spill.

Florida hurricanes, 2004. Hurricanes Charley, Frances, Ivan, and Jeanne hit the Florida coast in rapid succession between August 13 and September 25, 2004. Approximately 70 people died as a direct result of the hurricanes in Florida alone, and the property damage was estimated at more than $40 billion.

Hansin-Awaji earthquake. On January 17, 1995, an earthquake measuring 7.3 on the Richter scale hit the northern part of Awaji Island, near Kobe, Japan. More than 4,500 people died, and about 15,000 persons were injured in the earthquake.

Hurricane Andrew. On August 24, 1992, Hurricane Andrew hit south Florida, particularly the towns of Homestead, Florida City, and parts of Miami. The storm then continued northwest across the Gulf of Mexico and struck the Louisiana coastline. Forty people are believed to have died as a result of the storm, 250,000 people were left homeless, about 100,000 residents of south Dade County permanently left the area in the storm's wake, and in all it is estimated that the storm caused $30 billion in property damage.

Hurricane Hugo. Hurricane Hugo hit the Carolinas and Georgia as a category 4 hurricane on September 21, 1989. There were about 3,000 tornadoes embedded within the hurricane, accounting for extensive damage in some areas well outside the eye of the hurricane. Hurricane Hugo caused nearly $10 billion in damage in the United States and another $3 billion in damage in the Caribbean. Approximately 50 people were killed by hurricane Hugo.

Hurricane Katrina. At one point a rare Category 5 hurricane, Hurricane Katrina was a strong Category 3 hurricane when it struck the gulf coast of the United States on August 29, 2005. Katrina caused levees in New Orleans to fail, flooding much of the city. Damage to southern Mississippi was also catastrophic. Hurricane Katrina was the most costly and destructive natural disaster in the history of the United States and one of the most deadly. More than 1,600 people died, and more than 1,000,000 people were displaced.

Hurricane Mitch. One of the most powerful tropical cyclones ever observed, hurricane Mitch hit Central America between October 22 and November 5, 1998, killing more than 18,000 people. This was the deadliest hurricane in the region in more than 200 years and the second deadliest ever recorded. Most deaths were due to flooding. Thousands of homes were also damaged or destroyed during the hurricane.

Johnstown flood. The Great Flood of 1889, as it became known locally, occurred on May 31, 1889, in Pennsylvania. It was the result of several days of extremely heavy rainfall, greatly exacerbated by the failure of the South Fork Dam, 14 miles upstream from the town of Johnstown. More than 2,200 people were killed by the flood, and there was $17 million in damage. It was the first major U.S. disaster relief effort handled by the new American Red Cross.

Jupiter cruise ship sinking. On October 21, 1988, the *Jupiter* cruise ship, carrying some 500 children at the beginning of an 8-day cruise, was rammed by a tanker outside the Greek harbor of Piraeus. One child and three adults died in the crash.

Lockerbie Pan Am crash. On December 21, 1988, 12–16 ounces of plastic explosives were detonated in the cargo hold of Pan Am flight 103, resulting in the destruction of the plane over Lockerbie, Scotland. A total of 270 people from 21 countries died in the crash, including 11 people on the ground.

Loma Prieta earthquake. On October 17, 1989, an earthquake measuring 7.1 on the Richter scale struck the San Francisco Bay area, with the epicenter near Loma Prieta Peak in the Santa Cruz Mountains, about 10 miles northeast of Santa Cruz, California. The earthquake caused damage as far as 70 miles away. There were at least 66 deaths and approximately 3,800 injuries as a result of the earthquake. Most fatalities happened when a bridge portion of the Nimitz Freeway collapsed, crashing cars into the lower deck of the bridge. It is estimated that the earthquake caused $6 billion in property damage, making this the most costly natural disaster in U.S. history at the time.

Marmara, Turkey, earthquake. On August 17, 1999, a 7.8 Richter scale earthquake hit the Sea of Marmara, off the coast of Turkey near the town of Gölcük. Tsunamis secondary to the earthquakes hit the coast of Turkey, resulting in extensive flooding. Several aftershocks followed during subsequent days. It is estimated that 17,000 people died in the earthquakes, although the actual number of dead is likely higher.

Mexico City earthquakes. On September 19, 1985, Mexico City was struck by an earthquake that measured 8.1 on the Richter scale. Although official government estimates are that 5,000 people died, unofficial estimates range as high as 20,000. Up to 90,000 people were rendered homeless in the earthquake, and approximately $4 billion in damages was reported. An additional earthquake of 7.5 magnitude was recorded 36 hours after the initial earthquake.

Mississippi River flood. From May through September 1993, major and/or record flooding occurred across North Dakota, South Dakota, Nebraska, Kansas, Minnesota, Iowa, Missouri, Wisconsin, and Illinois. Fifty people died and damages approached $15 billion. Hundreds of levees failed along the Mississippi and Missouri rivers, and thousands of people were evacuated, some for months. At least 10,000 homes were totally destroyed, and hundreds of towns were affected. At least 75 towns were submerged at some point during the flooding.

Northridge earthquake. On January 17, 1994, a 6.9 Richter scale earthquake hit Northridge, about 30 kilometers northwest of Los Angeles. The earthquake damaged parking structures and freeway overpasses and triggered landslides. Fifty-seven people died in the Northridge earthquake, and about 9,000 people were injured.

Oklahoma City bombing. On April 19, 1995, a Ryder truck containing about 5,000 pounds of explosive material exploded in front of the Murrah Federal Building in Oklahoma City. A total of 168 people died in the bombing, more than 800 people were injured, and more than 300 buildings were destroyed or seriously damaged. By some estimates, more than one-third of the nearly half-million residents of Oklahoma City knew someone who was killed or injured in the bombing.

Piper Alpha explosion. The Piper Alpha, a North Sea oil production platform operated by Occidental Petroleum and Texaco, was destroyed by a natural gas explosion and the resulting fire on July 6, 1988. The explosion killed 167 men; only 67 crewmen survived the explosion.

San Diego High School shootings. On March 5, 2001, a 15-year-old student killed two classmates and wounded 13 others at a high school in Santee, California, about 10 kilometers away from San Diego. The perpetrator was arrested and later received a sentence of 50 years to life.

September 11, 2001, terrorist attacks. Two hijacked planes crashed into the twin towers of the World Trade Center in New York City in a coordinated terrorist attack. Approximately 2,800 people died in the World Trade Center towers, and transportation, commerce, and communication for large parts of the New York metropolitan area were disrupted for weeks thereafter. Those losing their lives included 343 firefighters and 87 police officers. Two other planes were also hijacked that day. One of them crashed into the Pentagon, in Washington, DC, killing 126 people. On the other plane, passengers resisted the hijackers and forced a crash landing in a Pennsylvania field, killing all on board.

Southeast Asian tsunami. An earthquake measuring 8.7 on the Richter scale, just off the coast of Sumatra, Indonesia, triggered a number of tsunamis that flooded parts of southeast Asia and eastern Africa, starting on December 26, 2004. As many as 280,000 people worldwide are believed to have died in the tsunamis, with most of the dead in Indonesia.

Spitak, Armenia, earthquake. An earthquake measuring 6.8 on the Richter scale took place on December 7, 1988, in the Spitak region of Armenia. Poor local housing infrastructure contributed to the deaths of an estimated 25,000 people. The entire city of Spitak was destroyed, and the earthquake also caused damage to many surrounding villages.

Three Mile Island nuclear accident. On March 28, 1979, equipment malfunction, design-related problems, and worker errors led to a partial meltdown of the Three Mile Island-2 reactor core. Although there was very little off-site release of radioactivity and there were no deaths or injuries to plant members or persons in the nearby community, the Three Mile Island nuclear accident brought about sweeping national changes in emergency response planning, reactor operator training, human factors engineering, radiation protection, and many other areas of nuclear power plant operations.

Times Beach contamination. Soil contamination from a pesticide plant owned by Syntex Agribusiness, Inc., resulted in the disincorporation and evacuation of the town of Times Beach, Missouri, in 1985. The town's entire population of 2,000 residents was evacuated. Subsequently, about 265,000 tons of soil and debris were burned, and the townsite was transformed into a park by the end of the 1990s.

Tungurahua volcano eruption, Ecuador. Mount Tungurahua is an active volcano dominating the Chimborazo and Tungurahua provinces in Ecuador. The volcano has had several periods of intense activity, with the most recent period between 1916 and 1925. On October 18, 1999, increasingly vigorous volcanic activity was recorded, including high levels of gas emissions, a volcano-tectonic earthquake below the earth, and continuous ash clouds rising above the summit. On October 19, 1999, ash clouds rose to 25,000 feet. As a result, 22,000 people were evacuated from the area surrounding the Tungurahua volcano. No deaths were reported as a direct result of this eruption.

Yungay, Peru, earthquake. On May 31, 1970, a 7.6 Richter scale earthquake hit Mount Huascaran in Peru. The earthquake broke loose a large amount of rock and ice from the west side of the Huascaran massif that rolled downhill at a speed of over 200 kilometers per hour onto the villages of Yungay and Ranrahirca in the mountain valley. Approximately 20,000 people were killed instantly in the earthquake, mostly in the village of Yungay. As many as 50,000 more people were killed in other parts of Peru as a result. This was the worst recorded natural disaster to hit South America.

APPENDIX 2

Searching the Traumatic Stress Literature

Fred Lerner

Anyone undertaking disaster mental health research needs to learn how to use the traumatic stress literature effectively. Selecting the wrong assessment instrument may diminish the value of the information obtained from research participants. Lack of familiarity with proper statistical methodology may render useless the conclusions drawn from field research. Similarly, a poorly designed literature search may provide a misleading picture of what is already known and lead to unproductive research activity. In this chapter, I discuss bibliographic resources available to disaster researchers and outline some of the ways that these resources can be used to identify those publications most useful to a particular inquiry.

The literature on traumatic stress is interdisciplinary in nature. Valuable papers are published not only in the psychiatry and psychology journals but also in those dealing with social work, sociology, criminology, law, public health, and general medicine. Typically, the literature for these different disciplines tends to be indexed in separate databases. The physician or psychologist whose concerns lie within the mainstream of his or her profession has little difficulty in searching the literature. The National Library of Medicine's MEDLINE database is readily accessible in a variety of formats; it may be searched free of charge; and it has an elaborate vocabulary of indexing terms that is updated annually. The American Psychological Association's PsycINFO database is highly regarded by librarians and psychologists for the extent of its indexing vocabulary and the accuracy of its staff-written abstracts.

There are well-regarded bibliographical databases covering other fields related to traumatic stress studies. *Social Work Abstracts, Sociological Abstracts*, and *Social Services Abstracts* index the social work literature. The literature of law is covered by the *Index to Legal Periodicals* and by the *Current Law Index* (also known as *LegalTrac* or *Legal Resource Index*). Public policy issues are indexed in the *PAIS International* database, produced by the Public Affairs Information Service.

Each of these databases has its own list of subject terms, which highly trained indexers use to characterize the content of each paper. These terms, along with authors' names, journal titles, and words occurring in the title or abstract of a paper, can be used to isolate references to publications likely to be relevant to a particular inquiry.

The terminology employed by indexers always lags behind the words that active scientists use in describing their research. Searching for recent papers that cited some particular previous paper offers a way of locating articles in a field too new or too specialized to be covered adequately by existing indexing vocabularies. Citation indexing is based on the assumption that the citation of one publication by a subsequent one implies an intellectual relationship between the content of the two papers. The Institute for Scientific Information's *Web of Science* includes the *Science Citation Index* and *Social Science Citation Index*, which allow one to specify a particular paper and identify those later publications in which it was cited. The ability to select those papers most frequently cited may help in determining where to begin one's review of an extensive literature.

Information scientists study the citation behavior of researchers to identify evolving trends and publishing patterns in scientific communication. Their experiments in creating graphical displays of these trends and patterns will lead to new ways of searching and using the traumatic stress literature and may suggest previously undiscovered research strategies.

CHOOSING A DATABASE

Given this bibliographical abundance, how does one decide where to begin a search of the literature? The most important factor is the coverage offered by the bibliographical service. A database that covers only material published after 1969 will be of limited use to someone interested in a historical approach to a field. One that is limited to English-language materials may serve the needs of a monolingual practitioner, but will not provide access to all the work of European, Asian, and Latin American writers.

Most bibliographical databases index only the journals included on a predetermined list. It often takes several years for a new journal to be selected: the *Journal of Traumatic Stress*, which published its first issue in January 1988, was not added to the list of serials indexed in MEDLINE until February 1994—and MEDLINE's coverage does not include pre-1994 issues.

The most important restriction on database coverage is the subject matter, which in many databases is defined by the list of sources from which documents are taken to be indexed. So, in deciding upon a database to search, the first question to ask is, "Does this database index the publications in which the information I am seeking is likely to be found?" Almost every database that confines its coverage to a predetermined list of publications issues a list of the titles it covers. In addition, many journals list in each issue the indexes and databases that cover their contents.

Not all databases restrict their coverage to a predetermined source list. Knowing how the producers of a bibliography define their subject coverage and determine which publications meet their criteria is an essential part of the decision whether to use it. In a printed bibliography, careful attention should be paid to any definitions of scope or approach contained or implied in the title or subtitle, and to any prefatory or introductory material. With a computerized database it is essential to read both on-screen and printed documentation. In many cases, several levels of documentation are offered, ranging from a one- or two-page list of basic search commands to a multivolume series of search manuals, vocabulary lists, and sample searches. Using a bibliography without consulting its documentation is like using a cookbook without reading the recipes carefully—in either case the results are likely to be unpalatable.

Database searching is a complex process, and the continual emergence of new information products, searching features, and communications systems means that keeping one's searching skills up to date is a full-time job. If a quick-and-dirty search yielding a few relevant papers is all that is needed, there is no reason why someone comfortable with database searching shouldn't perform his or her own search. But if an exhaustive or authoritative search of the literature is needed—if one is planning a course of treatment for a patient or writing a doctoral dissertation—it is always best, no matter what the subject matter under investigation or which database has been selected, to work with a reference librarian or other expert searcher to plan and execute a thorough search of the literature.

Anyone studying the mental health consequences of disasters should become familiar with the PILOTS Database, which offers many features to facilitate research and clinical work in all aspects of traumatic stress studies. The goal of the PILOTS Database is to index the world's literature on posttraumatic stress disorder (PTSD) and other forms of traumatic stress. The PILOTS Database is produced by the National Center for PTSD. No account or password is necessary, and there is no charge for using the database. Direct access to the database, and detailed instructions on using it, are available at the National Center's website at www.ncptsd.va.gov. PILOTS includes any published material dealing with posttraumatic stress disorder, any other mental disorders caused by or associated with direct or indirect exposure to an event perceived as traumatic, and any mental health-related consequences of such exposure. This focus includes not only those papers that explicitly discuss PTSD but also most of the literature on dissociative identity disorder and much of that on borderline personality disorder, both of which are often associated etiologically with childhood trauma. It also includes selected literature on anxiety disorders, eating disorders, mood disorders, sleep disorders, somatization disorders—all of which may occur as a result of, or in association with, exposure to a traumatic experience.

Seven percent of the papers indexed in the PILOTS Database deal directly with the aftermath of disasters. Many of the others contain findings that are applicable to disaster mental health. The design of the PILOTS Database facilitates searching for literature relevant to disasters in general, to particular types of disasters, or to specific incidents.

DEVELOPING A SEARCH STRATEGY

A database search is a three-step process: (1) putting together a search strategy, (2) executing the search, and (3) examining the results and modifying the search accordingly. Although this discussion concentrates on methods of searching the PILOTS Database, much of it is equally applicable to other bibliographical databases.

A database search is an exercise in pattern matching. The computer is given a pattern of letters, words, or phrases to seek, and it attempts to match that pattern with those it finds in the database. The computer can be told where in the database to look for a pattern and it can be instructed to search for a combination of patterns. The success of a search depends on the clarity of the pattern, the accuracy with which it is typed into the computer, and the skill and completeness of the database producer. Two out of the three are up to the searcher.

The PILOTS Database may be searched for the writings of a particular author, publications from a designated journal, papers in which a specific assessment instrument is used, material in a particular language, studies published in a designated year or period of time, and articles and chapters on a particular subject. There are two basic approaches to searching the PILOTS Database by subject: controlled vocabulary and natural language. In controlled vocabulary searching, the computer is instructed to match terms (descriptors) from a prescribed list (called a thesaurus) against terms assigned by indexers to the records contained in the database. In natural language searching, it is told to match words or phrases that might occur in the bibliographical records, regardless of whether they appear on a prescribed list of terms. Using either method, the occurrence of a match should indicate that the paper in which it is found discusses the subject indicated by the word, phrase, or term entered. Each method offers advantages and disadvantages. Many users will find that a combination of both types of searching will produce the best results.

Controlled vocabulary searching takes advantage of the work done by the database producer to standardize the terminology used by the thousands of authors and editors who produce the traumatic stress literature. This standardization is especially important in an interdisciplinary field, as there is no assurance that the terms used by psychiatrists will necessarily match those used by criminologists, or art therapists, or social workers. Even within a discipline, changes in terminology occur over time, or across geographic or ideological boundaries.

Natural language searching (sometimes called "free text" searching) allows the searcher to use the terms that he or she is most comfortable with; it does not require using the PILOTS Thesaurus. And it provides a way to locate material on subjects that are too new to be included in the Thesaurus, or that the Thesaurus does not cover well enough for a particular need. However, it is neither as precise nor as complete a way of searching as using a controlled vocabulary. Natural language searching offers too many opportunities to retrieve irrelevant material. For example, searching for the word "shifts" to discover papers on the effects of work schedules in exacerbating PTSD uncovered nothing on that subject—but it did turn up several articles discussing paradigm shifts in the sciences underlying traumatic stress studies. That same search would not find an article whose author disdained the word "shifts" in favor of "irregular work hours."

If one simply wants to find a few publications relevant to one's area of interest, natural language searching is an easy way to go about it. But if one needs to make a thorough study of the literature, and to be sure that important papers are not overlooked, one should not rely upon natural language searching alone.

In many databases (including the PILOTS Database) the thesaurus is integrated into the search software. This allows the searcher to select descriptors from an on-screen list instead of typing them into a search box, thus minimizing search failures caused by typing errors. The ability to "explode" a search—that is, to specify that a descriptor include all its narrower terms—can ensure that important papers are not missed because their subject matter embraces a narrower concept than that chosen by the searcher. For example, a PILOTS Database search exploding the descriptor "Disasters" will retrieve almost four times as many papers as an ordinary search using that descriptor, because it will also retrieve those papers indexed under "Earthquakes," "Floods," "Hurricanes," and other particular types of disasters. (But that search will not retrieve several hundred papers on "Terrorism," because that descriptor falls within "Crime" rather than "Disasters" in the PILOTS Thesaurus. In the PILOTS Database, as in any bibliographic database, it is essential to use the thesaurus and other documentation in preparing a search strategy.)

MODIFYING THE SEARCH STRATEGY

Database searching works best as an iterative process. It is unrealistic to expect to get definitive results on the first try; one should plan on doing an exploratory search and then modifying the search strategy according to the results obtained.

If a search produces an impossibly large number of citations, one should examine at least a few of them to see whether the topic was defined too broadly or if too broad a search strategy was employed. If almost all of them are indeed relevant, perhaps the objective should be redefined by choosing a narrower topic: for example, natural disasters rather than disasters in general. When many of the citations retrieved are irrelevant, it is necessary to refine the search strategy. If the same descriptor appears in all of the irrelevant citations, perhaps a search without using that descriptor (if it does not remove valuable citations as well as irrelevant ones) might bring the search results down to a more manageable size. Other methods to refine a search include restricting it by language, date, or format.

If a search has retrieved fewer citations than expected, perhaps there really are very few papers in the area (or at least very few that have found their way into the database). Or perhaps the search strategy was too narrow. Finding a citation that is directly relevant and seeing what descriptors were applied to it might suggest terms to add to the search strategy. It is also possible that a simple typing error is to blame. (Not all search systems are sophisticated enough to know that the searcher meant to type "alcohol" rather than "alvohol"!)

And what if the search returned no relevant citations? Is there a paper known to be relevant? A search for that paper by author and title can retrieve its citation, which will reveal how it was indexed in the PILOTS Database. That might suggest one or more descriptors to use in searching.

One should not be discouraged if the first search strategy does not work perfectly. Experts at database searching often have to modify their search techniques, especially when working with a database that is new to them.

OBTAINING COPIES OF MATERIALS FOUND IN A DATABASE SEARCH

Many online bibliographic databases provide links from their citations to the full text of the papers they index. What happens when the link is followed depends upon the searcher's relationship to the publisher. If the publisher's website recognizes the Internet address of a computer as one affiliated with a subscriber, it will give direct access to the full text (often giving a choice of formats in which to see or print the document). If it does not, an opportunity will usually be given to use a credit card to purchase access to the document. In some cases the publisher may offer free access to the document one is seeking.

If one cannot get online access to a particular publication, there are several other ways to get a copy. The first place to begin is a local library. Many public and academic libraries belong to networks that make the resources of large libraries available to the clients of smaller ones. In some cases materials can be provided free of charge; otherwise, a small fee may be charged for each article requested. (If a request does not come under the "fair use" provision of the copyright laws, there may also be a royalty fee payable to the publisher that the library will have to collect.) Librarians will know the fastest and cheapest ways to get the publications that users need.

There are several organizations and companies that specialize in providing rapid copies of publications. Information brokers offer a complete range of services, from searching databases to providing copies. Document delivery services offer copies of materials from their own resources and often from other library collections. They are operated by private companies, nonprofit organizations, and libraries. They usually offer a wide range of ordering and payment arrangements, accommodating users whose needs range from the single article to thousands of papers each year. Many are able to accept orders by electronic mail, and deliver copies by email, fax, or courier.

CONCLUSION

Any interdisciplinary literature, especially one in which exciting discoveries are continually being reported and controversial opinions frequently expressed, presents both a challenge and an opportunity to those working in the fields it covers. The challenge lies in the fact that the already difficult task of keeping up with the field one was trained in must be repeated in several other, less familiar, areas. The opportunity lies in the ability to apply the work of colleagues with an entirely different outlook to problems that often resist the solutions suggested by one's own background.

The ability to identify, evaluate, and benefit from the publications of those working in disciplines cognate to one's own is one of the most powerful tools with which a researcher or clinician can equip him- or herself. A basic understanding of the bibliographic infrastructure of medicine and the social sciences, and a knowledge of the many ways in which bibliographic databases can be searched, are necessary to use the literature effectively. The PILOTS Database offers an approach to the traumatic stress literature that has been designed particularly to meet the needs of those working in this fast-growing interdisciplinary field.

Index

Acute threats, 8–9
Age, and mental health effects of
   disasters, 32
   See also Children and disaster
   studies
Agentic theoretical framework, 295
AHRQ (Agency for Healthcare
   Research and Quality) Levels of
   Evidence for Clinical Research,
   211*t*
AIDS crisis, 9
Anthrax attacks, 181, 305
Ash Wednesday bushfires, 21, 305
Assessments, 95
   RAP (rapid assessment procedures),
   168–169
   strategies for children/adolescents in
   school settings, 147
   content, 147–148
   selection of participants, 148–149
   timing, 147
   See also Case studies; Focus group
   approach; In-person
   assessments; Interviews;
   Telephone-based research
   methods

B

Bali bombing (2002), 11, 12, 305
Behavioral genetics of stress-related
   disorders, 64–65
Behavioral Risk Factor Surveillance
   Survey (BRFSS), 120
Belmont Report, 82–83, 86
Beverly Hills Supper Club fire, 12, 306
Bhopal (India) disaster, 10, 306
Bioterrorism, classification difficulties, 11
Buffalo Creek dam collapse, 21, 306
"Buffer hypothesis," 68

C

Case studies, 165–166
Case–control design (epidemiological
      approach design option), 98–99
   case–control designs vs. cohort
      studies, 99–101
Centrifugal disasters, 12–13
Centripetal disasters, 12
Chornobyl nuclear disaster, 13, 306
   difficulties for unbiased study, 106–107
   epidemiological research design
      review, 96–98

Chi Chi earthquake (Taiwan), 21, 23, 304
Children and disaster studies, 141–142, 243–244
　conducting research (practical and logistical issues)
　　research in schools, 247–248
　　researcher communication, 246–247
　future directions, 250–251
　interventions for children and adolescents with PTSD, 218–219
　methodological issues
　　child abuse reporting, 248
　　developing/selecting instruments, 245–246
　　evaluation of interventions, 249
　　informed consent, 248
　　researcher/staff support, 249–250
　　study design, 244–245
　psychosocial interventions (research on), 214–215
　school-based approach, 142–145, 154–155, 247–248
　　challenges, 143–145
　　disaster types and suitability/unsuitability for study, 143
　study design issues
　　assessment strategies, 147–149
　　sampling strategies, 145–147
　study implementation issues
　　participant recruitment/retention, 149–152
　　research assistants (training considerations), 153–154
Chronic threats, 8
Cognitive-behavioral therapy (CBT), 219–220, 229–230
　intervention reviews, 210–211
　　early intervention, 212–214
　　later-stage intervention, 215–217
Cognitive perspective in stress research, 65–67
　current research trends, trauma recovery using social cognitive theory, 65–66

Collectively experienced traumas
　and collective efficacy, 66
　ecological assessment approaches, 31
　threats, 8–9
The Common Rule, 79
Computer-assisted telephone interviewing (CATI), 118–119, 122
Consent. See Voluntary informed consent
Conservation of resources (COR) theory, 27, 68–69
Coping (psychological), and mental health effects of disasters, 33–34
Cross-cultural traditions in stress research, 69–70
Cultural competence, 269
　See also Research with diverse/minority/marginalized communities
Current Population Survey (CPS), 120

D

Decisional capacity, 81–82
Depression and anxiety, as psychological response to disasters, 26
Descriptions in disaster research
　effects/estimates of effects of disasters, 48–49
　　qualitative and quantitative methods, mixed-method design, 170–171
　explanation, 50
　phenomena, 46
　populations, 46, 49
　qualitative and quantitative methods, 46, 158
　services and consumers, 48
　"thick description," 159
　See also Qualitative approaches/disaster effects studies
Diminishing threats. See Escalating threats

Disaster scaling, 14
  "disaster severity" concept
    (challenges of), 103–104
Disasters, 15, 17
  areas of the world at risk (based on
    statistical documentation), 6
  boundaries of, 8–9
  as collectively experienced event, 6
  commonalities with war/epidemics/
    mass displacements, 8
  and cultural idioms for expressing
    distress, 103
  definition, 3–4
    definitions based on collective
      impact, 6–7
    political definitions, 7
  dimensions, 11–12
    centripetal vs. centrifugal
      disasters, 12–13
    duration of the crisis, 13–14
    exposure severity/population and
      individual levels, 14–15
    and planning services and
      research, 15
    rapidity of onset, 13
    temporal, 9
  as potentially traumatic event, 4–5, 5f
  statistics on exposure to, 4
  typologies, 9–11
    vs. dimensional descriptions, 11
    interconnection of, 10
  See also Collectively experienced
    traumas; Human-caused
    disasters; Humanitarian crises;
    Mental health effects of
    disasters; Natural disasters;
    Phases of disaster

E

East County Ethnographic Study, 160,
    161
  and use of rapid assessment
    procedures (RAP), 168
Ecuador volcano eruption, 169, 310
El Al Boeing 747 crash, 105, 306
Emotional distress, 85

Epidemics, 11
Epidemiological approaches to disaster
    research, 95–96
  case–control designs, 98–99
  challenges, 101, 102t
    conceptual, 101–104
    dissemination of findings, 107
  epidemiology of trauma, 4
  and face-to-face assessment, 95, 101
    challenges, 102t
    rewards, 108t
  goal, 96
  retrospective cohort design, 96–98
Escalating threats, 8
Ethical issues in disaster research. See
    Research method selection/
    research goals/how (ethical/
    logistical/methodological issues)
Ethnicity, and mental health effects of
    disasters, 32
Ethnography, as strategy vs. method, 164
Evidence-based treatments (EBTs)/rapid
    deployment of, 226–227, 237
  EBT model, 230
  efficiencies/effectiveness in
    dissemination, 231
  future considerations, 296–297
  measurements
    evaluative, 232–233
    predictive, 232
  new-onset disorders from disasters,
    228–229
  pilot findings, 233–236, 234t
  postdisaster services delivery review
    (methodologies for), 236–237
  selection of EBT, 229–231
  surge capacity issues, 227–228
Exxon Valdez oil spill, 161, 306–307
Eye movement desensitization and
    reprocessing (EMDR) therapy,
    217

F

Farr, William, 178
Florida hurricanes, 144, 307
Focus group approach, 166

G

Gender, and mental health effects of disasters, 32
General adaption syndrome (GAS), 63–64
Global Burden of Disease report, 182
Global refugee crisis, and environmental hazards, 6–7
Gold standards for clinical research (Foa and Meadows), 211*t*

H

Hansin-Awaji earthquake (Japan), 21, 307
Health services research, 195
  directions to expand evidence-based knowledge about, 205–206
  political dimension, 202
    analyzing/communicating results, 204–205
    "evaluation culture" development/ getting usable data, 203–204
    evaluation design input, 203
  pragmatics, 197
    archival narrative records (content analysis of), 199
    archival quantitative data, 197–199
    client information, 200–202
    community surveys, 202
    program staff perspectives, 199–200
    research questions (and program theory), 195
    logic model elements, 195, 196f, 197
Hierarchical Linear modeling, 71
Human-caused disasters, 9
  mass violence, 9
    evidence of greater mental health consequences, 10–11
    imprecise definitions, 11
  technological accidents, 9, 10
    difficulty tolerating, 10
    equal effects to natural disasters, 10

Humanitarian crises, dimensions of, 7
Hurricane Andrew, 21, 52, 78, 143–144, 307
Hurricane Hugo, 21, 307
Hurricane Katrina, 105, 307
Hurricane Mitch, 29, 307–308

I

Impact ratio, 14
In-person assessments, 95, 101
  and challenges, 102t
  and rewards, 107–108, 108t
  vs. telephone-based assessments, 123–124
  See also Assessments
"Inoculation hypothesis," 64
International Federation of Red Cross and Red Crescent Societies, 6
International research, 278–279
  collaboration across borders, 279
    colleague facilitator, 279
    differences in training/research/ professional expectations, 280
    reward mechanisms, 279–280
  logistical challenges
    hidden costs, 285–286
    local staff, 286
    researcher as host-country guest, 286–287
    field morale, 288
    respect as reciprocal association, 287–288
    understanding of culturally determined priorities, 287
  study design and implementation challenges
    institutional review board and informed consent issues, 281–282
    language/language variations, 282–283
    local community engagement, 284–285
    participant compensation, 282
    validity (internal and external), 283–284

Interviews, semistructured, 164–165
  structured, 165
IRBs (institutional review boards), 79, 84
  risks/benefits evaluation, 84–86, 88

J

Johnstown (Pennsylvania) disaster, 10, 308
Jupiter cruise ship sinking, 12, 21, 308

K

Knowledge Networks, Inc. (KN), 135
Kosovo, 6

L

Latent growth curve (LGC) modeling, 71
Logic model, 195, 196f, 197
Loma Prieta earthquake, 78, 308

M

Major depressive disorder (MDD), 228
Marmara earthquake (Turkey), 21, 29, 215, 308
MEDLINE, 311, 312
Mental health effects of disasters
  best practices guidelines, 15, 16t, 34–36
  interventions (services) and research, 194–195
    expanding evidence-based knowledge about, 205–206
    political dimensions of, 202–205
    pragmatics, 197–202
    precepts, 195–202
  magnitude of effects, 27–28
    duration of effects, 30
    influence of methodological variables on, 29–30
    influence of substantive variables on, 28–29
  risk and protective factors, 30–31
    age, 32
    ethnicity, 32
    exposure severity, 31
    family factors, 33
    gender, 32
    predisaster functioning, 33
    psychological coping/resources, 33–34
    social support, 32
    socioeconomic status, 32–33
    See also Health services research; Psychosocial consequences of disaster; Question formulation/postdisaster mental health
Mental health measures, 54–56
  diagnostic assessment, 54–55
  screening tools, 55
Mexico City earthquakes, 21, 308
Mississippi River flood, 21, 49, 309
Mixed-method designs, 169–170

N

Natural disasters, 9
  equal effects to technological disasters, 10
  vs. human-caused, 9
  tolerance for (as "acts of God"), 10
NIMH Rapid Assessment Post-Impact of Disaster (RAPID) grants, 59
Northridge earthquake, 246, 309

O

Oklahoma City bombing, 21, 33, 53, 78, 80, 146, 309
  research approaches, 80

P

Pan Am 103 disaster, 308
  research, 112–113
Peaking threats. *See* Escalating threats
Peru earthquake (early 1970s), 310
  studies of, 159, 165
Pharmacotherapy, 214, 217–218
Phases of disaster, 15, 16t
Physiological perspective in stress research, 63–65
PILOTS Database, 313, 314, 317

Piper Alpha explosion, 21, 309
Political conflicts and mass
    displacements, 6
Population of interest in disaster
    research, 51
  age/ethnicity/other survivor
    characteristics selection criteria,
    54
  nature/severity of exposure selection
    criteria, 51
  communities/populations/schools,
    51–52
  rescue/recovery workers, 53–54
  victims/survivors, 52–53
  See also International research;
    Research with diverse/minority/
    marginalized communities;
    Research with military and
    uniformed services workers
Posttraumatic stress disorder (PTSD),
    35, 228
  and case–control studies, 101
  and effects of "catastrophizing," 67
  and gender, 32
  and health, 65
  interventions for children and
    adolescents, 218–219
  and place of disasters, 4
  as psychological consequence of
    disaster, 26
  research about, 55–56
  See also Eye movement
    desensitization and reprocessing
    (EMDR) therapy; Traumatic
    stress treatments
Primary/secondary appraisal, 65
Program theory, 195
Psychological debriefing, 211–212
Psychosocial consequences of disaster,
    20, 26–27, 56
  past research, 20–21
    frequency of studies by type/
    survivors' age ranges/locations,
    22–23, 22f
    study designs/sampling
    procedures, 23, 24t, 25–26,
    25f

updated empirical review (based
    on Norris and colleagues), 20–
    21
  research shortcomings, 35–36
  and resources decline, 27
  secondary stressors, 27
PsycINFO, 311
Public health surveillance, 177
  evolving concept of, 179–180
    focus on infectious disease
    monitoring, 179
    relationship to research, 179–180
    role of intervention, 179
  history of, 178
  prerequisites, 178–179
  types, 180
    disease-specific monitoring, 180–
    181
    syndromic surveillance systems,
    181
    systemic data collection and
    monitoring, 181–182
Public mental health surveillance, 191,
    295
  disaster context
    estimating postdisaster mental
    health burden, 184–185
    evaluating policies/interventions
    (and future planning), 185–186
    research advancement, 186–187
  key issues, 182
    analytic model development, 183–
    184
    case definitions (establishment of),
    182–183
    symptom linkage to morbidity/
    needs, 183
  strategy for (U.S.), 187
    current status of, 190–191
    features, 189–190
    purposes, 187–188
    stakeholders, 188
  See also Health services research
Public and research policy
    considerations/disaster mental
    health research, 300–302
  assessing disaster exposure, 292–293

ethical considerations, 299–300
evidence-based interventions, 296–297
    dissemination issues, 297–298
individual vs. social variables, 294–296
measurement considerations, 293–294
preparation and coordination, 298–299
temporal dimension, 292

Q

Qualitative approaches/disaster effects studies, 46, 158, 170–171
methods
    data analysis, 166–168
    data collection, 163–166
    sample selection, 162–163
mixed-method designs, 169–170
rapid assessment procedures (RAP), 168–169
rationale, 159–162
    clarification of values/meanings of people in disasters, 160–161
    exploratory research, 159
    local context understanding, 159–160
    "pilot data" collection, 161–162
    "thick description," 159
Question formulation/postdisaster mental health, 62–63, 73–74
stress theories/research perspectives, 63
    cognitive perspective, 65–67
    cross-cultural traditions, 69–70
    physiological perspective, 63–65
    social/ecological perspective, 67–69
time as critical frame of reference, 70–71

R

RAP. *See* Assessments
RAPID (NIMH Rapid Assessment Post-Impact of Disaster) grants, 59

Red Cross, *disaster* definition, 6
    See also International Federation of Red Cross and Red Crescent Societies
Research with diverse/minority/marginalized communities, 275
barriers, 269
    culture and linguistics, 268–269
    mistrust, 267–268
cultural competence model, 269–270, 270f
    addressing culture and linguistic challenges, 274–275
    barrier remedies, 271t
    expanding access (remedies), 273–274
    mistrust remedies, 270, 272–273
reasons for, 265–266
Research method selection/research goals, 45–46
how (ethical/logistical/methodological issues), 58–59, 88–91, 299–300
    decisional capacity of potential study participants, 81–82
    ethical considerations/guidelines, 89–90
    investigative collaboration and participant burden-reduction, 89
    and positive social goals, 78
    potential of traumatization in studies, 79
    regulations governing research, 79–80
    risk/benefits evaluation of research participation, 84–86
    voluntary informed consent issues, 86–88
    vulnerability of postdisaster participants, 82–84
what (variables), 54
    correlates of mental health, 56
    mental health measures, 54–56
when (and phase dependency), 57
    beginning research, 57–58
    research termination, 58

Research method selection/research
  goals, (*continued*)
  who (population of interest), 51
    age/ethnicity/other survivor
      characteristics criteria, 54
    nature/severity of exposure
      criteria, 51–54
  why (research goals), 46, 47t
    description, 46, 48–50
    influence, 50–51
    prediction, 50
  See also Descriptions in disaster
    research; Population of interest
    in disaster research; Stress
    prevention and mitigation
Research with military and uniformed
    services workers, 254–255,
    263–264
  access issues, 255–258
    "entry portal," 255, 256t
    establishing collaboration, 256–
      257
    relevant questions, 255, 257t
    respect for needs of disaster
      workers, 257–258
    working within jurisdictional
      boundaries, 255–256
  comparison groups, 260–261
  culture issues, 258–259
  feedback, 262–263
  recognition of participation, 261–
    262
  research plan development, 259
  and spouses/family as research
    participants, 261
  voluntary participation and
    confidentiality, 259–260
Research models and methods/disaster
    and terrorism studies,
    challenges of, 129–130, 291
  post-only designs, 131
  unpredictability issues, 130
  clinical research standards, 211t
  impact on of public mental health
    surveillance program, 186–187
  mixed-method designs, 169–170
  See also Epidemiological approaches

  to disaster research; Health
    services research; Psychosocial
    consequences of disaster/past
    research; Public and research
    policy considerations/disaster
    mental health research;
    Research method selection/
    research goals; Telephone-based
    research methods; Web-based
    research methods
Research regulations, federal, 79–80, 83
Resilience, neurobiology of, 64
Retraumatization, 85
Retrospective cohort design
    (epidemiological approach
    design option), 96–98
Rwanda genocide, 162, 169

S

Sampling, frame selection, 112
  methods, 112
    list-based, 113
    oversampling, 114
    random digit-dialing (RDD), 113–
      114
  probability samples, 132–133
  weights, 121
San Diego high school shootings, 160,
    309
SARS (severe acute respiratory
    syndrome), 11
Scientific inquiry, aims of, 159
Self-efficacy, 66
September 11, 2001, 11, 21, 78, 80,
    163, 309
  research approaches, 80
Severe acute respiratory syndrome
    (SARS), 11
Social support
  and mental health effects of
    disasters, 34
  received vs. perceived, 295–296
"Social support deterioration model,"
    27, 69
Social/ecological perspective in stress
    research, 67–69

Socioeconomic status, and mental
    health effects of disasters, 32–
    33
Somatization, 56
Southeast Asian tsunami, 221–222,
    309–310
Spitak (Armenia) earthquake, 21, 29,
    244, 310
STATA, 121
Stress, and decision-making capacity,
    81
  prevention and mitigation, 72–73
  stressor, 63
Stress inoculation training (SIT),
    220
Stress theories/research perspectives.
    See Question formulation/
    postdisaster mental health
Structural equation modeling (SEM),
    71
SUDAAN, 121

T

Telephone-based research methods,
    111
  advantages, 122–123
  conduct of surveys, 116–117
    calculation of outcome rates,
      119–121
    financial incentives, 117
    general principles, 115–116
    professional management of, 118–
      119
    sampling weights, 121
  design issues (sampling)
    sample frame selection, 112
    sample generation (list-based/
      random/oversampling), 112–
      114
    sampling telephones vs. people,
      114–115
  future directions, 125–126
  vs. in-person assessment, 123–124
  limitations, 124–125
  telephone sampling or telephone
    interviewing, 111

Telephone Consumer Protection Act
    (1991) (TCPA), 114
Template strategies, 167–168
Temporal perspective in stress
    research, 70–71
Terror and horror exposure, 14
Terrorism, and war, 11
Threats. See Acute threats; Chronic
    threats; Escalating threats
Three Mile Island (TMI) nuclear
    accident, 21, 78, 310
  plant workers/case–control study,
    100
  study foundation, 104–105
Time-delimited threats. See Acute
    threats
Times Beach contamination disaster,
    13, 310
Traumatic event, challenge to create
    narrative/integrate experience
    with other events, 15
  definition, 4
Traumatic stress literature, 311–312,
    317
  database selection, 312–314
  full text links, 316–317
  search strategy, 314–315
    as an iterative process, 315–316
Traumatic stress treatments,
    complication of symptom
    decline over time, 209
  early interventions (reviews of),
    210–211
    cognitive-behavioral therapy, 212–
      214
    pharmacotherapy, 214
    psychological debriefing, 211–212
    psychosocial intervention
      (children and adolescents), 214–
      215
  future research directions, 219–222
  later-stage interventions (reviews of),
    215
    children and adolescents with
      PTSD, 218–219
    cognitive-behavioral therapy, 215–
      217

Traumatic stress treatments,
later-stage interventions
(*continued*)
eye movement desensitization and
reprocessing, 217
pharmacotherapy, 217–218
limitations in literature about, 208–
209
and randomized clinical trials
(RCTs), 209
translational research issues, 209–
210
See also Evidence-based treatments
(EBTs)/rapid deployment of
Triangulation, 170

V

Villermé, Louis René, 178
Voluntary informed consent, 86–
88
Vulnerability, 82–84

W

War, and terrorism, 11
Web-based research methods, 129–130
data collection (mechanics of), 136–
137
future directions, 137–138
Internet usage for disaster study
design, 131–132
advantages and challenges, 134–
136
longitudinal design, 134
probability samples, 132–133
psychometrically sound
assessment/primary outcomes,
133–134
West Nile virus, 180
World Disasters Report, 6

Y

Yungay. *See* Peru earthquake (early
1970s)